Covid-19 in Children

Editors

ELIZABETH SECORD
ERIC J. MCGRATH

T0200460

PEDIATRIC CLINICS
OF NORTH AMERICA

www.pediatric.theclinics.com

Consulting Editor
BONITA F. STANTON

October 2021 • Volume 68 • Number 5

ELSEVIER

1600 John F. Kennedy Boulevard • Suite 1800 • Philadelphia, Pennsylvania, 19103-2899

http://www.theclinics.com

THE PEDIATRIC CLINICS OF NORTH AMERICA Volume 68, Number 5
October 2021 ISSN 0031-3955, ISBN-13: 978-0-323-83518-3

Editor: Kerry Holland
Developmental Editor: Axell Ivan Jade M. Purificacion

The Pediatric Clinics of North America (ISSN 0031-3955) is published bimonthly by Elsevier Inc., 360 Park Avenue South, New York, NY 10010-1710. Months of issue are February, April, June, August, October, and December. Periodicals postage paid at New York, NY and additional mailing offices. Subscription prices are $250.00 per year (US individuals), $984.00 per year (US institutions), $315.00 per year (Canadian individuals), $1048.00 per year (Canadian institutions), $376.00 per year (international individuals), $1048.00 per year (international institutions), $100.00 per year (US students and residents), $100.00 per year (Canadian students and residents), and $165.00 per year (international residents and students). To receive students/resident rare, orders must be accompanied by name of affiliated institution, date of term, and the signature of program/residency coordinator on institution letterhead. Orders will be billed at individual rate until proof of status is received. Foreign air speed delivery is included in all *Clinics* subscription prices. All prices are subject to change without notice. **POSTMASTER:** Send address changes to *The Pediatric Clinics of North America*, Elsevier Health Sciences Division, Subscription Customer Service, 3251 Riverport Lane, Maryland Heights, MO 63043. **Customer Service: 1-800-654-2452 (US and Canada). From outside of the US and Canada: 1-314-447-8871. Fax: 1-314-447-8029. For print support, E-mail: JournalsCustomerService-usa@elsevier.com. For online support, E-mail: JournalsOnlineSupport-usa@elsevier.com**.

Reprints. For copies of 100 or more, of articles in this publication, please contact the Commercial Reprints Department, Elsevier Inc., 360 Park Avenue South, New York, NY 10010-1710. Tel.: 212-633-3874; Fax: 212-633-3820; E-mail: reprints@elsevier.com.

The Pediatric Clinics of North America is also published in Spanish by McGraw-Hill Inter-americana Editores S.A., Mexico City, Mexico; in Portuguese by Riechmann and Affonso Editores, Rua Comandante Coelho 1085, CEP 21250, Rio de Janeiro, Brazil; and in Greek by Althayia SA, Athens, Greece.

The Pediatric Clinics of North America is covered in *MEDLINE/PubMed (Index Medicus), Excerpta Medica, Current Contents, Current Contents/Clinical Medicine, Science Citation Index, ASCA, ISI/BIOMED,* and *BIOSIS*.

PROGRAM OBJECTIVE
The goal of the *Pediatric Clinics of North America* is to keep practicing physicians and residents up to date with current clinical practice in pediatrics by providing timely articles reviewing the state-of-the-art in patient care.

TARGET AUDIENCE
All practicing pediatricians, physicians and healthcare professionals who provide patient care to pediatric patients.

LEARNING OBJECTIVES
Upon completion of this activity, participants will be able to:
1. Review the physical and mental impact the COVID-19 pandemic had on children and adolescents.
2. Discuss Multisystem Inflammatory Syndrome in Children (MIS-C), as well as treatment options.
3. Recognize the role telehealth technology played in connecting chronically ill children and adolescents to health care services during the COVID-19 pandemic.

ACCREDITATIONS
Physician Credit

The Elsevier Office of Continuing Medical Education (EOCME) is accredited by the Accreditation Council for Continuing Medical Education (ACCME) to provide continuing medical education for physicians.

The EOCME designates this journal-based activity for a maximum of 13 *AMA PRA Category 1 Credit*(s)™. Physicians should claim only the credit commensurate with the extent of their participation in the activity.

All other healthcare professionals requesting continuing education credit for this this journal-based activity will be issued a certificate of participation.

ABP Maintenance of Certification Credit

Successful completion of this CME activity, which includes participation in the activity and individual assessment of and feedback to the learner, enables the learner to earn up to 13 MOC points in the American Board of Pediatrics' (ABP) Maintenance of Certification (MOC) program. It is the CME activity provider's responsibility to submit learner completion information to ACCME for the purpose of granting ABP MOC credit.

DISCLOSURE OF CONFLICTS OF INTEREST
The EOCME assesses conflict of interest with its instructors, faculty, planners, and other individuals who are in a position to control the content of CME activities. All relevant conflicts of interest that are identified are thoroughly vetted by EOCME for fair balance, scientific objectivity, and patient care recommendations. EOCME is committed to providing its learners with CME activities that promote improvements or quality in healthcare and not a specific proprietary business or a commercial interest.

The planning committee, staff, authors and editors listed below have identified no financial relationships or relationships to products or devices they or their spouse/life partner have with commercial interest related to the content of this CME activity:

Matthew Adams, MD; Colleen Buggs-Saxton, MD, PhD; Ciara Cannoy, MA; Regina Chavous-Gibson, MSN, RN; Hey Chong, MD, PhD; Heather Chow, DO; Adriana Diakiw, MD; Pezad N. Doctor, MBBS; Nivine El-Hor, MD; Adam J. Esbenshade, MD, MSCI; Christopher Failing, MD; Gloria Fall, BA; David Frame, PharmD; Ramon Galindo, MD; Samuel Gnanakumar; William Christopher Golden, MD; Tuhina Govil-Dalela, MD; Shipra Gupta, MD; Kerry Holland; Jacob Hoofman, MS; Deepak Kamat, MD, PhD; Leslie H. Lundahl, PhD; Rajkumar Mayakrishnann; Eric John McGrath, MD; Jill Meade, PhD; Aishwarya Navalpakam, MD; Milind Pansare, MD; Abigail C. Radomsky, BS; Ashley Rapp, MPH; Chokechai Rongkavilit, MD; Sara Santarossa, PhD; Elizabeth A. Secord, MD; Lalitha Sivaswamy, MD; Layne Smith, PharmD; Lynn C. Smitherman, MD; Beena G. Sood, MD, MS; Jennifer R. Walton, MD, MPH

The planning committee, staff, authors and editors listed below have identified financial relationships or relationships to products or devices they or their spouse/life partner have with commercial interest related to the content of this CME activity:

James A. Connelly, MD: Consultant/advisor: Horizon Therapeutics, X4 Pharmaceuticals, Inc.

Kelly Walkovich, MD: Consultant/advisor: Horizon Therapeutics, Pharming, Sobi AB

UNAPPROVED/OFF-LABEL USE DISCLOSURE

The EOCME requires CME faculty to disclose to the participants:

1. When products or procedures being discussed are off-label, unlabelled, experimental, and/or investigational (not US Food and Drug Administration [FDA] approved); and
2. Any limitations on the information presented, such as data that are preliminary or that represent ongoing research, interim analyses, and/or unsupported opinions. Faculty may discuss information about pharmaceutical agents that is outside of FDA-approved labelling. This information is intended solely for CME and is not intended to promote off-label use of these medications. If you have any questions, contact the medical affairs department of the manufacturer for the most recent prescribing information.

TO ENROLL

To enroll in the *Pediatric Clinics of North America* Continuing Medical Education program, call customer service at 1-800-654-2452 or sign up online at http://www.theclinics.com/home/cme. The CME program is available to subscribers for an additional annual fee of USD 324.00.

METHOD OF PARTICIPATION

In order to claim credit, participants must complete the following:

1. Complete enrolment as indicated above.
2. Read the activity.
3. Complete the CME Test and Evaluation. Participants must achieve a score of 70% on the test. All CME Tests and Evaluations must be completed online.

In order to claim MOC points, participants must complete the following:

1. Complete steps listed above for claiming CME credit
2. Provide your specialty board ID#, birth date (MM/DD), and attestation.
3. Online MOC submission is only available for the American Board of pediatrics' (ABP) Maintenance of Certification (MOC) program

CME INQUIRIES/SPECIAL NEEDS

For all CME inquiries or special needs, please contact elsevierCME@elsevier.com.

Contributors

CONSULTING EDITOR

BONITA F. STANTON, MD
Professor of Pediatrics and Founding Dean, Robert C. and Laura C. Garrett Endowed Chair, Hackensack Meridian School of Medicine, President, Academic Enterprise, Hackensack Meridian Health, Nutley, New Jersey

EDITORS

ELIZABETH SECORD, MD
Professor of Pediatrics, Division Chief for Allergy and Immunology, Wayne State University School of Medicine, Professor, Pediatric Allergy and Immunology, Wayne State University, Wayne Pediatrics, Detroit, Michigan

ERIC J. MCGRATH, MD
Professor of Pediatrics, Division of Pediatric Infectious Diseases and Prevention, Department of Pediatrics, Wayne State University School of Medicine, Detroit, Michigan

AUTHORS

MATTHEW ADAMS, MD
Assistant Professor of Pediatrics, Division Chief for Pediatric Rheumatology, Wayne State University School of Medicine, Wayne Pediatrics, Detroit, Michigan

COLLEEN BUGGS-SAXTON, MD, PhD
Assistant Professor, Department of Pediatrics, Pediatric Endocrinology, Wayne Pediatrics, Wayne State University School of Medicine, Detroit, Michigan

CIARA CANNOY, MA
Clinical Psychology PhD Candidate, Department of Psychology, Wayne State University, Detroit, Michigan

HEY CHONG, MD, PhD
Associate Professor, Pediatric Allergy and Immunology, UPMC Children's Hospital of Pittsburgh, Pittsburgh, Pennsylvania

HEATHER CHOW, DO
Department of Pediatrics, UCSF Fresno, Fresno, California

JAMES A. CONNELLY, MD
Assistant Professor, Pediatric Hematology/Oncology, Monroe Carell Jr Children's Hospital, Vanderbilt University, Nashville, Tennessee

ADRIANA DIAKIW, MD
Assistant Professor, General Pediatrics, West Virginia University School of Medicine, Morgantown, West Virginia

PEZAD N. DOCTOR, MBBS
Department of Pediatrics, Children's Hospital of Michigan, Detroit, Michigan

NIVINE EL-HOR, MD
Department of Internal Medicine and Pediatrics, Children's Hospital of Michigan, Detroit, Michigan

ADAM J. ESBENSHADE, MD, MSCI
Associate Professor, Pediatric Hematology/Oncology, Monroe Carell Jr Children's Hospital, Vanderbilt University, Nashville, Tennessee

CHRISTOPHER FAILING, MD
Assistant Professor, Pediatric Rheumatology, Essentia Health, Fargo, North Dakota

GLORIA FALL, BA
Department of Public Health Sciences, Henry Ford Health System, Detroit, Michigan

DAVID FRAME, PharmD
Assistant Professor, School of Pharmacy, University of Michigan, Ann Arbor, Michigan

RAMON GALINDO, MD
Department of Pediatrics, UCSF Fresno, Fresno, California

WILLIAM CHRISTOPHER GOLDEN, MD
Associate Professor, Eudowood Neonatal Pulmonary Division, Department of Pediatrics, Johns Hopkins School of Medicine, Baltimore, Maryland

TUHINA GOVIL-DALELA, MD
Departments of Pediatrics and Neurology, Children's Hospital of Michigan, Wayne State University, Department of Pediatric Neurology, Children's Hospital of Michigan Specialty Center, Detroit, Michigan

SHIPRA GUPTA, MD
Assistant Professor, Pediatric Infectious Diseases, West Virginia University School of Medicine, Morgantown, West Virginia

JACOB HOOFMAN, MS2
Wayne State University School of Medicine, Detroit, Michigan

DEEPAK KAMAT, MD, PhD
Department of Pediatrics, UT Health Science Center, UT Health San Antonio, San Antonio, Texas

LESLIE H. LUNDAHL, PhD
Associate Professor, Department of Psychiatry and Behavioral Neurosciences, Wayne State University School of Medicine, Detroit, Michigan

JILL MEADE, PhD
Assistant Professor, Department of Pediatrics, Wayne State University, Psychologist, Children's Hospital of Michigan, Detroit, Michigan

AISHWARYA NAVALPAKAM, MD
Fellow-in-Training, Division of Allergy and Immunology, Department of Pediatrics, Pediatric Specialty Center, Children's Hospital of Michigan, Detroit, Michigan

MILIND PANSARE, MD
Associate Professor, Department of Pediatrics, Division of Allergy and Immunology, Pediatric Specialty Center, Children's Hospital of Michigan, Central Michigan University, Detroit, Michigan

ABIGAIL C. RADOMSKY, BS
Wayne State University, School of Medicine, Detroit, Michigan

ASHLEY RAPP, MPH
Department of Public Health Sciences, Henry Ford Health System, Detroit, Michigan

CHOKECHAI RONGKAVILIT, MD
Department of Pediatrics, UCSF Fresno, Fresno, California

SARA SANTAROSSA, PhD
Department of Public Health Sciences, Henry Ford Health System, Detroit, Michigan

ELIZABETH SECORD, MD
Professor of Pediatrics, Division Chief for Allergy and Immunology, Wayne State University School of Medicine, Professor, Pediatric Allergy and Immunology, Wayne State University, Wayne Pediatrics, Detroit, Michigan

LALITHA SIVASWAMY, MD
Department of Pediatric Neurology, Children's Hospital of Michigan Specialty Center, Detroit, Michigan; Departments of Pediatrics and Neurology, Central Michigan University, Pleasant, Michigan

LAYNE SMITH, PharmD
West Virginia University School of Pharmacy, Morgantown, West Virginia

LYNN C. SMITHERMAN, MD
Associate Professor, Vice Chair of Medical Education, Department of Pediatrics, Wayne State University School of Medicine, Detroit, Michigan

BEENA G. SOOD, MD, MS
Department of Pediatrics, Wayne State University School of Medicine, Detroit, Michigan

KELLY WALKOVICH, MD
Associate Professor, Pediatric Hematology/Oncology, C.S. Mott Children's Hospital, University of Michigan, Ann Arbor, Michigan

JENNIFER R. WALTON, MD, MPH
Assistant Professor, Division of Developmental Behavioral Pediatrics, Department of Pediatrics, Nationwide Children's Hospital, The Ohio State University College of Medicine, Columbus, Ohio

Contents

> Research confirms that children and adolescents are experiencing signif-
> icant anxiety and depression during the coronavirus disease 2019
> pandemic. Adolescents may be at greater risk, particularly females. So-
> cial isolation, loneliness, lack of physical exercise, and family stress
> may contribute to these problems. Children who feel unsafe with regards
> to coronavirus disease 2019 may be more likely to experience somatic
> symptoms, depression, and anxiety. Parental stress and mental health
> problems may put children at an increased risk for maltreatment. Medical
> and behavioral health professionals should routinely screen for depres-
> sion and anxiety. Increased access to mental health services will be
> critical.

> Children usually present with milder symptoms of COVID-19 as compared
> with adults. Supportive care alone is appropriate for most children with
> COVID-19. Antiviral therapy may be required for those with severe or crit-
> ical diseases. Currently there has been a rapid development of vaccines
> globally to prevent COVID-19 and several vaccines are being evaluated
> in children and adolescents. Currently, only the Pfizer–BioNTech
> messenger RNA vaccine is approved for emergency authorization use in
> the pediatric population ages 12 years and older.

> Studies have yielded mixed findings regarding changes in adolescent sub-
> stance use during the COVID-19 pandemic; some report increased alcohol
> and cannabis use, others show less binge drinking and vaping behaviors,
> and others no change. In 2019, only 8.3% of the 1.1 million adolescents
> with a substance use disorder received specialized treatment. Treatment
> rates for 2020 have not yet been published. Stay-at-home orders and so-
> cial distancing guidelines put into place in March 2020 caused the partial
> closure of many outpatient substance use clinics. The implications of this

treatment suspension and special considerations for working with adolescents during stay-at-home orders are discussed.

The present study is systematic rapid review on the nature of the relationship between the COVID-19 pandemic and child maltreatment. Database searches on December 28, 2020, identified 234 unique citations; 12 were ultimately included in our analysis. Included articles measured child maltreatment inclusive of physical, psychological, and sexual abuse, and child neglect during the COVID-19 pandemic. Compared with the prepandemic period, 5 articles found an increase in child maltreatment, 6 articles found a decrease, and 1 study found no difference. There existed variation in geography of study location, age of child maltreatment victims, and types of child maltreatment assessed.

A multisystem inflammatory syndrome (MISC) can result from COVID-19 infection in previously healthy children and adolescents. It is potentially life threatening and is treated initially with intravenous immunoglobulin and aspirin but may require anti-inflammatory monoclonal antibody treatment in severe cases. SARS-CoV-2 infection can cause macrophage activation syndrome , chilblains, and flares of existing rheumatologic diseases. The pandemic has led to later presentation of some rheumatologic conditions as parents and patients have avoided health care settings. PubMed and Google scholar have been utilized to review the literature on the rheumatologic conditions resulting from COVID-19 and the current treatment options.

Although living with the threat of severe infection is a constant worry for many pediatric immunocompromised patients, the pandemic begotten by the severe acute respiratory syndrome coronavirus-2 (SARS-CoV-2) created new fears and challenges for families and health care providers. As people around the world through government directive or independent choice moved into protective isolation, immunosuppressed children who routinely require medical management were challenged with necessary public ventures to health care facilities. Medical centers adapted by developing new approaches to care for immunocompromised children such as expanding telemedicine services and conversion to athome immune therapies to reduce infectious exposure. Testing of asymptomatic patients for SARS-CoV-2 before medical therapies became routine in most modern health care units, and development of highly sensitive assays was critical to avoid patient and staff exposure as well as initiation of new immunosuppressive treatment in positive patients. As the prevalence of coronavirus disease (COVID-

19) amplified and infected immunocompromised patients became more common, questions quickly arose including how aggressively to treat the infection with most agents still in clinical trials. In addition, how should chronic immunosuppressant drugs that may interfere with the ability to clear the virus be adjusted? Finally, what if the infection leads to excessive immune responses or flares of the underlying disorder? In this review, we explore the impact of the COVID-19 pandemic on immunocompromised children during the first year, summarizing what is known and yet to be discovered, approaches to testing and treatment of SARS-CoV-2, considerations in management of underlying immune suppressive medications, outcomes published to date, and strategies for vaccinating this unique population.

COVID-19 has afflicted the health of children and women across all age groups. Since the outbreak of the pandemic in December 2019, various epidemiologic, immunologic, clinical, and pharmaceutical studies have been conducted to understand its infectious characteristics, pathogenesis, and clinical profile. COVID-19 affects pregnant women more seriously than nonpregnant women, endangering the health of the newborn. Changes have been implemented to guidelines for antenatal care of pregnant women, delivery, and newborn care. We highlight the current trends of clinical care in pregnant women and newborns during the COVID-19 pandemic.

COVID-19 has changed education for learners of all ages. Preliminary data project educational losses at many levels and verify the increased anxiety and depression associated with the changes, but there are not yet data on long-term outcomes. Guidance from oversight organizations regarding the safety and efficacy of new delivery modalities for education have been quickly forged. It is no surprise that the socioeconomic gaps and gaps for special learners have widened. The medical profession and other professions that teach by incrementally graduated internships are also severely affected and have had to make drastic changes.

The COVID-19 pandemic has spread rapidly across the world in 2020, affecting both adults and, to a lesser extent, children. In this article, the authors describe the neurologic manifestations of COVID-19 in children, including the epidemiology, pathogenesis, clinical features, laboratory and imaging findings, and treatment options. The management of patients with concomitant neuroimmunologic disorders and drug interactions between medications used to treat COVID-19 and other neurologic disorders (especially immune-modifying drugs) is also discussed.

higher rates of COVID-19 infections and deaths than their population percentages in the United States. Unique populations of children, including children with developmental disabilities, children in the foster care system, children with chronic medical problems, and children who are homeless are particularly vulnerable to COVID-19 infection. This article explores how the COVID-19 pandemic superimposed on health disparities directly and indirectly affects children, adolescents, and their caregivers.

PEDIATRIC CLINICS OF NORTH AMERICA

SERIES OF RELATED INTEREST

Clinics in Perinatology
http://www.perinatology.theclinics.com/
Advances in Pediatrics
http://www.advancesinpediatrics.com/

THE CLINICS ARE AVAILABLE ONLINE!
Access your subscription at:
www.theclinics.com

Foreword

COVID-19 Pandemic, Children, Pediatricians, and the Future

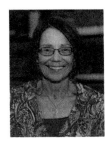

Bonita F. Stanton, MD
Consulting Editor

Severe acute respiratory syndrome coronavirus 2 (more widely known as COVID-19) appears to have made its global debut in December 2019 in China.[1] To date (July 4, 2021), 172,612 publications regarding COVID-19 have been recognized by the United States National Library of Medicine (accessible through PubMed). To put into perspective the massive amount of work that this represents over such a short time, let us turn to the publications regarding the human immunodeficiency virus (HIV), also a pandemic of enormous and continuing global recognition, importance, and cost. This disease was first recognized in June 1981. To date, after forty years, there have been only 462, 827 publications regarding HIV,[2] which is only 2.6 fold the number of publications concerning COVID-19 after only 1.5 years.[2] What makes COVID-19 especially concerning?

There are many reasons. First, it is difficult to identify a segment of the world's population that has not been impacted by the COVID-19 Pandemic. It is difficult to identify a professional group that has not been impacted by the COVID-19 Pandemic. It is difficult to imagine a curriculum, a technology, or a local, state, national, or global health policy that has not in some way been impacted by COVID-19. Indeed, the lives of virtually every person in every country across the world have been fundamentally uprooted by COVID-19, and may remain so for many more years to come.

Second, it is important to specifically address the consequences of the pandemic on all subpopulations, but most especially on children. Children's many needs, both preventive and treatment, include but are not limited to medical, economic, educational, emotional, and developmental domains. Moreover, until the emergence of some of the more recent mutations of COVID-19, children were misperceived as being less impacted by COVID-19 than were adults, especially elderly adults. While this perception may have accurately assessed the likelihood of serious biologic trauma inflicted on children by COVID-19, it was never a correct characterization of children's

Pediatr Clin N Am 68 (2021) xv–xvii
https://doi.org/10.1016/j.pcl.2021.07.002
0031-3955/21/© 2021 Published by Elsevier Inc.

vulnerabilities to all the consequences of the disease. Children are susceptible to many of these consequences, some of which can last for years. Moreover, as COVID-19 variants emerge, serious illness among children has been increasing.[3]

In recognition of the need to specifically address the needs of children in the context of a global pandemic, this issue of *Pediatric Clinics of North America* offers a panoramic view of the possible impact of COVID-19 among children, including potential aggravation of preexisting health disparities; mental health and substance abuse effects; vaccine effects (both desired and undesired); changes in the approach to pediatric care, including vaccinations; impact of COVID-19 on other major pediatric health issues, including diabetes, asthma, neurologic disorders, and such; and differences in broad public health preventive measures between children and adults.

We recognize that each of the descriptions provided in this issue of *Pediatric Clinics of North America* only reflect our understanding of the pandemic up to a specific moment in time. Some of the causal relationships we describe in this issue may already have undergone reanalysis by the time of printing, and many more will change in the future. Both the disease itself and/or our understanding of the factors that mitigate or aggravate the disease or its impact in certain circumstances will vary over time or by population. We have already seen evidence that many treatments and ameliorative agents that initially appeared promising did not ultimately retain this ability over time. We are also well aware that the virus mutates quickly and effectively, thereby impacting the potential of the affect the vaccine.

Finally, we know that population groups varying by race, nationality, income, educational background, and so forth may have very different understandings of the safety and efficacy of the potential treatments and prevention options available. It is our responsibility as pediatricians and other child health care advocates to recognize these differences in their acceptance of existing and future drugs and vaccines and to work with the families, parents, and children expressing such views to help them understand our perspectives and help us understand their perspectives. We must let them know that to the degree possible, our perspectives and recommendations will be specific to each of their children and may change over time as we gain greater understanding of the disease and as more options become available. For now, we believe that among the available vaccines, drugs, and other treatments currently available, the approaches that we are recommending are what we believe to be in the best interest of their child, and in many cases these options are very effective with little or no risk to the child.

Bonita F. Stanton, MD
Hackensack Meridian
School of Medicine
Academic Enterprise
Hackensack Meridian Health
123 Metro Boulevard
Nutley, NJ 07110, USA

E-mail address:
Bonita.Stanton@hackensackmeridian.org

REFERENCES

1. AJM C Staff. Available at: A timeline of COVID-19 developments in 2020. Available at: https://www.ajmc.com/view/a-timeline-of-covid19-developments-in-2020. Accessed January 1, 2021.

2. HIV Gov. Overview: history—a timeline of HIV and AIDS. Available at: https://www.hiv.gov/hiv-basics/overview/history/hiv-and-aids-timeline. Accessed May 24, 2021.
3. Global Data Healthcare. Covid-19 is killing infants and young children in Brazil. Available at: https://www.clinicaltrialsarena.com/comment/covid-19-infants-young-children-brazil/. Accessed May 24, 2021.

Preface

How Do We Take Care of Children During this COVID-19 Pandemic?

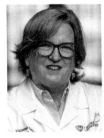 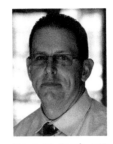

Elizabeth Secord, MD   Eric J. McGrath, MD
Editors

On March 10, 2021, a colleague of mine posted the following on Facebook, "A year ago today we were living the last normal week of our lives, and we had no idea." He was, of course, correct that we have shared a very life-altering and very difficult year due to COVID-19. In the United States alone, over half a million have died of COVID-19; many jobs have been lost, and our way of life has been grossly altered due to loss, social distancing, and pandemic precautions.

The pandemic has affected children and adolescents in different ways than it has affected adults, and in different ways than we anticipated. Our asthmatics had a break from the emergency room and hospital because of decreased exposure to all viruses while staying home. School was transformed into a screen. Obesity secondary to lack of exercise and food insecurity plagued many children and adolescents. Children did not suffer the morbidity and mortality that their elders realized, but a newly described severe inflammatory syndrome associated with COVID-19 multisystem inflammatory syndrome in children (MIS-C) began to affect children. Treatments for COVID-19 in children and treatments for MIS-C lagged behind treatments for adults, as did vaccine opportunities for children and adolescents. Pediatricians and pediatric subspecialists mobilized through telehealth visits to reach chronically ill children and adolescents who were unable to access health care during the pandemic, and mental health issues worsened secondary to isolation and anxiety. And, of course, not all children and adolescents were equally affected, and children of color, children with disabilities, and children of lower socioeconomic classes, as usual, lost the most.

We have tried to cover the major aspects of what we learned this year. We have covered safety precautions, treatment, vaccines, educational adaptations, special

Pediatr Clin N Am 68 (2021) xix–xx
https://doi.org/10.1016/j.pcl.2021.07.001
0031-3955/21/© 2021 Published by Elsevier Inc.

populations (eg, substance abuse disorder, diabetes, and immunocompromised children), and mental health issues. There is, as in every review, much we do not yet know.

Elizabeth Secord, MD
Wayne Pediatrics
400 Mack Avenue
Detroit, MI 48201, USA

Eric J. McGrath, MD
Wayne Pediatrics
400 Mack Avenue, Suite 1E
Detroit, MI 48201, USA

E-mail addresses:
esecord@med.wayne.edu (E. Secord)
emcgrath@med.wayne.edu (E.J. McGrath)

Mental Health Effects of the COVID-19 Pandemic on Children and Adolescents

A Review of the Current Research

Jill Meade, PhD

KEYWORDS

- COVID-19 • Child • Adolescent • Mental health • Psychological • Anxiety
- Depression

KEY POINTS

- Research is ongoing regarding mental health effects of the coronavirus disease 2019 pandemic on children and adolescents.
- Early studies show children and adolescents experiencing increased anxiety and depression.
- Isolation, loneliness, lack of physical activity, family stress, and racism may contribute to the effects of the coronavirus disease 2019 pandemic on child and adolescent mental health.

BACKGROUND

Coronavirus disease 2019 (COVID-19) has created unimaginable challenges for children, adolescents, and their families around the world. This virus, which was first identified in Wuhan, China, in December 2019,[1] has led to 23,440,774 cases of COVID-19 in the United States (as of January 16, 2021) and has caused more than 390,938 total US deaths.[2] Pandemic-related school and business closings and community lockdowns have had significant effects on families. The earliest world-wide lockdowns that started in China around January 23, 2020,[3] included restrictions on schools and gatherings, and resulted in children being transitioned to online school. In the United States, many school districts began transitioning to online school in March 2020 in conjunction with community closures.[4] Since then, individual communities and states within the United States have continued to impose and lift restrictions in response to COVID-19 outbreaks. This situation has been and continues to be a constantly changing situation, with new stressors occurring constantly.

Children's Hospital of Michigan, Department of Psychiatry/Psychology, Box 137, 3901 Beaubien Boulevard, Detroit, MI 48201, USA
E-mail address: jmeade@med.wayne.edu

Pediatr Clin N Am 68 (2021) 945–959
https://doi.org/10.1016/j.pcl.2021.05.003
0031-3955/21/© 2021 Elsevier Inc. All rights reserved.

COVID-19–RELATED SOURCES OF STRESS FOR CHILDREN AND ADOLESCENTS

Everyday life for children and adolescents has been significantly disrupted by the COVID-19 pandemic. Potential stressors for children and adolescents during this challenging time could include:

- Increased social isolation
- Heightened concerns over safety and health
- Increased stress of parents and caregivers owing to work, financial, or other impacts
- Increased family conflict, parent–child conflict, and/or child abuse
- Placements with friends or relatives owing to parent work situation
- Loss of prosocial activities (school, sports, social activities, hobbies)
- Adjustment to online schooling processes and demands
- Increased screen time and sedentary behaviors
- Decreased access to medical and mental health care, including exacerbated health disparities

ADDED EFFECTS OF SOCIOPOLITICAL EVENTS

In addition to the pandemic-related changes discussed, co-occurring sociopolitical stressors during this time also likely impact the mental health of children and adolescents. Given that the first cases of COVID-19 were identified China,[1] some American politicians began referring to it as the "Wuhan virus" or the "Chinese virus," which led to reports of a racism pandemic against Asian Americans in the United States.[5] Early research on this topic demonstrated that nearly one-half of Chinese American parents and their children ages 10 to 18 who were surveyed reported being targeted by or witnessing COVID-19 racial discrimination.[6]

Additional racial-based stressors occurred in the United States beginning May 25 with the death of George Floyd at the hands of the police.[7] Through media coverage and a video of his death, many children were exposed to examples of violence and/or racism. Outrage over police violence focused the country on issues of racial justice and resulted in months of protests and demonstrations, peaking in June 2020.[8] It is difficult to disentangle the effects of the COVID-19 pandemic stressors from these sociopolitical events in the United States.

EARLY REVIEWS ON COVID-19 AND CHILD MENTAL HEALTH

The earliest identified reviews of original research looking at COVID-19 effects on child and adolescent mental health identified concerns about increasing levels of depression and anxiety[9] as well as post-traumatic symptoms.[10] A review by Fong and Iarocci[11] published in November 2020 combined past pandemic research with newly available COVID-19 findings and concluded that pandemic-related social isolation and quarantining is resulting in significant anxiety, post-traumatic stress disorder (PTSD), and fears in children and adolescents. The authors emphasized the importance of reducing barriers to mental health services for children and families.

CURRENT STUDIES

The purpose of this article is to provide an updated review of the current body of research findings to date on the specific impacts of COVID-19 on the mental health functioning of children and adolescents. Original data studies examining mental health outcomes in the general population of children and adolescents during COVID-19 were identified through search engines and publications. **Table 1** provides a summary of studies reviewed, including authors, country of origin, month(s) of data collection, number and ages of subjects, and major findings with regards to child and adolescent mental health. These studies present a snapshot in time, and it will be important that research be ongoing in order to understand the short- and long-term effects of the pandemic on children and adolescents.

Changes in Mental Health Owing to COVID-19

To investigate changes in child/adolescent mental health functioning in relation to the pandemic, studies have examined parent and youth retrospective symptoms reports and have compared current data to that from previous years. Longitudinal data analyses would be ideal, but are not yet available.

Parent and child report of changes

The worsening of child mental health during the pandemic has been reported by parents and children. A US study of 1000 parents with at least 1 child under age 18 years found that 14.3% of parents reported observing worsening in child's behavioral health after March, with little difference in racial, ethnic, income, or education groups.[23] Reported declines in parent and child mental health for these families were linked to having younger children, loss of child care, and reported increased food insecurity. Canadian researchers collected data from both clinical and community samples of youth ages 14 to 28 approximately 1 month after pandemic onset. Both groups reported significant declines in mental health compared with prepandemic functioning, with the community sample reporting the greatest decline. Interestingly, this primarily college-aged sample reported decreased substance use from before to after the onset of the pandemic, possibly owing to a return to parents' homes.

Suicide statistics across times periods

Studies examining large health-related datasets have been able to compare changes in suicide-related behaviors from year to year. Hill and colleagues[17] examined the outcomes of routine screening for suicide in 18,247 youth ages 11 to 21 years in a large US city hospital emergency department (ED), comparing percentage of youth seen reporting recent suicidal ideation and recent attempts from March through July 2020 with the same months in 2019. They found higher rates of both suicidal ideation in March and July 2020 (compared with 2019), and higher rates of recent suicide attempts in February through April and July 2020 (compared with 2019), suggesting that events in 2020 were leading to these increases. In contrast, in Japan researchers used public data to compare rates of completed suicides in youth under age 20 years for March through May of 2019 and the same months in 2020.[18] Although they found that youth suicide in Japan did increase from March to May each year, rates were not worse in 2020. Researchers hypothesized that youth remaining at home with family (owing to COVID-19 restrictions) may have been a protective factor.

Mental health emergency visit rates

Hospital emergency departments are often the site for crisis mental health evaluations of children and adolescents. Using data from the Centers for Disease Control and Prevention reporting general mental health-related visits for children less than 18 years of age at hospital emergency departments across 47 US states, Leeb and colleagues[20] examined rates of visits for the period of January through October in 2019 and 2020. When examining proportion of mental health-related visits per 100,000 emergency department visits, sharp increases were found after March 2020, and these increases

Table 1
Research examining mental health impacts of COVID-19 on children and adolescents

Author	Country (Data Collection Dates)	Participants	Findings Regarding Child and Adolescent Mental Health
Cheah et al,[6] 2020	United States (March 14 to May 31, 2020)	543 parents in the United States who identify as Chinese and 320 of their children, ages 10–18 y	Majority of parents and children reported directly experiencing or witnessing racial discrimination against Chinese or Asian Americans owing to COVID-19. Both parent report of poorer child well-being and child report of anxiety linked to experiences of racial discrimination.
Chen et al,[12] 2020	Guiyang, China (April 2020)	1036 children, ages 6–15 y	11.78% rate of depression, 18.92% rate of anxiety, and 6.56% rate of both. Factors linked with depression: being female, being older teen, lower parent education, no companion on weekdays, and less physical exercise. Factors linked with anxiety: being female, no companion on weekdays, and less physical exercise. Some belief physical exercise serves a protective factor.
Duan et al,[13] 2020	20 provinces in mainland China (article submitted in April 2020)	3613 children ages 7–18 y	22.28% of sample reported depressive symptoms above clinical threshold. Anxiety in children was 23.87% and 29.27% in adolescents. Increased anxiety linked to being aged 13–18, female, living in urban area, emotion-focused coping style, Increased depression linked to smartphone addiction, Internet addiction. Problem-focused coping and fewer hours on the Internet before pandemic related to decreased depressive symptoms.

Study	Location (Date)	Sample	Findings
Fitzpatrick et al,[14] 2020	United States (April to July 2020)	133 caregivers of at least 1 child aged 1–19 y	Parents reported top mental health problems in their most challenging child; Results grouped by age: 1–5 y: misbehavior, social isolation, boredom, needing attention, anxiety; 6–12 y: academics, misbehavior, anxiety, social isolation, depression; 13–19 y: depression, anxiety, misbehavior, social isolation, inattention or impulsivity
Gassman-Pines et al,[15] 2020	United States (Feb to April 2020)	645 parents of children 5–7 y	In children of hourly service-industry workers, more COVID-related hardships (job loss, loss of income, caregiver burden) resulted in increased children's uncooperative and worry behaviors.
Hawke et al,[16] 2020	Canada (April 2020)	Clinical sample of 276 youth, and community sample of 346 youth, majority Caucasian, ages 14–28 y	Significant mental health decline reported by participants across groups. Internalizing disorder: 68.4% of clinical sample and 39.9% youth in the community sample had high likelihood of meeting criteria. Externalizing disorders: 40.2% of clinical and 16.9% of community sample had high likelihood.
Hill et al,[17] 2020	United States (February to July 2020)	11- to 21-year-old youth seen at a city emergency department	City ED screened youth for reported recent suicidal ideation and suicide attempts; rates were higher in several months of February to July 2020 compared with same period in 2019

(continued on next page)

Table 1
(continued)

Author	Country (Data Collection Dates)	Participants	Findings Regarding Child and Adolescent Mental Health
Isumi et al,[18] 2020	Japan (March to May, 2018, 2019, 2020)	Nationwide suicides among youth <20 y	Concluded pandemic did not have significant effect on suicide rates compared with previous years or pre–post school closure. Discussed possible positive connections, cohesion, and social support for children.
Jiao et al,[19] 2020	Shaanxi Province, China (February 2020)	320 parents of children and adolescents, ages 3–18 y	Younger children (3–6 y) had more clinginess and fear about safety of family members from COVID (compared with older children). Older children (6–18 y) had more inattention and "obsessive request of updates." Most common symptoms in entire sample were clinging, inattention, and irritability.
Leeb et al,[20] 2020	United States (January to October, 2019 and 2020)	Examined data from the CDC's National Syndromic Surveillance Program regarding ED visits among children <18 y	Children had fewer total mental health ED visits after lockdown, but percentage of visits that were for mental health-related sharply increased in late March and continued through October. Percentage of mental health-related visits in late March through October was significantly higher than during same months in 2019. Ages 5–11 y: 24% increase in percentage. Ages 12–17 y 31% increase in percentage.

Liu et al,[21] 2020	China (February to March 2020)	Grades 5–6 (estimated ages 10–11 y) and college students (estimated ages 17–22y)]	In primary school children, concerns regarding threat to life and health (endorsed by 39.7%) was related to somatic symptoms and anxiety but not depression. Overall rates were low, however.
Liu et al,[22] 2021	Wuhan and Huangshi, China (February to March 2020)	1264 children ages 7–12 y and their parents.	Higher inattention-hyperactivity and problems with prosocial behaviors when children did little or no physical exercise. Children in Wuhan at higher risk for peer problems and overall behavior difficulties vs Huangshi.
Patrick et al,[23] 2020	United States (June 2020)	1000 parents with ≥1 child <18 y households	14.3% reported worsening in child's behavioral health with little difference in racial, ethnic, income, or education groups. Worsening of mental health in parent and child linked to having younger children, loss of child care, and reported increased food insecurity.
Tang et al,[24] 2021	China (March 2020)	4342 Primary and secondary school students, ages 6–17 y	Higher reported depression, anxiety, and stress among senior secondary students, those who saw quarantine having more problems vs benefits, and those whose parents had not discussed COVID with them.

(continued on next page)

Table 1
(continued)

Author	Country (Data Collection Dates)	Participants	Findings Regarding Child and Adolescent Mental Health
Xie et al,[3] 2020	Wuhan and Huangshi, China (February to March 2020)	1784 children, Chinese grades 2–6 (approx. ages: 7–12 y)	Rates of anxiety and depression higher than previous population studies in China. Higher depression scores found in children from Wuhan vs Huangshi, those who rated themselves as "quite worried" about being affected by COVID-19, or those who rated themselves as "not optimistic about the epidemic."
Yeasmin et al,[25] 2020	Bangladesh (April to May 2020)	384 parents of children ages 5–15 y	Severity of depressive, anxiety, and sleep symptoms was higher for children in urban area, who had more COVID + family/neighbors, and whose parents had higher education, needed to go to workplace, who smoked, or were at risk of losing job.
Yue et al,[26] 2020	China (February 2020)	1360 children and parents; average child age 10.56 y (SD = 1.79)	Anxiety and PTSD symptoms in children related to spending more time on COVID media reports.
Zhou et al,[27] 2020	China (March 2020)	8079 teens ages 12–18 y	Found higher depressive and anxious symptoms in females, in rural areas, and in higher grades. Protective factors included: knowing more about COVID, taking safety precautions, and being optimistic about pandemic

Abbreviations: CDC, Centers for Disease Control and Prevention; ED, emergency department.

continued through October. Additionally, the proportion of mental health-related visits in late March through October was significantly higher than during same months in 2019. More specifically, the proportion of such visits for ages 5 to 11 demonstrated a 24% increase from 2019 to 2020 (from 783 per 100,000 visits to 972 per 100,000), and the proportion of adolescents aged 12 to 17 years presenting for mental health-related visits increased 31% (from 3098 per 100,000 emergency department visits to 4051 per 100,000). These increases may well reflect increased distress among children and adolescents owing to pandemic-related stressors. Additionally, the authors raised the possibility that these increases are related to the public's difficulties accessing mental health services in the community.[20]

Predominant COVID-19–Related Mental Health Concerns by Age

Across studies reviewed, rates of mental health symptoms during COVID-19 have varied by age. Findings here are grouped for younger children, school-aged children, and adolescents.

Younger children

Studies examining the most significant mental health concerns in younger children (eg, <7 years of age) during the pandemic have found reports of more clinginess and fear about safety,[19] increased uncooperative and worry behaviors,[15] and misbehavior, boredom, needing attention, and anxiety.[14] Young children of hourly service workers who experienced significant COVID-related stressors displayed increased uncooperative and worry behaviors.[15]

School-aged children

Children of elementary school age (approximately 7–13 years) have been reported to display rates of anxiety and depression that are higher than normal during the COVID-19 pandemic.[3] Rates of significant depressive symptoms in studies of children during this time have ranged from 2.2%[26] to 11.78%.[12] Rates of significant anxiety symptoms have ranged from 1.8%[26] to 18.92%[12] to 23.87%.[13] The rate of PTSD was reported as 3.16%.[26] The most problematic behaviors have been reported to be increased inattention and need for reassurance,[19] as well as difficulties with academics, misbehavior, anxiety, social isolation, and depression.[14]

Adolescents

Parents have reported that the most significant behavioral concerns in adolescents during the pandemic have included depression, anxiety, misbehavior, social isolation, (poor) attention, and impulsivity.[14] Self-report rates of significant anxiety symptoms have been found to range from 10.4%[27] to 29.27%.[13] Rates of significant depressive symptoms have been reported to range from 17.3%[27] to 22.28%[13] and were found to be higher in female adolescents compared with males.[12,13,27] Several studies indicated that high school seniors (as compared with younger children) demonstrated the highest ratings for depression,[27] anxiety, and stress.[24] Mental health-related emergency department visits were more common in ages 12 to 17 during the postpandemic months (March to October, 2020) with females having the higher proportion of visits.[20] In a community sample of primarily college-aged youth, 39.9% reported symptoms of an internalizing disorder (eg, depression or anxiety), and 16.9% reported symptoms of an externalizing disorder (eg, aggression, oppositionality).[16] Another study of college age youth indicated high rates of somatic symptoms (34.85%), particularly when worried about necessities of daily life.[21]

Factors Found to Contribute to Mental Health Symptoms

Research on mental health and psychosocial functioning has identified multiple factors that seem to affect rates of mental health symptoms in children and adolescents.

Social isolation

Research has shown that social isolation and loneliness increase the risk of depression and possibly anxiety, with duration of loneliness having the biggest impact on child mental health.[28] The COVID-19 studies reviewed here did indeed link social isolation to increased depression and anxiety, including children who were unhappy with home quarantine,[24] those whose parents went to work while children stayed at home,[25] and children who had no companion on weekdays.[12] Sexual minority youth may be particularly vulnerable to the mental health effects of social isolation. A study by Fish and colleagues[29] with lesbian, gay, bisexual, transgender, and youth questioning sexual orientation (LGBTQ) youth identified the challenges of youth being homebound with unsupportive families, as well as loss of in-person support and socialization. Researchers stressed the importance of assisting LGBTQ youth in maintaining social supports and mental health through electronic connections.

Screen time

The use of phones and the Internet have become integral parts of coping with the COVID-19 pandemic. Although some parents reported successfully using media entertainment to soothe children during the initial weeks of the pandemic,[19] a large study of children and adolescents linked smartphone and Internet addiction (defined as excessive use) to increased depression.[13]

Lack of physical activity

Children engaging in regular physical activity during the pandemic seemed to fare better, demonstrating less hyperactive–inattentive behavior and more prosocial behaviors.[22] Conversely, a lack of physical exercise during COVID-19 has been linked to higher levels of depression and anxiety, and investigators suggest that physical activity may serve as a protective factor.[12] Mittal and colleagues[30] raised concerns about significant negative effects of sedentary behavior on children's mental health, noting that children's play is crucial to meet developmental milestones. They emphasized the importance of alternatives such as zoom to continue physical activity, as well as community and academic partnerships to ensure that children remain active.

Perceived COVID-19 risk

Child and adolescent mental health has been found to vary directly with perceived risks of COVID-19. Two studies examined negative effects of living near high rates of COVID-19 (ie, City of Wuhan compared with other areas in China). Children living near Wuhan displayed higher levels of depression,[3] more peer problems, and overall behavior difficulties.[31] Consistent with this finding, primary school children were found to have increased somatic symptoms and anxiety when experiencing higher concerns regarding threats to their life and health.[21] Yeasmin and colleagues[25] found that children with a greater severity of sleep problems had more COVID-positive family members or neighbors. Fitzpatrick and colleagues[14] examined the effects of community COVID-19 rates and restrictions, finding that number of COVID-19 cases in a family's geographic region was significantly associated with child and adolescent internalizing problems. More leniency in community restrictions was associated with greater child and adolescent internalizing, as well as externalizing problems, suggesting that children felt safer and had better mental health outcomes when community restrictions were in place.

Exposure to COVID-19 information

Some evidence has been found that exposure to COVID-related information can affect mental health. In a large study 1 month after quarantine, grade school children who reported spending more time on COVID-19 media reports also reported higher levels of anxiety and PTSD symptoms. In the same study, the amount of attention paid to such reports was related to PTSD symptoms only.[26] In contrast, a separate study found that children seemed to benefit from discussions about COVID-19 with parents; those whose parents did not discuss COVID-19 with them reported higher levels of depression, anxiety, and stress.[24] A large study of adolescents found that those reporting greater knowledge about COVID-19, more optimism about it, and engaging in more safety steps reported lower levels of depressive and anxious symptoms.

Parenting stress

It is difficult to separate child and parent well-being from each other. Studies examining parent well-being during the COVID-19 pandemic found that it was directly related to hardships such as decreases in work, incomes and increased caregiving burden.[15] In a US study of 1000 parents, 26.9% reported worsening of their own mental health since onset of the pandemic, especially in mothers, unmarried parents, and families with younger children.[23] Such stressors can lead to increased risks of domestic violence and child abuse.[32] Studies during COVID-19 have found that parental depression, job loss, and previous maltreatment predicted higher rates of maltreatment for children ages 4 to 10 years of age.[33] A study examining parenting of a wider range of children (<18 years) found that greater received support and perception of control resulted in parents being less likely to maltreat.[34] Rodriguez and colleagues noted that the pandemic serves as a perfect storm, given the economic hardships, effects on parental mental health, and the increased time families are spending together during the COVID-19 restrictions.[35] The authors call for investment in primary prevention, rather than a reactive approach, to support and educate families and communities to protect children.

DISCUSSION

Experts have cautioned that the high number of deaths, continued experience of grief and loss, and exacerbation of current mental health disorders mean that a "second wave" of mental health consequences from this pandemic is "imminent."[36] Consequently, the need for effective social supports and mental health interventions is crucial.

Kaslow and colleagues[37] proposed a behavioral health response continuum to "flatten the emotional distress curve," which was inspired by the Centers for Disease Control and Prevention's pandemic intervals framework. Through strategic planning, behavioral health experts can mobilize and provide large-scale interventions such as education on coping strategies, social connectedness, and other behavioral health education. Continued data gathering and research would then help to identify continued needs and provide information on program effectiveness. Using a public health model to address the mental health needs of a population is a promising approach.

Going forward, the need for accessible mental health services for children and families has never been greater. Decreasing financial and insurance barriers to access will be essential, including continued development of parity for mental health care. The increase in telehealth mental health services in the United States has been dramatic[38] and offers one way to expand access to families with distance, safety, or transportation barriers. The disproportionate effect of COVID-19 on communities of Black,

Latino, and Native American families requires collaborative behavioral health care in which experts build capacity around the needs of these communities.[39]

Medical settings are often the front line with regard to identifying mental health needs. Professionals in these settings will want to assess for depression and anxiety in children and adolescents during this continued pandemic. Standardized, empirically based mental health screening measures can quickly identify those in need of further assessment and/or referrals for mental health services. The American Academy of Pediatrics provides recommended screening measures (Mental Health Tools) within their Mental Health Initiatives website, which can be found here: https://www.aap.org/en-us/advocacy-and-policy/aap-health-initiatives/Mental-Health/Pages/Primary-Care-Tools.aspx.[40] The site provides information on the measures, as well as information on obtaining them. Integrating mental health professionals within medical care can be ideal for assessing and treating overall psychosocial functioning of patients.

As we approach the 1-year anniversary of COVID-19 pandemic, continued research will be critical to understand ongoing impacts to child and adolescent mental health. There is a need for more research within communities disproportionally affected by COVID-19 such as the Black, Latino, and Native American populations. There is also a need for further research of COVID-19 impacts on children and adolescents with disabilities. There is a need to identify effective prevention strategies and treatment interventions.

SUMMARY

Research on the mental health effects of the COVID-19 pandemic on children and adolescents confirms the presence of significant anxiety and depression, as well as increases in these symptoms compared with prepandemic levels. Research reviewed suggests that teenagers, especially females and high school seniors, may suffer the most. There is evidence that social isolation and sedentary behaviors contribute to these mental health problems. Children who feel unsafe with regard to COVID-19 may be more likely to experience somatic symptoms, depression, and anxiety. Exposure to excessive information about COVID without parental communication on the topic may lead to higher anxiety and PTSD symptoms.

Many parents are experiencing significant economic and personal stress along with increasing mental health symptoms, especially single parents and parents of young children. It is clear that parental stress and mental health problems directly affect their children, and some children may be at increased risk for child maltreatment owing to pandemic-related stressors and situations.

Increasing access to mental health services for children and families will be vital. Integrating mental health care into medical settings would be ideal to provide frontline and comprehensive care. Research on the continuing effects of COVID-19 will be necessary as the situation continues to change, and studies of effective prevention and treatments strategies are also needed.

CLINICS CARE POINTS

- Professionals are just beginning to understand how the ongoing COVID-19 pandemic has significantly impacted the lives and mental health of children and adolescents.
- Current research shows children are displaying increased anxiety and depression, and that social isolation and a lack of physical activity may worsen these factors.

- Racial minority children and adolescents may be at even greater risk, given the additive effects of racism on health.
- Health care professionals should screen patients routinely for unmet mental health needs and provide links to care when indicated. Increasing access to mental health care is crucial.

DISCLOSURE

The author has nothing to disclose.

REFERENCES

1. CDC. About COVID-19. CDC: Centers for Disease Control and Prevention. 2020. Available at: https://www.cdc.gov/coronavirus/2019-ncov/cdcresponse/about-COVID-19.html. Accessed January 16, 2021.
2. CDC. COVID Data Tracker: United States COVID-19 Cases and Deaths by State. Centers for Disease Control and Prevention (CDC). 2021. Available at: https://covid.cdc.gov/covid-data-tracker/#cases_casesper100klast7days. Accessed January 16, 2021.
3. Xie X, Xue Q, Zhou Y, et al. Mental Health Status Among Children in Home Confinement During the Coronavirus Disease 2019 Outbreak in Hubei Province, China. JAMA Pediatr 2020;174(9):898–900.
4. Taylor DB. A Timeline of the Coronavirus Pandemic. New York Times. 2021. Available at: https://www.nytimes.com/article/coronavirus-timeline.html. Accessed January 16, 2021.
5. Gee GC, Ro MJ, Rimoin AW. Seven Reasons to Care About Racism and COVID-19 and Seven Things to Do to Stop It. Am J Public Health 2020;110(7):954–5.
6. Cheah CSL, Wang C, Ren H, et al. COVID-19 racism and mental health in Chinese American families. Pediatrics 2020;146(5). https://doi.org/10.1542/peds.2020-021816.
7. Taylor DB. George Floyd protests: a timeline. New York Times. Available at: https://www.nytimes.com/article/george-floyd-protests-timeline.html. Accessed January 16, 2021.
8. Buchanan L, Bui Q, Patel JK. Black Lives Matter May Be the Largest Movement in U.S. History. New York Times. 2020. Available at: https://www.nytimes.com/interactive/2020/07/03/us/george-floyd-protests-crowd-size.html. Accessed January 16, 2020.
9. Racine N, Cooke JE, Eirich R, et al. Child and adolescent mental illness during COVID-19: a rapid review. Psychiatry Res 2020;292:113307.
10. Marques de Miranda D, da Silva Athanasio B, Sena Oliveira AC, et al. How is COVID-19 pandemic impacting mental health of children and adolescents? Int J Disaster Risk Reduction 2020;51:101845.
11. Fong VC, Iarocci G. Child and family outcomes following pandemics: a systematic review and recommendations on COVID-19 policies. J Pediatr Psychol 2020;45(10):1124–43.
12. Chen F, Zheng D, Liu J, et al. Depression and anxiety among adolescents during COVID-19: a cross-sectional study [Letter to the Editor]. Brain Behav Immun 2020;88:36–8.
13. Duan L, Shao X, Wang Y, et al. An investigation of mental health status of children and adolescents in China during the outbreak of COVID-19. J Affect Disord 2020;275:112–8.

14. Fitzpatrick O, Carson A, Weisz JR. Using mixed methods to identify the primary mental health problems and needs of children, adolescents, and their caregivers during the coronavirus (covid-19) pandemic. Child Psychiatry Hum Dev 2020. https://doi.org/10.1007/s10578-020-01089-z.

15. Gassman-Pines A, Ananat EO, Fitz-Henley J II. COVID-19 and parent-child psychological well-being. Pediatrics 2020;146(4). https://doi.org/10.1542/peds. 2020-007294.

16. Hawke LD, Barbic SP, Voineskos A, et al. Impacts of COVID-19 on youth mental health, substance use, and well-being: a rapid survey of clinical and community samples: Répercussions de la COVID-19 sur la santé mentale, l'utilisation de substances et le bien-être des adolescents : un sondage rapide d'échantillons cliniques et communautaires. Can J Psychiatry 2020;65(10):701–9.

17. Hill RM, Rufino K, Kurian S, et al. Suicide ideation and attempts in a pediatric emergency department before and during CoViD-19. Pediatrics 2020;147(3). e2020029280.

18. Isumi A, Doi S, Yamaoka Y, et al. Do suicide rates in children and adolescents change during school closure in Japan? The acute effect of the first wave of COVID-19 pandemic on child and adolescent mental health. Child Abuse Neglect 2020;110(Part 2). https://doi.org/10.1016/j.chiabu.2020.104680.

19. Jiao WY, Wang LN, Liu J, et al. Behavioral and Emotional Disorders in Children during the COVID-19 Epidemic. J Pediatr 2020;221:264–6.e1.

20. Leeb RT, Bitsko RH, Radhakrishnan L, et al. Mental Health-Related Emergency Department Visits Among Children Aged <18 Years During the COVID-19 Pandemic - United States, January 1-October 17, 2020. MMWR Morb Mortal Wkly Rep 2020;69(45):1675–80.

21. Liu S, Liu Y, Liu Y. Somatic symptoms and concern regarding COVID-19 among Chinese college and primary school students: a cross-sectional survey. Psychiatry Res 2020;289:113070.

22. Liu Q, Zhou Y, Xie X, et al. The prevalence of behavioral problems among school-aged children in home quarantine during the COVID-19 pandemic in China. J Affect Disord 2021;279:412–6.

23. Patrick SW, Henkhaus LE, Zickafoose JS, et al. Well-being of parents and children during the COVID-19 pandemic: a national survey. Pediatrics 2020;146(4). https://doi.org/10.1542/peds.2020-016824.

24. Tang S, Xiang M, Cheung T, et al. Mental health and its correlates among children and adolescents during COVID-19 school closure: the importance of parent-child discussion. J Affect Disord 2021;279:353–60.

25. Yeasmin S, Banik R, Hossain S, et al. Impact of COVID-19 pandemic on the mental health of children in Bangladesh: a cross-sectional study. Child Youth Serv Rev 2020;117:105277.

26. Yue J, Zang X, Le Y, et al. Anxiety, depression and PTSD among children and their parent during 2019 novel coronavirus disease (covid-19) outbreak in China. Curr Psychol 2020. https://doi.org/10.1007/s12144-020-01191-4.

27. Zhou S-J, Zhang L-G, Wang L-L, et al. Prevalence and socio-demographic correlates of psychological health problems in Chinese adolescents during the outbreak of covid-19. Eur Child Adolesc Psychiatry 2020. https://doi.org/10. 1007/s00787-020-01541-4.

28. Loades ME, Chatburn E, Higson-Sweeney N, et al. Rapid systematic review: the impact of social isolation and loneliness on the mental health of children and adolescents in the context of COVID-19. J Am Acad Child Adolesc Psychiatry 2020; 59(11):1218–39.

29. Fish JN, McInroy LB, Paceley MS, et al. 'I'm kinda stuck at home with unsupportive parents right now': LGBTQ youths' experiences with COVID-19 and the importance of online support. J Adolesc Health 2020;67(3):450–2.

30. Mittal VA, Firth J, Kimhy D. Combating the dangers of sedentary activity on child and adolescent mental health during the time of COVID-19. J Am Acad Child Adolesc Psychiatry 2020;59(11):1197–8.

31. Liu D, Baumeister RF, Zhou Y. Mental health outcomes of coronavirus infection survivors: a rapid meta-analysis. J Psychiatr Res 2020. https://doi.org/10.1016/j.jpsychires.2020.10.015.

32. Fegert JM, Vitiello B, Plener PL, et al. Challenges and burden of the Coronavirus 2019 (COVID-19) pandemic for child and adolescent mental health: a narrative review to highlight clinical and research needs in the acute phase and the long return to normality. Child Adolesc Psychiatry Ment Health 2020;14:20.

33. Lawson M, Piel MH, Simon M. Child maltreatment during the COVID-19 pandemic: consequences of parental job loss on psychological and physical abuse towards children. Child Abuse Neglect 2020;110(Part 2). https://doi.org/10.1016/j.chiabu.2020.104709.

34. Brown SM, Doom JR, Lechuga-Peña S, et al. Stress and parenting during the global COVID-19 pandemic. Child Abuse Neglect 2020;110(Part 2). https://doi.org/10.1016/j.chiabu.2020.104699.

35. Rodriguez CM, Lee SJ, Ward KP, et al. The perfect storm: hidden risk of child maltreatment during the Covid-19 pandemic. Child Maltreat 2020. https://doi.org/10.1177/1077559520982066. 1077559520982066.

36. Simon NM, Saxe GN, Marmar CR. Mental health disorders related to COVID-19–Related Deaths. JAMA 2020;324(15):1493–4.

37. Kaslow NJ, Friis-Healy EA, Cattie JE, et al. Flattening the emotional distress curve: a behavioral health pandemic response strategy for COVID-19. Am Psychol 2020;75(7):875–86.

38. Patients with Depression and Anxiety Surge as Psychologists Respond to the Coronavirus Pandemic. November 2020, 2020.

39. Fortuna LR, Tolou-Shams M, Robles-Ramamurthy B, et al. Inequity and the disproportionate impact of COVID-19 on communities of color in the United States: the need for a trauma-informed social justice response. Psychol Trauma Theor Res Pract Policy 2020;12(5):443–5.

40. Pediatrics AAo. Mental health initiatives: primary care tools. Available at: https://www.aap.org/en-us/advocacy-and-policy/aap-health-initiatives/Mental-Health/Pages/Primary-Care-Tools.aspx. Accessed January 16, 2021.

COVID-19 in Children

Clinical Manifestations and Pharmacologic Interventions Including Vaccine Trials

Ramon Galindo, MD[1], Heather Chow, DO[1], Chokechai Rongkavilit, MD*

KEYWORDS

• COVID-19 • SARS-CoV-2 • Coronavirus • Children • Infant • Treatment • Vaccine

KEY POINTS

- COVID-19 in children usually presents with milder symptoms as compared with adults.
- Supportive care alone is appropriate for most children with COVID-19.
- There has been a rapid development of vaccines globally to prevent COVID-19.
- As of June 2021, only Pfizer–BioNTech BNT162b2 mRNA vaccine is approved for emergency authorization use in the pediatric population age 12 years and older.
- A serious hyperinflammatory process after COVID-19 in children known as multisystemic inflammatory syndrome in children has been described. Its clinical features can overlap with Kawasaki disease.

INTRODUCTION

There have been reports of severe acute respiratory syndrome coronavirus-2 (SARS-CoV-2) infecting children in all age groups; however, children still comprise a small percentage of the total number of cases of coronavirus disease 2019 (COVID-19). As low as 2% of 80,900 COVID-19 cases during the case surge in China were pediatric cases.[1] Similarly, a systematic review showed that children accounted for 1% to 5% of reported COVID-19 cases.[2] Interestingly, the proportion of children with COVID-19 seems to be higher in the United States. By the end of 2020, 2,128,587 COVID-19 cases in US children have been reported, and children represented 12% of all reported cases in the United States. The overall rate was 2828 cases per 100,000 US children.[3] The difference in prevalence among different geographic locations could be due to multiple factors, including the case definition used, access to testing, varied sensitivity

Department of Pediatrics, University of California San Francisco-Fresno Branch Campus, 155 North Fresno Street, Suite 219, Fresno, CA 93701-2302, USA
[1] The first author and the second author contributed equally to this article.
* Corresponding author.
E-mail address: chokechai.rongkavilit@ucsf.edu

Pediatr Clin N Am 68 (2021) 961–976
https://doi.org/10.1016/j.pcl.2021.05.004
0031-3955/21/© 2021 Elsevier Inc. All rights reserved.

of the tests used, differences in anatomic respiratory sampling sites, variability in sample collection by personnel, levels of case surge within communities, and other as yet unknown host and pathogen factors.

CLINICAL MANIFESTATIONS IN CHILDREN
COVID-19 Symptoms in Children Are Milder Compared with Those in Adults

It has been observed since early in the pandemic that children seem to experience milder symptoms when compared with adults. Correspondingly, in a large case series of 2135 pediatric patients with COVID-19 in China, 55% of cases were asymptomatic or had only mild symptoms.[4] Only 6% of pediatric cases were classified as severe and critical cases. This number is fewer compared with the number of severe and critical cases in the adult population, which was found to be about 18.5%. In a report from the US Centers for Disease Control and Prevention (CDC), 73% of pediatric COVID-19 cases had symptoms of fever, cough, or shortness of breath compared with 93% of adults aged 18 to 64 years during the same reporting period, and only 6% of all pediatric cases required hospitalization.[5] Thus, the majority of pediatric COVID-19 cases are either asymptomatic or mild in disease severity.

Theories for the milder symptoms and lower prevalence in children

Multiple theories have been suggested to explain why children may contribute to such a small percentage of reported COVID-19 cases and why children may have a milder clinical presentation than adults. In a systematic review and meta-analysis including 32 studies, children and adolescents younger than 20 years had a 44% lower odds of infection with SARS-CoV-2 compared with adults 20 years and older, and the finding was most marked in those younger than 10 to 14 years.[6]

Davies and colleagues[7] generated a modeling study to determine the manifestation of clinical symptoms based on susceptibility of infection in children versus adults. Their data suggested an "age gradient," in which the risk for severe disease increases with advancing age. More specifically, they found that 79% of pediatric patients in the 10- to 19-year-old group are asymptomatic, and that individuals 20 years and older are 2 times more susceptible to COVID-19 than those younger than 20 years of age.

Several potential causes have been implicated in creating this distribution across the different age groups. Having more mild symptoms or being asymptomatic may contribute to reporting bias and account for the low number of reported cases of COVID-19 in children. Those with less noticeable symptoms are less likely to seek medical care, and in turn the cases are less likely to be confirmed and reported.

Second, because children get frequent viral upper respiratory tract infections including coronaviruses that cause common cold, it has also been proposed that infections from other coronaviruses offer some immunity to children, rendering children less susceptible to infection by SARS-CoV-2. This phenomenon may be due to either cross-protection from other types of previous coronavirus infections or nonspecific protection from other respiratory viruses. Coinfection with another virus could also compete with SARS-CoV-2 and decrease its replication, and thus result in a milder illness.[8]

Third, SARS-CoV-2 uses its spike protein to bind with human angiotensin-converting enzyme 2 (ACE-2) receptor for host cell entry.[9] In a cohort study of 305 individuals aged 4 to 60 years, ACE-2 gene expression in the nasal epithelium was lowest in children less than 10 years of age and it increased with advancing age.[10] Low ACE-2 expression could limit SARS-CoV-2 entry into host cells. This factor could lead to a lower risk of infection and a milder clinical presentation in children. Moreover, the lower prevalence of comorbidities such as diabetes, chronic lung disease, and cardiovascular disease in children may contribute to a milder clinical course as compared with adults.[11]

Many pediatric COVID-19 cases have been found to be linked to a family member. In a study with 34 confirmed pediatric cases, 13 (38%) patients were found to have an exposure to COVID-19 from a family member.[12] It has been suggested that if an adult transmits SARS-CoV-2 to a child, the infection would be caused by a second or third generation of virus, and the infection may be milder owing to decreased pathogenicity. A retrospective review analyzed the data collected from 9 children and their 14 adult family members.[13] It was found that 3 children had symptoms of fever or cough, and 6 were asymptomatic. Four children (44%) had abnormal chest radiograph findings, whereas 71% of the adults had abnormal radiograph studies. Thus, this concept of family clusters may also explain why pediatric patients have a milder presentation.[8,11]

Clinical Manifestations

The most common symptoms in children include fever, upper respiratory symptoms, and gastrointestinal symptoms. Because SARS-CoV-2 attaches to human cells via ACE-2 receptors, the expression of ACE-2 receptors on epithelial cells in the lung and the intestines may account for the manifestations of respiratory and gastrointestinal symptoms, respectively.[8]

In a review of 333 pediatric patients, the most common symptoms included cough with a prevalence of 48%, fever (42%), and sore throat (42%). Moreover, 35% of cases were reported to be asymptomatic.[11] Similarly, in a study in Wuhan, China, that examined 171 children with confirmed COVID-19, 49% of children had cough, 42% had fever, and 46% had pharyngitis.[2] Other symptoms that have been reported include rhinorrhea, nasal congestion, myalgia, fatigue, shortness of breath, dyspnea, abdominal pain, diarrhea, vomiting, nausea, headache, dizziness, decreased oral intake, and rash. **Fig. 1** provides a compilation of clinical symptom data from 3 review articles that altogether include 26 studies for a total of 1793 children with COVID-19.[1,11,14] Fever

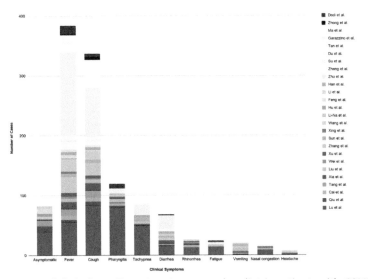

Fig. 1. Summary of clinical manifestations in reported pediatric patients with COVID-19.

and cough were by far the most prevalent symptoms (see **Fig. 1**). Recovery occurred within 1 to 2 weeks after the onset of symptoms.[8]

In adults, anosmia and ageusia have been reported in COVID-19 cases. These symptoms have been reported less frequently in children. Coronaviruses as a family of viruses invade the olfactory bulb, leading to loss of smell. Parisi and colleagues[15] emphasizes the importance of further evaluation in pediatric patients with COVID-19 complaining of loss of smell. Nasal endoscopy and smell tests, such as the Pediatric Smell Wheel, can be used to help identify the degree of olfactory loss.[15]

Severe and Critical Disease in Children

Although most children with COVID-19 are mildly symptomatic or asymptomatic, there have been reported cases of severe infection and even death, albeit few. Reported symptoms of severe and critical disease include hypoxia defined as an oxygen saturation of less than 92%, acute respiratory distress syndrome, shock, and various organ failure such as encephalopathy, heart failure, abnormal coagulation, and acute kidney injury.[4] According to a review by Zimmerman and colleagues, 9 (3%) of 333 children required admission to pediatric intensive care units, and two of these children had preexisting conditions, namely, leukemia and hydronephrosis.[11]

The adult and elderly population have experienced more COVID-19–related deaths than the pediatric population.[1] The presence of comorbidities such as cancer, diabetes, cardiovascular disease, chronic lung disease, and a weaker immune system has been implicated in the greater prevalence of deaths in adults. One study of 44,672 COVID-19 cases found that 26% had comorbidities.[2] Additionally, there were 965 deaths, and only one of these deaths was a pediatric patient. No information was provided on the 14-year-old boy in this study. By March 2020, this case was 1 of the 2 deaths reported in children with COVID-19. The other child was a 10-month-old girl with intussusception, encephalopathy, septic shock, and multiorgan failure.[2,11]

In a review of 29 studies with 4300 children included, 19% were asymptomatic and 37% had no radiographic abnormalities.[16] A small proportion of 0.1% required admission to intensive care units and 4 deaths were reported. Among 208 hospitalized children with complete medical chart reviews by the US COVID-19-Associated Hospitalization Surveillance Network, 33% were admitted to an intensive care unit, 6% required invasive mechanical ventilation, and 1 child (0.5%) died.[17] The comorbid conditions included obesity (38%), chronic lung disease (18%), and prematurity (15%). Overall, children with COVID-19 have a good prognosis. However, a serious postinfectious hyperinflammatory process known as multisystemic inflammatory syndrome in children has been described. See details in Chapter 5 in this issue.

COVID-19 Symptoms in Newborns and Infants

COVID-19 in neonates has also been reported. In China, between early December 2019 and February 2020, 9 infants (1–11 months of age) were hospitalized. Four had fever, 2 had mild upper respiratory tract infections, 1 was asymptomatic, and there was no information on 2 infants.[18] Another review reported 3 neonatal cases.[2] One had fever and cough, one had rhinorrhea and vomiting, and the third had respiratory distress. Neonatal complications from COVID-19–infected mothers have been reported as well. In 67 neonates born to 65 mothers who had COVID-19 during pregnancy, 12 had respiratory distress or pneumonia (18%), 9 were born with low birth weight (13%), 2 developed a rash (3%), 2 developed disseminated intravascular coagulation (3%), 1 had asphyxia (2%), and 2 died (3%).[11]

Inverse Relationship between Severity and Age in Pediatrics

Even though severity of COVID-19 seems to increase with advancing age in the general population overall, severity in the pediatric population seems inversely related to age, as depicted by the study performed by Dong and colleagues.[4] Infants were the most susceptible to severe illness, with 10.6% of infants less than 1 year of age presenting with severe or critical disease. A decreasing frequency of severity with advancing age was demonstrated, with severe illness being reported in 7.3% in the 1- to 5-year-old group, 4.2% in the 6- to 10-year-old group, 4.1% in the 11- to 15-year-old group, and 3.0% in the 16 or older group. In the United States, infants less than 1 year old accounted for the highest percentage (estimated range, 15%–62%) of hospitalizations among pediatric patients with COVID-19.[5]

PHARMACOLOGIC INTERVENTIONS, INCLUDING VACCINE TRIALS
Pharmacologic Interventions

Antivirals
Remdesivir. The antiviral that has perhaps received the most attention is remdesivir. Remdesivir has a broad spectrum antiviral activity that was first developed to treat hepatitis C and respiratory syncytial virus and subsequently repurposed to treat the Ebola virus.[19] SARS-CoV-2 is part of the Coronaviridae family characterized by positive sense single-stranded RNA that requires the function of an RNA-dependent RNA polymerase for replication. Remdesivir is a nucleoside analog capable of inhibiting the RNA polymerase via chain termination and has demonstrated in vitro activity against SARS-CoV-1 and Middle Eastern respiratory syndrome coronavirus.[20–22] The efficacy of remdesivir in treating adults with lower respiratory tract infection with COVID-19 was assessed in a double-blinded placebo-controlled trial with the primary outcome being time to recovery. The results demonstrated that a 10-day course of remdesivir resulted in a shorter time to recovery with a median of 10 days versus 15 days with placebo. Despite the shorter recovery, the study did not demonstrate a reduction in mortality.[23] At present, a phase II/III study evaluating safety, tolerability, pharmacokinetics, and efficacy of remdesivir in the pediatric population is ongoing. Despite the lack of clinical trial data, there have been reported cases of its use in children.[24,25] The most recent guidelines regarding antiviral therapy in children has been set forth by a panel of pediatric infectious disease physicians and pharmacists in the United States. Their suggestion is that supportive care alone is appropriate for most cases given the mild course of COVID-19 in children in general. For children with severe or critical illness, as defined by the need for supplemental oxygen, noninvasive or invasive mechanical ventilation, or extracorporeal membrane oxygenation, remdesivir should be considered. A treatment duration of 5 days is appropriate for most children.[26] Although approved for use in children with COVID-19 by the US Food and Drug Administration (FDA) through an Emergency Use Authorization (EUA), the safety and efficacy of remdesivir have not been evaluated fully in pediatric patients aged less than 12 years or weighing less than 40 kg. Other medications including chloroquine, hydroxychloroquine, azithromycin, or lopinavir/ritonavir are not recommended for the treatment of COVID-19.[27]

Corticosteroids
The use of corticosteroids for COVID-19 is based primarily on the results of the multicenter, randomized, open-label RECOVERY trial.[28] Mortality at 28 days was lower among adult patients on invasive mechanical ventilation who received up to 10 days of dexamethasone 6 mg once daily (29.3%) than among those who received the standard of care (41.4%). This benefit was also observed in patients who required

supplemental oxygen. No mortality benefit was seen in those who required no supplemental oxygen. According to the National Institutes of Health guidelines, if dexamethasone is not available, alternatives such as prednisone, methylprednisolone, or hydrocortisone can be used.[27] The safety and effectiveness of dexamethasone or other corticosteroids for COVID-19 treatment have not been sufficiently evaluated in children. However, dexamethasone may be beneficial in children who require mechanical ventilation. The use of dexamethasone for those who require supplemental oxygen support should be considered on a case-by-case basis.

Monoclonal antibodies

Bamlanivimab (LY-CoV555). Bamlanivimab is an antispike neutralizing monoclonal antibody that was discovered from the convalescent plasma of a patient with COVID-19. This antibody was shown to bind the receptor-binding domain of the trimeric spike protein in both its up (active) or down (resting) state. This finding generated interest because the up state has been shown to be required for ACE-2 binding and viral fusion for cell entry. In a study in nonhuman primates, the administration of this antibody in rhesus monkeys decreased SARS-CoV-2 replication in both the upper and lower respiratory tracts.[29] In the outpatient setting, the administration of bamlanivimab to adults with mild to moderate COVID-19 was shown to decrease the viral load from baseline compared with placebo and to decrease hospitalizations or emergency department visits.[30] Unfortunately, the administration of bamlanivimab among hospitalized adults did not result in a decrease in the clinical severity or in the time to recovery compared with placebo.[31] At this time, there are no published data on the efficacy of bamlanivimab in children; however, the BLAZE-1 trial (NCT04427501) is currently planned to assess the efficacy of bamlanivimab in children greater than 12 years of age with high-risk medical conditions. Despite the lack of published data in persons less than 18 years of age, the FDA issued an EUA in November 2020 granting the use of bamlanivimab for both adults and high-risk children older than 12 years of age who have mild to moderate COVID-19 and who are at high risk of progression to severe COVID-19 and/or hospitalization.

REGN-COV2 (casirivimab and imdevimab). The REGN-COV2 cocktail is composed of 2 fully humanized antibodies that were generated from genetically humanized immune systems of mice. The pair of monoclonal antibodies known as casirivimab and imdevimab bind noncompetitively to the receptor-binding domain of the SARS-CoV-2 spike protein.[32] The idea behind using pairs rather than a single antibody is to help decrease the emergence of escape mutations and in fact REGN-COV2 cocktail was shown to prevent the emergence of spike protein mutants in vitro.[33] In rhesus macaques, the use of the REG-COV2 cocktail was shown to successfully prevent and treat SARS-CoV2 infection.[34] The results of the phase III randomized double-blinded placebo-controlled trial demonstrated that the use of the antibody cocktail in nonhospitalized persons greater than 18 years of age with COVID-19 produced a modest decrease in SARS-CoV-2 viral load levels from baseline as compared with placebo at day 7 of infection.[35] This effect was observed among those who had a high baseline viral load. Secondary end points such as hospitalization or emergency room visits were similar between the placebo group and the antibody treated groups. On November 21, 2020, the FDA issued an EUA for casiravimab and imdevimab to be used together in the treatment of mild to moderate COVID-19 in both ambulatory adults and pediatric patients older than 12 years of age who are at high risk for a poor outcome.[27]

Currently, there is no evidence for the safety and efficacy of monoclonal antibody therapy for treatment of COVID-19 in children or adolescents. Moreover, there is evidence for potential harm associated with monoclonal antibody infusion reactions or anaphylaxis. As of December 2020, the pediatric expert panel suggested against the routine administration of monoclonal antibody therapy (bamlanivimab, or casirivimab and imdevimab) for the treatment of COVID-19 in children or adolescents, including those designated by the FDA as being at high risk of progression to hospitalization or severe disease.[36]

Convalescent plasma
Convalescent plasma has been used for centuries to treat infectious diseases; however, to date the use of convalescent plasma has only been shown to be of clear value in the treatment of Argentine hemorrhagic fever.[37] There are reported cases (n = 4) of improvement after convalescent plasma use in children with severe COVID-19.[38] However, to date no clinical studies have systematically evaluated the efficacy of convalescent plasma in pediatrics. In a placebo-controlled trial in adults with severe COVID-19 with evidence of radiologically confirmed pneumonia and signs of respiratory distress, the use of convalescent plasma did not improve the clinical outcome at 7, 14, or 30 days when compared with placebo, nor did it decrease mortality (11.0% in convalescent plasma group vs 11.4% in placebo).[39] Of note, there was no statistically significant difference in transfusion-related adverse events between the convalescent plasma and the placebo group.

SARS-CoV-2 vaccines
The emergence of SARS-CoV-2 has prompted international efforts to develop effective vaccines at an unprecedented rate. As of January 2021, just 11 months after the announcement of the COVID-19 pandemic by the World Health Organization, 64 vaccines are under clinical evaluation and 173 in preclinical evaluation.[40] The United States has directed more than $10 billion to help streamline the production and distribution of promising antivirals and vaccines in a strategy known as Operation Warp Speed. This operation is a large-scale collaboration between the Department of Health and Human Services, the CDC, the US National Institutes of Health, and the Biomedical Advanced Research and Development Authority along with the Department of Defense.[41] **Table 1** lists the 6 vaccines whose data have shown promise against COVID-19 as of January 2021.

To better appreciate the latest development of COVID-19 vaccines, a brief discussion on messenger RNA (mRNA)-based vaccines is merited, especially because 2 of the 6 vaccines to be discussed elsewhere in this article use this new mRNA-based vaccine technology. Although the technology has been around since the 1990s,[42] its use in the development of vaccines has largely been hindered by its poor stability, unpredictable immune response, and inefficient delivery methods when used in vivo. As a result, vaccine approaches have largely relied on traditional methods using subunits, live attenuated, or inactivated pathogens. In the past decade, however, major advancements through the use of modified nucleosides, synthetic cap analogues, the incorporation of regulatory genetic elements, and purification techniques have resulted in an increased stability of mRNA and improved control over its immunogenicity. Furthermore, the use of lipid nanoparticle technology has greatly enhanced the delivery of mRNA into target cells. In 2017, the first successful use of an mRNA-based vaccine was shown to protect mice against Zika virus.[43] Since then, multiple clinical trials have been initiated to test the efficacy of mRNA-based vaccines against rabies and influenza in humans.[44,45] A review on the latest advancements of mRNA-based vaccine technology is well beyond the scope of this article, but has been excellently reviewed elsewhere.[46] In summary, mRNA-based vaccines have been touted to

Table 1
Current SARS-CoV-2 vaccines (as of January 11, 2021)

Company	Vaccine	Key Component	Series	Efficacy	Storage
Pfizer–BioNTech	BNT162b2	mRNA lipid particle encoding SARS-CoV-2 S-P2 spike protein	2 doses 21 d apart	95%	Storage between −80 °C to −60 °C
Moderna	mRNA-1273	mRNA lipid particle encoding SARS-CoV-2 S-P2 spike protein	2 doses 28 d apart	94.1%	Short-term storage: 2 °C–8 °C. Long-term storage: −20 °C
Oxford–AstraZeneca	ChAdOx1 nCov-19	Replication-deficient chimpanzee adenovirus vector expressing SARS-CoV2 Spike gene	2 doses 28 d apart	70.4%	Storage between 2 °C and 8 °C
Janssen	Ad26.COV2.S	Replication-deficient adenovirus vector serotype 26 encoding full length stabilized SARS-CoV2 spike protein	Single dose vs double dose being studied	Pending	Short-term storage: 2 °C–8 °C. Long-term storage: −20 °C
Novavax	NVX-CoV2373	Purified recombinant SARS-CoV-2 spike glycoprotein and Matrix-M1 adjuvant.	2 doses, 21 d apart	Pending	Storage between 2 °C and 8 °C

have superiority over traditional vaccines via their improved safety profile, efficacy at delivery, and relatively rapid and low-cost production. However, the need for costly laboratory-grade freezers for storage could hinder the widespread use of mRNA-based vaccines in real-world settings.

Pfizer–BioNTech BNT162b2 mRNA vaccine. The Pfizer–BioNTech vaccine consists of a nucleoside-modified mRNA molecule enveloped within a lipoprotein nanoparticle that encodes the SARS-CoV-2 spike protein in a prefusion state. The phase I/II trials were conducted in Germany and the United States and initially involved testing 2 vaccine candidates (BNT162b1 and BNT162b2) for safety and immunogenicity. The molecular difference between these vaccine candidates is that the BNT162b1 mRNA encodes a soluble trimerized SARS-CoV-2 receptor-binding domain protein, whereas the BNT162b2 mRNA encodes a full-length membrane-anchored SARS-CoV-2 spike protein in a prefusion conformation. The phase I/II trial in the United States involved healthy adults 18 to 55 and 65 to 85 years of age. The administration of a primer dose and a booster dose spaced apart by 21 days demonstrated equally robust IgG responses against the S1-binding domain of the spike protein in both vaccine candidates and in all age groups.[47] Furthermore, the immunogenicity was greatly enhanced after the booster dose. One notable difference between BNT162b1 and BNT162b2 was that the latter was associated with a lower incidence of severe systemic reactions such as fever, fatigue, and chills in adults older than 65 years of age. It is worth mentioning that no participants reported a fever of greater than 40 °C or systemic events requiring emergency department visit or hospitalization. Meanwhile the phase I/II trial in Germany demonstrated that the vaccine elicited a strong humoral and cell-mediated immune response as demonstrated by the activation of $CD4^+$ and $CD8^+$ T cells and release of immune-modulatory cytokines such as interferon-gamma, suggesting that the vaccine not only elicited an antibody response, but also an appropriate T-helper type-1 T-cell mediated response.[48] Owing to the preferred safety profile of BNT162b2, it went on to phase III clinical trials. This is a double-blinded randomized trial of 43,448 persons ages 16 years or older who either received a 2-dose placebo or a 2-dose 30 µg BNT162b2 vaccine spaced apart by 21 days.[49] The results demonstrated a 95% efficacy at preventing symptomatic COVID-19. The adverse effects included short-term, mild-to-moderate pain at the injection site along with systemic signs of fatigue, fever, and headache. The incidence of serious adverse events was low and was similar to placebo. The vaccine received FDA EUA for persons ages 16 years and older on December 11, 2020 and subsequently on May 10, 2021 for persons ages 12 years and older. Since the rollout of Pfizer–BioNTech vaccine, there have been 21 reported cases of anaphylaxis among the 1,893,360 first doses (ie, 11.1 cases per million doses given).[50] At the time of this writing according to the CDC, a history of immediate or severe allergic reactions after either mRNA-based COVID-19 vaccine or its components is a contraindication to vaccination with either Pfizer–BioNTech or Moderna COVID-19 vaccine.[51] A history of any immediate allergic reaction to any other vaccine or injectable therapy not related to a component of mRNA COVID-19 vaccines or polysorbate is a precaution but not a contraindication to vaccination.

Moderna mRNA-1273 vaccine. Moderna mRNA-based vaccine also known as mRNA-1273 is composed of a nucleoside-modified mRNA molecule encapsulated within a lipoprotein nanoparticle. The mRNA encodes an anchored transmembrane SARS-CoV-2 S-2P spike protein. The mRNA has been modified such that 2 consecutive prolines are inserted at positions 986 and 987 during translation of the S-2P mRNA. This change maintains the trimeric spike protein in a prefusion state also known as the down or inactive state. To place this in context, viral cell entry via fusion requires that the spike protein to be in the up or active state to facilitate binding to human ACE-2 receptor.[52] This phase I trial involved healthy participants more than 18 years of age being randomized to receive 2 doses of either placebo, 25 μg mRNA-1723 vaccine, or 100 μg mRNA-1723 vaccine given 28 days apart. Both doses of the vaccines elicited robust antispike antibody response in a dose-dependent manner. The level of binding and neutralizing antibody titers generated were greater than antibody titers observed from convalescent serum of patients recovered from COVID-19 and the titers remained elevated at 119 days after the first dose of the vaccine.[53] In addition to eliciting a strong humoral response, the 100 μg dose was shown to preferentially stimulate T-helper type-1 $CD4^+$ cells over T-helper type-2 $CD4^+$ cells, suggesting that the vaccine not only induced a humoral immune response, but also stimulated cell-mediated immunity. Last, the results from the phase I study demonstrated that the most common adverse events consisted of headache, fatigue, myalgia, chills, and pain at the injection site, all of which were reported to be mild to moderate with the majority resolving within 1 day.[54,55] The Moderna mRNA-1273 vaccine entered phase III trials in July 2020. This is a double-blinded study with more than 30,000 participants 18 years of age or older being randomized to receive 2 doses of either placebo or 100 μg mRNA-1273 vaccine given 28 days apart.[56] The vaccine showed 94.1% efficacy at preventing COVID-19 illness including severe COVID-19 disease. Aside from transient local and systemic reactions, no safety concerns were identified.[57] The vaccine received FDA EUA for persons ages 18 years and older on December 18, 2020.

Oxford–AstraZeneca ChAdOx1 nCov-19 vaccine. Unlike Pfizer's and Moderna's mRNA-based vaccines, the University of Oxford–AstraZeneca vaccine known as ChAdOx1 nCov-19 (AZD1222) uses a replication-deficient adenovirus vector to express the SARS-CoV-2 trimeric spike protein. The adenovirus, which causes the common cold in chimpanzees, is modified so as to not replicate in humans. An interim analysis of the randomized controlled trials in the United Kingdom and Brazil demonstrated a vaccine efficacy of 62.1% among participants who received 2 standard doses and 90.0% among participants who received a half dose followed by a standard dose. The overall vaccine efficacy across both groups was 70.4%.[58] Although the overall efficacy was not as high as the mRNA-based vaccines, this vaccine has some advantages, namely, the low cost per dose and no requirement for ultralow temperature storage.[59] These factors makes it attractive for resource-limited settings. It is important to keep in mind that the US FDA and World Health Organization require a vaccine to be at least 50% efficacy for licensure. This vaccine has been authorized for emergency use for persons 18 years and older in the United Kingdom on December 30, 2020.

Janssen Ad26.COV2.S (JNJ-78436725). Similar to the Oxford–AstraZeneca vaccine, the Janssen Ad26.COV2.S vaccine is built on a replication-deficient adenovirus serotype 26 vector that has been modified so as to not replicate in humans. The adenovirus vector was used by Janssen during the design of Ebola virus vaccine. Like the previous vaccines discussed, the adenovirus vector encodes a prefusion stabilized spike protein that is membrane bound and contains a mutation at the furin cleavage site along with 2 protein stabilizing mutations at positions 986 and 987. The basis behind the prefusion conformation is 2-fold. First, the prefusion state facilitated the initial crystallography of this highly glycosylated spike protein,[60] Second, the prefusion conformation has been shown to illicit the highest binding and neutralizing antibody titers when compared with other spike protein variants.[61] The preclinical findings demonstrated that the Ad26.COV2.S vaccine is capable of inducing a humoral immune response in rhesus macaques and that the immunogenicity provided protection when animals were challenged with SARS-CoV-2.[62] One potential benefit of this vaccine is that it could induce immunogenicity (ie, neutralizing antibodies) after a single dose up to day 71 after vaccination as observed in the phase I/IIa trials.[63] This feature would be a benefit over the 2-dose vaccine regimen, particularly in the real-world setting. At the time of this writing, it has entered a phase III (ENSEMBLE) study.

Novavax NVX-CoV2373. Unlike the previous vaccines discussed thus far, the Novavax NVX-CoV2373 vaccine contains purified recombinant full-length trimeric SARS-CoV-2 spike proteins. The recombinant spike protein is modified such that it is resistant to proteolytic cleavage and stabilized to maintain the prefusion conformation. In addition, the vaccine also contains a patented saponin-based Matrix-M adjuvant that enhances immune response and thereby produces high levels of neutralizing antibodies. In a phase I/II study in healthy persons 18 to 59 years of age, the 2-dose 5-µg adjuvanted regimen induced geometric mean antispike IgG antibody and neutralization responses that were greater than those observed in convalescent serum of COVID-19 patients.[64] Reactogenicity was absent or mild. At the time of this writing, it is undergoing phase III trials in the United Kingdom, Mexico, and the United States.

Sanofi–GlaxoSmithKline COVID-19 vaccine. This is an adjuvanted recombinant protein-based vaccine. The phase I/II study involved adults ages 18 to 49 years of age. The vaccine demonstrated immune responses comparable to those who had recovered from COVID-19.[65] Unfortunately, there was a lower immune response observed among those older than 50 years of age. A phase IIb study using an amended formulation is planned for early 2021.

VACCINE CONSIDERATIONS

At the time of this writing, there are currently 64 COVID-19 vaccines in clinical trials and 173 in preclinical development[40]; thus, it is important we do not overlook the usefulness of other upcoming vaccines. This process is ever more important because scientists have discovered the presence of SARS-CoV-2 mutated variants in the United Kingdom, Brazil, and South Africa that have a potential to spread rapidly.[66–68] Published data are lacking on whether immunogenicity from current vaccines can prevent infections by these variants. Our armamentarium against variant strains may rely on the swift identification of new mutations and the rapid development of diverse vaccine candidates.

It is also critical to point out that the clinical trials have not focused specifically on children thus far. It is imperative that we do not delay the development of vaccines for this population. Although children are less likely to suffer from severe COVID-19, children particularly those 10 years of age and older could readily spread COVID-19 as effectively as adults. Furthermore, approximately 12% of all COVID-19 cases are seen in children and some have succumbed to a severe disease.[3] In addition, children have been greatly affected by the pandemic, with large disruptions to in-person school, limited peer interactions, and decreased access to activities that helps to develop their physical and emotional well-being. Thus, the development of COVID-19 vaccines must not only target the adult population, but also the pediatric population. It is encouraging that at the time of this writing, Pfizer has enrolled children to the age of 6 months and its EUA for vaccine indications down to the age of 12 years was approved. Moderna is initiating a similar study, as is Janssen. AstraZeneca vaccine has an approval to enroll children ages 5 to 12 years in the United Kingdom.

SUMMARY

The COVID-19 pandemic has significantly impacted a large number of children worldwide. Although most children present with no or mild symptoms from COVID-19, more data are needed regarding its long-term effects in children. Antivirals and immune-based therapies may play a role in management of those with severe diseases; however, such interventions have not been evaluated fully in pediatric patients to date. The development of vaccines is rapidly evolving, and several vaccine candidates are being assessed in the pediatric population.

CLINICS CARE POINTS

- COVID-19 in children is usually mild, and COVID-19–related deaths in the pediatric population are extremely rare.
- Cases in children have been linked to having a family member with COVID-19.
- Severity in the pediatric population seems to be related inversely with age, with infants being most susceptible to severe COVID-19.
- Supportive care alone is sufficient for most children and antiviral remdesivir may be appropriate for those with severe or critical illness.
- Several vaccine candidates are being evaluated in pediatrics. At this time, only the Pfizer–BioNTech mRNA vaccine is approved for emergency authorization use in the pediatric population ages 12 years and older.

DISCLOSURE

All contributing authors declare no conflicts of interest.

REFERENCES

1. Lok Tung Ho C, Oligbu P, Ojubolamo O, et al. Clinical characteristics of children with COVID-19. AIMS Public Health 2020;7(2):258–73.
2. Ludvigsson JF. Systematic review of COVID-19 in children shows milder cases and a better prognosis than adults. Acta Paediatr 2020;109(6):1088–95.
3. American Academy of Pediatrics and the Children's Hospital Association. Children and COVID-19: state-level data report. Available at: https://services.aap.org/en/pages/2019-novel-coronavirus-covid-19-infections/children-and-covid-19-state-level-data-report/. Accessed January 6, 2021.
4. Dong Y, Mo X, Hu Y, et al. Epidemiology of COVID-19 among children in China. Pediatrics 2020;145(6):e20200702.
5. CDC COVID-19 Response Team, CDC COVID-19 Response Team, Bialek S, et al. Coronavirus disease 2019 in children — United States, February 12–April 2, 2020. MMWR Morb Mortal Wkly Rep 2020;69(14):422–6.
6. Viner RM, Mytton OT, Bonell C, et al. Susceptibility to SARS-CoV-2 infection among children and adolescents compared with adults: a systematic review and meta-analysis. JAMA Pediatr 2020;25. https://doi.org/10.1001/jamapediatrics.2020.4573.

7. CMMID COVID-19 Working Group, Davies NG, Klepac P, et al. Age-dependent effects in the transmission and control of COVID-19 epidemics. Nat Med 2020; 26(8):1205–11.

8. Balasubramanian S, Rao NM, Goenka A, et al. Coronavirus disease 2019 (COVID-19) in children - what we know so far and what we do not. Indian Pediatr 2020;57(5):435–42.

9. Hoffmann M, Kleine-Weber H, Schroeder S, et al. SARS-CoV-2 cell entry depends on ACE2 and TMPRSS2 and is blocked by a clinically proven protease inhibitor. Cell 2020;181(2):271–80.e8.

10. Bunyavanich S, Do A, Vicencio A. Nasal gene expression of angiotensin-converting enzyme 2 in children and adults. JAMA 2020;323(23):2427–9.

11. Zimmermann P, Curtis N. Coronavirus infections in children including COVID-19: an overview of the epidemiology, clinical features, diagnosis, treatment and prevention options in children. Pediatr Infect Dis J 2020;39(5):355–68.

12. Zhang C, Gu J, Chen Q, et al. Clinical and epidemiological characteristics of pediatric SARS-CoV-2 infections in China: a multicenter case series. Persson LÅ. PLoS Med 2020;17(6):e1003130.

13. Su L, Ma X, Yu H, et al. The different clinical characteristics of coronavirus disease cases between children and their families in China – the character of children with COVID-19. Emerg Microbes Infect 2020;9(1):707–13.

14. Martins MM, Prata-Barbosa A, Magalhães-Barbosa MC de, et al. Clinical and laboratory characteristics of SARS-COV-2 infection in children and adolescents. Rev Paul Pediatr 2021;39:e2020231.

15. Parisi GF, Brindisi G, Indolfi C, et al. Upper airway involvement in pediatric COVID-19. Eigenmann P. Pediatr Allergy Immunol 2020;31(S26):85–8.

16. Liu C, He Y, Liu L, et al. Children with COVID-19 behaving milder may challenge the public policies: a systematic review and meta-analysis. BMC Pediatr 2020; 20(1):410.

17. Kim L, Whitaker M, O'Halloran A, et al. Hospitalization Rates and Characteristics of Children Aged <18 Years Hospitalized with Laboratory-Confirmed COVID-19 - COVID-NET, 14 States, March 1-July 25, 2020. MMWR Morb Mortal Wkly Rep 2020;69(32):1081–8.

18. Hong H, Wang Y, Chung H-T, et al. Clinical characteristics of novel coronavirus disease 2019 (COVID-19) in newborns, infants and children. Pediatr Neonatol 2020;61(2):131–2.

19. Warren TK, Jordan R, Lo MK, et al. Therapeutic efficacy of the small molecule GS-5734 against Ebola virus in rhesus monkeys. Nature 2016;531(7594):381–5.

20. Sheahan TP, Sims AC, Leist SR, et al. Comparative therapeutic efficacy of remdesivir and combination lopinavir, ritonavir, and interferon beta against MERS-CoV. Nat Commun 2020;11(1):222.

21. Sheahan TP, Sims AC, Graham RL, et al. Broad-spectrum antiviral GS-5734 inhibits both epidemic and zoonotic coronaviruses. Sci Transl Med 2017;9(396). https://doi.org/10.1126/scitranslmed.aal3653.

22. Gordon CJ, Tchesnokov EP, Feng JY, et al. The antiviral compound remdesivir potently inhibits RNA-dependent RNA polymerase from Middle East respiratory syndrome coronavirus. J Biol Chem 2020;24. https://doi.org/10.1074/jbc.AC120.013056. jbc.AC120.013056.

23. Beigel JH, Tomashek KM, Dodd LE, et al. Remdesivir for the Treatment of Covid-19 - Final Report. N Engl J Med 2020. https://doi.org/10.1056/NEJMoa2007764.

24. Frauenfelder C, Brierley J, Whittaker E, et al. Infant With SARS-CoV-2 Infection Causing Severe Lung Disease Treated With Remdesivir. Pediatrics 2020;146(3). https://doi.org/10.1542/peds.2020-1701.

25. Patel PA, Chandrakasan S, Mickells GE, et al. Severe Pediatric COVID-19 Presenting With Respiratory Failure and Severe Thrombocytopenia. Pediatrics 2020;146(1):e20201437. https://doi.org/10.1542/peds.2020-1437.

26. Chiotos K, Hayes M, Kimberlin DW, et al. Multicenter interim guidance on use of antivirals for children with COVID-19/SARS-CoV-2. J Pediatr Infect Dis Soc 2020; 12. https://doi.org/10.1093/jpids/piaa115.

27. The US National Institutes of Health. Coronavirus Disease 2019 (COVID-19) Treatment Guidelines. National Institutes of Health. Available at: https://www.covid19treatmentguidelines.nih.gov/. Accessed January 22, 2021.

28. Dexamethasone in Hospitalized Patients with Covid-19 — Preliminary Report. N Engl J Med 2020. https://doi.org/10.1056/NEJMoa2021436.

29. Jones BE, Brown-Augsburger PL, Corbett KS, et al. LY-CoV555, a rapidly isolated potent neutralizing antibody, provides protection in a non-human primate model of SARS-CoV-2 infection. bioRxiv 2020. https://doi.org/10.1101/2020.09.30.318972.

30. Chen P, Nirula A, Heller B, et al. SARS-CoV-2 Neutralizing Antibody LY-CoV555 in Outpatients with Covid-19. N Engl J Med 2020. https://doi.org/10.1056/NEJMoa2029849.

31. ACTIV-3/TICO LY-CoV555 Study Group, Lundgren JD, Grund B, et al. A Neutralizing Monoclonal Antibody for Hospitalized Patients with Covid-19. N Engl J Med 2020. https://doi.org/10.1056/NEJMoa2033130.

32. Hansen J, Baum A, Pascal KE, et al. Studies in humanized mice and convalescent humans yield a SARS-CoV-2 antibody cocktail. Science 2020;369(6506):1010–4.

33. Baum A, Fulton BO, Wloga E, et al. Antibody cocktail to SARS-CoV-2 spike protein prevents rapid mutational escape seen with individual antibodies. Science 2020;369(6506):1014–8.

34. Baum A, Ajithdoss D, Copin R, et al. REGN-COV2 antibodies prevent and treat SARS-CoV-2 infection in rhesus macaques and hamsters. Science 2020;370(6520):1110–5.

35. Weinreich DM, Sivapalasingam S, Norton T, et al. REGN-COV2, a Neutralizing Antibody Cocktail, in Outpatients with Covid-19. N Engl J Med 2020. https://doi.org/10.1056/NEJMoa2035002.

36. Wolf J, Abzug MJ, Wattier RL, et al. Initial Guidance on Use of Monoclonal Antibody Therapy for Treatment of COVID-19 in Children and Adolescents. J Pediatr Infect Dis Soc 2021. https://doi.org/10.1093/jpids/piaa175.

37. Maiztegui J, Fernandez N, Damilano AD. Efficacy of immune plasma in treatment of Argentine hæmorrhagic fever and association between treatment and a late neurological syndrome. Lancet 1979;314(8154):1216–7.

38. Diorio C, Anderson EM, McNerney KO, et al. Convalescent plasma for pediatric patients with SARS-CoV-2-associated acute respiratory distress syndrome. Pediatr Blood Cancer 2020;67(11):e28693.

39. Simonovich VA, Burgos Pratx LD, Scibona P, et al. A Randomized Trial of Convalescent Plasma in Covid-19 Severe Pneumonia. N Engl J Med 2020. https://doi.org/10.1056/NEJMoa2031304.

40. Draft landscape of COVID-19 candidate vaccines. Available at: https://www.who.int/publications/m/item/draft-landscape-of-covid-19-candidate-vaccines. Accessed January 21, 2021.

41. Explaining operation Warp Speed. :7.
42. Wolff JA, Malone RW, Williams P, et al. Direct gene transfer into mouse muscle in vivo. Science 1990;247(4949 Pt 1):1465–8.
43. Richner JM, Himansu S, Dowd KA, et al. Modified mRNA Vaccines Protect against Zika Virus Infection. Cell 2017;168(6):1114–25.e10.
44. Alberer M, Gnad-Vogt U, Hong HS, et al. Safety and immunogenicity of a mRNA rabies vaccine in healthy adults: an open-label, non-randomised, prospective, first-in-human phase 1 clinical trial. Lancet Lond Engl 2017;390(10101):1511–20.
45. Bahl K, Senn JJ, Yuzhakov O, et al. Preclinical and Clinical Demonstration of Immunogenicity by mRNA Vaccines against H10N8 and H7N9 Influenza Viruses. Mol Ther 2017;25(6):1316–27.
46. Pardi N, Hogan MJ, Porter FW, et al. mRNA vaccines — a new era in vaccinology. Nat Rev Drug Discov 2018;17(4):261–79.
47. Walsh EE, Frenck RW, Falsey AR, et al. Safety and immunogenicity of two RNA-based Covid-19 vaccine candidates. N Engl J Med 2020. https://doi.org/10.1056/NEJMoa2027906.
48. Sahin U, Muik A, Derhovanessian E, et al. COVID-19 vaccine BNT162b1 elicits human antibody and T H 1 T cell responses. Nature 2020;586(7830):594–9.
49. Polack FP, Thomas SJ, Kitchin N, et al. Safety and Efficacy of the BNT162b2 mRNA Covid-19 Vaccine. N Engl J Med 2020;383(27):2603–15.
50. CDCMMWR. Allergic reactions including anaphylaxis after receipt of the first dose of Pfizer-BioNTech COVID-19 vaccine — United States, December 14–23, 2020. MMWR Morb Mortal Wkly Rep 2021;70. https://doi.org/10.15585/mmwr.mm7002e1.
51. Interim clinical Considerations of Use of MRNA COVID-19 vaccines currently authorized in the United States. Available at: https://www.cdc.gov/vaccines/covid-19/info-by-product/clinical-considerations.html. January 21, 2021.
52. Wrapp D, Wang N, Corbett KS, et al. Cryo-EM structure of the 2019-nCoV spike in the prefusion conformation. Science 2020;367(6483):1260–3.
53. Widge AT, Rouphael NG, Jackson LA, et al. Durability of Responses after SARS-CoV-2 mRNA-1273 Vaccination. N Engl J Med 2020. https://doi.org/10.1056/NEJMc2032195.
54. Jackson LA, Anderson EJ, Rouphael NG, et al. An mRNA Vaccine against SARS-CoV-2 — Preliminary Report. N Engl J Med 2020;383(20):1920–31.
55. Anderson EJ, Rouphael NG, Widge AT, et al. Safety and Immunogenicity of SARS-CoV-2 mRNA-1273 Vaccine in Older Adults. N Engl J Med 2020. https://doi.org/10.1056/NEJMoa2028436.
56. ModernaTX, Inc. A Phase 3, Randomized, Stratified, Observer-Blind, Placebo-Controlled Study to Evaluate the Efficacy, Safety, and Immunogenicity of MRNA-1273 SARS-CoV-2 Vaccine in Adults Aged 18 Years and Older. clinical-trials.gov. 2020. Available at: https://clinicaltrials.gov/ct2/show/NCT04470427. Accessed December 28, 2020.
57. Baden LR, El Sahly HM, Essink B, et al. Efficacy and Safety of the mRNA-1273 SARS-CoV-2 Vaccine. N Engl J Med 2020. https://doi.org/10.1056/NEJMoa2035389.
58. Voysey M, Clemens SAC, Madhi SA, et al. Safety and efficacy of the ChAdOx1 nCoV-19 vaccine (AZD1222) against SARS-CoV-2: an interim analysis of four randomised controlled trials in Brazil, South Africa, and the UK. Lancet 2020. https://doi.org/10.1016/S0140-6736(20)32661-1.
59. Knoll MD, Wonodi C. Oxford–AstraZeneca COVID-19 vaccine efficacy. Lancet 2020. https://doi.org/10.1016/S0140-6736(20)32623-4.

60. Kirchdoerfer RN, Cottrell CA, Wang N, et al. Pre-fusion structure of a human co-ronavirus spike protein. Nature 2016;531(7592):118–21.

61. Bos R, Rutten L, van der Lubbe JEM, et al. Ad26 vector-based COVID-19 vaccine encoding a prefusion-stabilized SARS-CoV-2 Spike immunogen induces potent humoral and cellular immune responses. NPJ Vaccin 2020;5(1):1–11.

62. Mercado NB, Zahn R, Wegmann F, et al. Single-shot Ad26 vaccine protects against SARS-CoV-2 in rhesus macaques. Nature 2020;586(7830):583–8.

63. Sadoff J, Le Gars M, Shukarev G, et al. Interim Results of a Phase 1-2a Trial of Ad26.COV2.S Covid-19 Vaccine. N Engl J Med 2021;13. https://doi.org/10.1056/NEJMoa2034201.

64. Keech C, Albert G, Cho I, et al. Phase 1–2 Trial of a SARS-CoV-2 Recombinant Spike Protein Nanoparticle Vaccine. N Engl J Med 2020;383(24):2320–32.

65. Sanofi's two vaccine candidates against COVID-19. Available at: https://www.sanofi.com/en/about-us/our-stories/sanofi-s-response-in-the-fight-against-covid-19. Accessed January 21, 2021.

66. Korber B, Fischer WM, Gnanakaran S, et al. Tracking changes in SARS-CoV-2 spike: evidence that D614G increases infectivity of the COVID-19 virus. Cell 2020;182(4):812–27.e19.

67. Tegally H. Emergence and rapid spread of a new severe acute respiratory syndrome-related coronavirus 2 (SARS-CoV-2) lineage with multiple spike muta-tions in South Africa. Available at: https://www.medrxiv.org/content/10.1101/2020.12.21.20248640v1. Accessed January 21, 2021.

68. Leung K, Shum MH, Leung GM, et al. Early transmissibility assessment of the N501Y mutant strains of SARS-CoV-2 in the United Kingdom, October to November 2020. Euro Surveill Bull Eur Sur Mal Transm Eur Commun Dis Bull 2021;26(1). https://doi.org/10.2807/1560-7917.ES.2020.26.1.2002106.

COVID-19 and Substance Use in Adolescents

Leslie H. Lundahl, PhD[a],*, Ciara Cannoy, MA[b]

KEYWORDS

- Adolescence • Substance use • COVID-19 • Review

KEY POINTS

- The impact of the COVID-19 pandemic on adolescent substance use is not clear, because emerging studies have yielded inconsistent results.
- The COVID-19 pandemic has significantly disrupted daily life for adolescents, leading to increased stress, social isolation, boredom, anxiety, and depression, all of which are risk factors for adolescent substance use.
- Stay-at-home and social distancing orders might create unexpected benefits for reducing adolescent use.
- The full impact of partial clinic closures on substance abuse treatment for adolescents is currently unknown. Special considerations should be taken by clinicians working remotely with adolescents.
- Although substance abuse treatment may be affected by clinic shutdowns, health care workers may use adolescents' lack of access to substances as a means for setting substance cessation goals.

Adolescence is a critical period for social and emotional development. Important tasks during this time include fashioning a social identity, developing a degree of emotional and personal independence from parents and caregivers, and moving toward self-reliance.[1] The coronavirus disease 2019 (COVID-19) pandemic has caused tremendous upheaval and disruption of this process. Since March 2020, most teens have been unable to go to school in person, interact with peers, or engage in sports and extracurricular activities. Traditional milestone events like prom, graduation, and going away to college have been missed. Many teens have had to take on childcare duties, such as caring for younger siblings while their parents work. Remote schooling requires hours of screen time and remaining engaged and motivated can be difficult. Sheltering in place is a drastic shift for adolescents who are accustomed to spending much of their time with peers, teachers, coaches, and others. The loss of routine and few

[a] Department of Psychiatry & Behavioral Neurosciences, Wayne State University School of Medicine, 3901 Chrysler Service Drive, Tolan Park Medical Building, Suite 2A, Detroit, MI 48201, USA; [b] Department of Psychology, Wayne State University, 5057 Woodward Avenue, Detroit, MI 48202, USA
* Corresponding author.
E-mail address: llundahl@med.wayne.edu

Pediatr Clin N Am 68 (2021) 977–990
https://doi.org/10.1016/j.pcl.2021.05.005
pediatric.theclinics.com

opportunities to take healthy risks or to express developmentally appropriate independence may be slowing the individuation process that is a critical part of adolescence.[2] It is unsurprising that pandemic-related isolation, uncertainty, and fear are leading to increased depression, anxiety, stress, and boredom and it is possible that a new cohort of adolescents may be at heightened risk for developing substance use disorders.[3,4]

SUBSTANCE USE PREVALENCE BEFORE THE COVID-19 PANDEMIC

Experimentation with alcohol and drugs often begins during adolescence,[5] and in non-pandemic times alcohol and drug use by adolescents are quite common. The Monitoring the Future (MTF) survey, administered annually to middle and high school students across the United States, asks about substance use and attitudes toward various drugs. According to results from the 2019 MTF survey by the time teens reached their senior year of high school more than 50% reported alcohol use, more than 40% had vaped, and about 36% had used cannabis in the past year. The use of other substances was fairly low. **Table 1** shows the percentage of twelfth graders reporting past year use of various substances in 2020 compared with 2019.[6]

From 2019 to 2020, there were nonsignificant increases in alcohol, LSD, over-the-counter cold and cough medications, and heroin use.[7] However, it is not clear whether these changes are related to the COVID-19 pandemic, because annual surveys on substance use also have been impacted by the pandemic. For example, the MTF generally is administered from February through May, with results released later in the year. Because of the pandemic, schools closed in-person operations in mid-March 2020 and only one-quarter of the usual sample had completed the survey.[8] These 2020 data are considered nationally representative, however, and indicate that the rates of vaping of both nicotine and marijuana had leveled off somewhat compared with the alarming increases in previous years. The use of drugs like cocaine, MDMA, and heroin remained relatively low among twelfth graders. Whether these trends will continue throughout the pandemic will not be known until this year's MTF survey data are available in late 2021.

The National Survey on Drug Use and Health (NSDUH) is another major national survey that provides data on the use of alcohol, tobacco products, and illicit drugs. According to results of the 2019 survey, 13.2% of adolescents (12–17 years of age)

Table 1
Past-year prevalence rates of various substances reported by twelfth graders in the 2019 and 2020 MTF surveys

Substance	2019	2020	2019–2020 Change
Alcohol	52.1	55.3	+3.2
Vaping	40.6	39.0	−1.6
Cannabis	35.7	35.2	−0.5
Any prescription drug	8.6	7.6	−1.1
LSD	3.6	3.9	+0.3
Over-the-counter cold or cough medicine	2.5	3.2	+0.7
Cocaine	2.2	2.9	+0.7
MDMA	2.2	1.8	−0.4
Heroin	0.4	0.3	−0.1

reported cannabis use in the past year, and 9.4% reported past year alcohol use.[9] Of note, 1.4 million teens initiated cannabis use in 2019, which equates to 3700 teens a day starting cannabis use. The overall use rates differ between the MTF and NSDUH surveys owing to differing methodologies, different age groupings (ie, the NSDUH groups 12- to 17-year-olds together and puts 18-year-olds, who generally have high rates of use, in an 18- to 25-year-old group, whereas the MTF groups by grade level). In addition, the NSDUH interviews are conducted in homes, where a lack of privacy might result in adolescents underreporting their drug use.[10] The NSDUH 2020 results will not be available until fall 2021.

EFFECTS OF THE COVID-19 PANDEMIC ON ADOLESCENT SUBSTANCE USE

Although data are lacking, it seems that adult substance use has increased in response to the stress and isolation associated with months of lockdown and social distancing.[8] This point may be true for adolescents, as well; data from the Centers for Disease Control and Prevention indicated that 10% of individuals aged 18 to 24 in their sample of 5412 online survey respondents increased their substance use in the past month (the survey was completed during June 2020), with the greatest increases observed at the younger ages within the cohort.[11] However, this study did not include teens under the age of 18 years. The only studies published to date that specifically examined the effects of the pandemic on substance use in younger adolescents include online surveys conducted in Canada and an online survey on vaping from Stanford University.[12–14] The results of these studies indicate that the impact of the pandemic on adolescent substance is far from clear.

An online survey was administered to 1054 Canadian teens (aged 14–18 years) who provided information about their alcohol, cannabis, and vape use in the 3 weeks before and 3 weeks after the start of the COVID-19 stay-at-home orders. The results indicated that, overall, fewer teens reported binge drinking, vaping, or using cannabis after COVID compared with before COVID, and alcohol use was unchanged. However, among teens who did use substances, the mean number of days they used alcohol (0.76–0.96 days) and cannabis (0.94–1.1 days) were significantly greater after COVID compared with before COVID.[12]

Interestingly, use patterns changed after COVID as well. Substance use by these respondents was most often solitary (49%), followed by with parents (42%), with friends via technology (32%), and face-to-face with peers (24%). Given that adolescent substance use is a highly social behavior, the proportion of teens who reported solitary substance use rather than virtual or face to face with friends is fairly unexpected. Solitary use was associated both with increased fears about COVID-19 and depressive symptomatology. The authors posited that teens who tend to use substances to cope with negative affect may increase their use in response to pandemic-related stress and isolation.[12] This finding is in contrast with previous reports that teens are less likely to use drugs to cope with stress and less likely to use them alone.[15,16] This change in use patterns is particularly concerning, because solitary teen substance use has been linked with poorer mental health,[17]

Similarly, the rather large percentage of teens who reported using alcohol with their parents is surprising and distressing, particularly because 26% of them reported binge drinking with their parents. Through this behavior, parents not only are communicating approval of alcohol use by their teens, which is a known risk factor for risky substance use,[18] but they also are presumably providing alcohol to their teens. Although teens tend to use alcohol moderately when using with their parents, they are also more likely to engage in higher risk drinking outside of the home.[18,19]

Conversely, it is not surprising that teens would use substances with peers via video chat or post photos on social media of themselves engaged in substance use, because these behaviors offer a means of feeling more connected during social distancing. Finally, and somewhat alarmingly, 24% of teens reported using substances face to face with peers, apparently not adhering to emergency stay-at-home orders. It is not clear from the study whether parents were aware of or permitting social interaction with peers. It may be that adolescents do not consider themselves to be at high risk for developing severe coronavirus symptoms and were more willing to take chances with their health. Although this study was conducted very early in the pandemic and patterns of use may not have been established, results provide preliminary information on COVID-19–related substance use trends.

Other studies have demonstrated decreased substance use during the pandemic. Some evidence suggests that decreased commercial availability and access to vape products may have decreased rates of vaping.[20] A survey on self-reported vaping habits was conducted in May 2020, 2 months after stay-at-home orders were issued. Data from 2167 e-cigarette users aged 13 to 24 years indicated that 67% of the 1442 participants who were 21 years and younger reported quitting or decreasing their use of vaping products in the 2 months since the pandemic started. Among reasons given for this change included concerns about lung function, an inability to purchase products, and worry about parents finding out. Because adolescents typically report obtaining e-cigarettes from friends or brick-and-mortar retail stores and not online, stay-at-home orders that closed vape shops and decreased social contact prevented many teens from obtaining vape products from stores or friends, resulting in decreased rates of vaping.[21]

Social distancing was offered as an explanation for the decrease in substance use during the first 2 weeks after closure of nonessential services in Canada, according to data collected using an online survey of 622 youth and young adults in established clinical and community settings.[13] Unfortunately, no information was provided on the types of the substances used or the frequency or quantity of use, and the findings were not reported by age groups.

ADDITIONAL COVID-19–RELATED FACTORS LIKELY TO IMPACT ADOLESCENT SUBSTANCE USE

Until it is possible to fully characterize the effects of the pandemic on adolescent substance use patterns, we can look to well-known risk and protective factors for substance use to anticipate potential use and plan for current and future treatment needs, even in these exceptional circumstances. For example, factors typically associated with an increased risk for use include drug availability, association with peers who use drugs, a lack of parental supervision, boredom, and coping with negative affect, among others. In contrast, parental monitoring, a lack of negative peer influence, academic achievement, and strong family and community attachments are considered protective factors. Although the pandemic might cause the rates of substance use to increase as teens seek relief from stress, isolation, or boredom, it is also possible that pandemic-related restrictions will decrease known risk factors and decrease substance use.[2,22]

Certainly, the COVID-19 pandemic has disrupted daily life and contributed to higher levels of stress and anxiety in both adults and adolescents. Adult drinking has increased substantially during the pandemic, resulting in greater teen exposure to parent alcohol use and possibly greater accessibility to alcohol and other drugs in the home.[23] In turn, adolescents who have access to a variety of substances within their homes may be at risk for increased substance use. In 2019, 87% of reports made to poison control centers in the United States involving exposures among individuals 13 to 19 years old occurred in the home. The most common substances these adolescents were exposed to included prescription or nonprescription pain relievers, antidepressants, sedatives, hypnotics, antipsychotics, antihistamines, and stimulants or street drugs. More than 60% of these exposures were reported as intentional.[24] A related potential risk factor involves parents modeling substance use to relieve stress, which increases the risk that teens will use substances to relieve stress, manage negative affect, and cope with feeling isolated. Similarly, older siblings in the home may also be facilitating use by their younger siblings through co-use or providing their younger siblings with access.[22] Additional reasons for post-COVID increases in alcohol and cannabis use could include an increase in unstructured time resulting from asynchronous remote learning and a lack of extracurricular and other leisure activities, as well as social isolation, boredom, and life stress, which may all have increased for adolescents during stay-at-home orders.[4,25]

Conversely, several factors likely contribute to a decreased risk of substance use during the pandemic.[2] Perhaps the greatest risk reduction comes from the increased time that parents are at home with their children. Not only are families eating meals together and participating in shared activities, which might decrease the risk of engaging in unhealthy behaviors like substance use, but parental and caregiver monitoring is likely increased, as well. Having parents and caregivers home much of the time might curtail activities conducive to binge drinking, such as parties, and make it much more difficult for teens to obtain and use vaping products and other substances.[26] Similarly, stay-at-home orders have limited opportunities for teens to spend time with peers who engage in unhealthy behaviors like substance use, which is significant, because the time spent with substance-using peers is a major risk factor for substance use.[27]

For teens who experienced academic or social pressure at school, remote or hybrid learning offer less anxiety and stress. This decreased stress may have decreased substance use by teens who use drugs to cope with stress and negative affect. In addition, remote learning does not require early morning start times, thus alleviating the sleep deprivation that is a risk factor for substance use.[2]

Finally, for teens who have not yet started substance use, fewer opportunities to engage in risky behavior and restricted access to alcohol and drugs that result from parents being at home and social distancing may translate into delayed initiation of substance use. Delaying the onset of substance use is a primary target of prevention strategies, given the effects of substances on the developing adolescent brain.[28] In addition, the earlier the onset of use, the greater the risk of developing substance use disorder in adulthood.[29] Thus, social distancing may be offsetting the first use of substances, which may decrease the risk of future problematic use.[2]

EFFECTS OF SUBSTANCE USE ON COVID-19 SUSCEPTIBILITY AND SEVERITY

Although it seems that younger people are less likely to contract COVID-19 than older adults, it is not clear whether using substances or having a substance use disorder makes an individual more susceptible to coronavirus transmission or increase the likelihood of severe infection.[30] Alcohol and/or other drug use can lead to changes in immune, pulmonary, and respiratory function that affect the ability to fight infection.[31,32] For example, alcohol consumption can impact the immune system and heavy use can lead to chronic weakening of lung function over time, increasing the risk of developing pneumonia.[33] Stimulants like cocaine and methamphetamine act as vasoconstrictors that can cause pulmonary and cardiovascular damage. Opioids, particularly at high doses, can slow breathing and cause hypoxia, putting users at risk of overdose. Drugs that are administered via smoking or inhalation, such as nicotine or cannabis, can worsen respiratory conditions like asthma and may increase risk of severe illness from COVID-19, even for adolescents. Emerging evidence indicates that smoking and vaping can cause lung irritation, inflammation, and damage to lung tissue, which can increase the risk of viral infection.[34–36] Youth who smoke or vape may be more likely to develop complications from coronavirus, such as pneumonia or acute respiratory distress. Behaviors associated with smoking and vaping also increase the risk of viral transmission. For example, teens often exhale forcefully when vaping and cannot wear masks while they are using. In addition, smoking and vaping behaviors typically include the sharing of joints, blunts, and vaping devices, which increases opportunities for exposure.[37]

Gaiha and colleagues[14] conducted the first (and only, to date) population-based, cross-sectional online survey study to investigate associations among smoking, e-cigarettes, and COVID-19. A total of 4351 adolescents and young adults (13–24 years) completed the survey, and the results indicated that youth who used e-cigarettes were 5 times more likely to become infected with COVID-19 illness compared with nonusers, and those who co-used e-cigarettes and tobacco cigarettes were 7 times more likely to become infected.[14] The high rates of vaping in teens combined with links between smoking and vaping and increased risk for COVID-19 illness underscore the need for health care providers to screen all youth and COVID-19–infected youth for cigarette and e-cigarette use.[6,7,14]

ADOLESCENT SUBSTANCE USE TREATMENT

According to the most up-to-date NSDUH, approximately 1.1 million adolescents in the United States met diagnostic criteria for a substance use disorder in 2019, a significant increase from 2018.[38] Despite a greater number of adolescents using substances, there was no significant increase in the number of adolescents engaged in treatment for a substance use disorder. Only 8.3% of these adolescents received substance abuse treatment in the year leading up to the survey.[38] Among those who did not receive any treatment, approximately 98.5% reported that they felt they did not need treatment, despite meeting criteria for a substance use disorder diagnosis (Substance Abuse and Mental Health Services Administration, 2020).[38] Thus, clinicians working with adolescents with a substance use disorder must consider the needs of the adolescent as well as their level of motivation to change when choosing a specific intervention. The following evidence-based treatment approaches have been found to be efficacious for treatment of substance use disorders among adolescents with varying needs and levels of readiness for treatment.[39]

Behavioral Interventions

Cognitive behavioral therapy (CBT), motivational interviewing (MI), contingency management (CM), and motivational enhancement therapy are all approaches to treating substance use that, according to Division 12 of the American Psychological Association, have strong research support. The National Institute on Drug Abuse has also recognized the adolescent community reinforcement approach (A-CRA) and 12-step facilitation therapy as acceptable treatments for adolescents with substance use problems.[39]

CBT for substance use encourages adolescents to monitor their emotions, recognize thought distortions, and identify substance use triggers. CBT therapists attempt to teach adolescents to anticipate high-risk substance use situations and to develop coping strategies for those situations.[39] MI is used to enhance a person's motivation for and commitment to change, largely using change talk facilitated by the therapist. It can be particularly helpful for adolescents who are ambivalent about their substance use.[40] Motivational enhancement therapy is based on the principles of MI and incorporates individual assessment feedback. The goal of motivational enhancement therapy for adolescent substance use is to help patients to develop a motivation and desire to engage in treatment. Generally, both MI and motivational enhancement therapy are not used as standalone treatment methods, but are combined with CBT.[39,40]

CM uses the principles of reinforcement for decreasing substance use. CM for substance abuse usually involves monitoring drug use behaviors and reinforcing desired behaviors (treatment participation, achieving specified goals, not using drugs, etc) using tangible rewards. CM is typically used as an adjunct to other psychosocial treatment.[39,40]

A-CRA is a treatment that attempts to replace reinforcements for substance use in the patient's life with more effective family, social, educational, or vocational reinforcers. Finally, the aim of 12-step facilitation therapy is to increase the likelihood that an adolescent receiving treatment for substance use will become involved in a 12-step program such as Narcotics Anonymous.[39]

Family-Based Interventions

Family-based therapeutic interventions involve the adolescent's family in their substance abuse treatment. These approaches often address problems beyond the adolescent's substance use, and may address issues regarding family conflict, co-occurring disorders, and school problems. Interventions that involve the family may be particularly useful for adolescents because most of them live with at least 1 parent or guardian and are subject to their rules and supports.[39]

Several iterations of family-based interventions have been shown to be efficacious for the treatment of substance abuse among adolescents. Brief strategic family therapy views problem behaviors as stemming from unhealthy family interactions and seeks to resolve negative interaction patterns among family members. Family behavior therapy combines the principles of CM with behavioral contracting to decrease problem behaviors, including substance use. Functional family therapy combines the principles of brief strategic family therapy and family behavior therapy; problem behaviors are viewed as a response to unhealthy family functioning, and behavioral techniques are used to increase family communication and problem solving. Functional family therapy also incorporates principles of CM.[39]

Multidimensional family therapy combines family- and community-based interventions for adolescents with substance use problems. The goal of multidimensional family therapy is to foster collaboration between the adolescent's family and the school and/or justice system. For juvenile detainees, 'Multidimensional family therapy is often used to facilitate their reintegration into their community. Similarly, multisystemic therapy incorporates the principles of family- and community-based interventions. In this model, the adolescent's substance use is not only viewed in terms of the adolescent and their family, but also in terms of peers, school, and neighborhood qualities.39

COVID-19 IMPACT ON TREATMENT

The majority of adolescents who were in treatment for a substance use disorder in 2019 received care in an outpatient setting; only 9.1% received nonhospital inpatient care, and 1.3% received inpatient care in a hospital setting.[38] These percentages are similar to reports spanning 2009 to 2017. Although 2020 treatment data have not yet been published, it is likely that outpatient services will continue to be the most common setting for adolescents in treatment for substance use disorder.

Following the stay-at-home orders and social distancing guidelines that were put into place in March 2020, many outpatient substance abuse clinics experienced partial closures and were forced to suspend certain types of treatment. Group therapies may have been halted to comply with social distancing, and in some instances therapeutic interventions have moved to online formats such as video conferencing. Recent studies have indicated that telehealth interventions show promise in treating substance use disorder among adult patients. For example, the Houston Emergency Opioid Engagement System (HEROES) has transitioned to telehealth services for substance use disorder. Initial studies indicate that this system has maintained patient engagement and has actually experienced an increase in attendance at some virtual recovery group meetings.[41]

Other researchers have been in the process of creating various digital platforms aimed at supporting individuals with substance use disorder, such as RAE (Realize, Analyze, Engage). RAE is a digital treatment for substance use disorder that includes a wearable device that measures biomarkers of stress and craving. The platform also includes several levels of dialectical behavior therapy interventions, connection to a clinician when a need for help is indicated, and a clinician-facing portal that delivers client information to a treatment team. Clinical trials are set to take place throughout 2021 to better understand the efficacy of this type of platform.[42]

It is important to note that these studies only included adult samples. There may be unique considerations for using telehealth services to treat adolescents with a substance use disorder. Unlike adults, most adolescents live with a parent or guardian as well as other family members, which may result in limited privacy within their homes. Adolescents may be less likely to be open and honest with health care workers if they fear being overheard by others in the household. Additionally, adolescents with a substance use disorder are more likely to have a parent or caregiver who also has a substance use disorder and 1 in 8 children live with at least 1 parent with a substance use disorder.[4,43] An adolescent who is seeking treatment for a substance use disorder but who has a parent with an active substance use disorder may feel particularly unsafe engaging in treatment from the confines of their own home. Community-based interventions may be particularly helpful for an adolescent in this position, but the lack of in-person outpatient services may hamper service providers' ability to integrate an adolescent patient with community supports. Alternatively, adolescents may feel reluctant to seek out any form of in-person treatment for fear of COVID-19 exposure.

Adolescents who are members of at-risk groups likely face additional barriers to receiving treatment during the COVID-19 pandemic. Impoverished and homeless youth, for example, appear to be facing even greater resource insecurity during the pandemic than pre-pandemic. Many of these adolescents are likely unable to engage in telehealth services owing to a lack of internet, phone, or computer access. Additionally, the halt of in-person services and decreased admissions to community service providers/shelters may also create barriers to obtaining mental health and substance use disorder treatment. Not only do health risks associated with both homelessness/poverty and substance use disorder put these adolescents at heightened risk for COVID-19 infection, but lack of treatment may result in an increase in engaging in risky behaviors to obtain substances.[44]

Lesbian, gay, bisexual, transgender, and gender and sexuality questioning (LGBTQ) youth represent another at-risk group that may be disproportionately affected by the COVID-19 pandemic. Adolescents who identify as LGBTQ are at an increased risk for physical and sexual abuse; stay-at-home orders may inadvertently increase contact with abusers in the home and having an abuser in the home would likely decrease engagement in telehealth treatment. LGBTQ adolescents are already at a higher risk for a multitude of psychological disorders, including substance use disorder; this risk, coupled with the potential for increased victimization, may contribute to an increase in substance use.[44]

Finally, adolescents have not been spared from the opioid epidemic. From 1999 to 2016, overdose deaths owing to prescription opioids, heroin, and fentanyl increased by 95%, 405%, and 2925%, respectively, in youth under the age of 20.[45] Recent findings indicate that opioid overdoses have increased during the COVID-19 pandemic[46] with disproportionate increases observed among Black Americans.[47] Data from the Centers for Diseaswe Control and Prevention[48] from more than 42 states show that nonfatal opioid-related overdoses have also risen dramatically since the pandemic was identified in March 2020. Heroin overdose rates peaked in May 2020 and have gradually decreased, although the rate in September 2020 (the most recent month with available data) remained elevated compared with almost all of 2019. Similarly, nonfatal overdoses from opioids peaked in July and slightly decreased in August and September, although the rate in September is greater than prepandemic 2020 and any month in 2019.[48] Although these COVID-19–related results did not examine adults and youth separately, the significant increases in adolescent opioid overdoses observed in prepandemic years largely mirrored those seen in adults. Thus, it is reasonable to suspect that the number of fatal and nonfatal opioid-related overdoses have also increased significantly in adolescents during COVID-19. The increase in opioid overdoses may be due to several factors, including disruption to treatment, an increase in mental health stressors, and an increased prevalence of solitary substance use, leading to a decrease in readily available assistance.

IMPLICATIONS FOR TREATMENT

Although an increase in substance use among adolescents during the COVID-19 pandemic is not definitive, treatment providers may benefit from preparing for an increase in the number of adolescents who need treatment for a substance use disorder as services begin to return to in person. Pediatricians and primary care providers should screen for substance use during routine checkups and may want to consider administering urine drug screens to concerning patients.[4] Additionally, clinicians who are providing general psychological services to adolescents should consider incorporating substance-related programming into their services; even adolescents who do not meet criteria for a substance use disorder may benefit from some substance-related treatment.[39] Treatment providers who service impoverished, homeless, or LGBTQ adolescents in particular may experience an increase in demand for in-person services owing to barriers to telehealth treatment, as discussed elsewhere in this article.

In the meantime, there are steps that both families and clinicians can take during this time to help adolescents with substance use problems. Stay-at-home orders provide a unique opportunity for parents and caregivers to create and maintain structure in the home. For example, they may implement a morning routine, encourage activities that build connection among family members, and facilitate nonjudgmental open communication within the home to support adolescent recovery efforts. Parents and caregivers should also monitor the adolescent for signs of ongoing substance use or withdrawal symptoms. A publication by J. Wolfe offers some examples of substance use signs that parents and caregivers might report to health care professionals.[49] Both withdrawal as well as continued substance use during social isolation may result in difficulty controlling emotions or extreme mood swings among adolescents. Attempts to isolate oneself in the home may also be a sign that an adolescent is hiding efforts to obtain or use substances. Isolation may look like sleeping throughout the day, staying locked in one's room, or simple avoidance of interaction with family. Additionally, multiple arguments about leaving the home to be with friends or sneaking out behavior may indicate that the adolescent is attempting to obtain or use substances. Last, strange smells coming from the adolescent or the adolescent's room may also indicate ongoing substance use. For example, marijuana has a distinct skunk-like smell when smoked. Unusually sweet scents may result from the use of a vape or from sweet drinks mixed with alcohol. Additionally, an excessive use of air fresheners, perfume, or cologne may be a tactic used to cover up the smell of substances. If a parent or caregiver is concerned that their adolescent is engaging in substance use, they may consider reaching out to their pediatrician for advice about treatment options.

Service providers who conduct remote services for adolescents with a substance use disorder should make efforts to check-in with the patient about their safety and difficulties they may be experiencing at home. If possible, health care workers should also encourage adolescents to seek out a private space from which to engage in remote treatment. If an adolescent is unable to openly discuss problems they are having because of lack of privacy or fear of safety, providers may want to consider resuming in-treatment services while following social distancing guidelines (ie, staying 6 feet apart, wearing masks, and washing hands and surfaces).

Health care workers may also see this time as an opportunity for encouraging complete cessation of substance use behaviors, including smoking and vaping. Adolescents may be experiencing increased difficulty in accessing various substances, including cigarettes and vapes owing to stay-at-home orders. Thus, treatment providers may use this time to increase motivation to quit; pediatricians or other health care professionals may also consider prescribing nicotine replacement treatments to help with craving or withdrawal symptoms experienced by adolescents.[50] Last, many 12-step support groups such as Alcoholics Anonymous and Narcotics Anonymous have transitioned some of their meetings to an online platform. Their respective websites now have entire pages devoted to providing information about virtual meetings, including how to find and join a virtual meeting. Adolescents with substance use problems may benefit from receiving this type of support, particularly if they have experienced a disruption in their in-person treatment.

FUTURE DIRECTIONS

Exploring the various impacts of the COVID-19 pandemic on adolescent substance use provides a unique opportunity to understand factors that both increase and decrease the risk of future substance use among teens. Some pandemic-related life changes, such as social isolation and boredom, seem to exacerbate the risk of substance use. Other changes seem to mitigate some of the risk, including increased family time, parental monitoring, and decreased access to substances.

Longitudinal studies are needed to monitor shifts in substance use patterns over time as the pandemic evolves to fully characterize the impact of pandemic-related stresses on teen substance use, motivations for use, and mental health correlates. Given the key role of peer pressure and social group dynamics in determining drug experimentation and use in teens, important factors to examine include the long-term consequences of school closures, remote and hybrid learning, social distancing, and quarantining. Studies also are needed to understand how the pandemic changed opportunities for teens, and their family members, to engage in substance use, and whether these changes increased or decreased use.

Studies should also examine the parental permissiveness that allowed for the parent–teen drinking and binge drinking behavior reported in the early weeks of the pandemic in the study by Sumas and associates.[12] Although some parents may have relaxed some rules in the face of the exceptionally challenging circumstances created by the shutdown, perhaps considering alcohol use with parents at home relatively safer for their teens than sneaking out and drinking with friends, there may be lasting effects of this co-use drinking behavior, because parental permissiveness has been linked to higher rates of substance use.[22,51]

SUMMARY

Currently, it is not clear whether substance use by teens has increased or decreased since the state of emergency was declared in mid-March 2020. Stressors such as uncertainty, fears about contracting the virus, social isolation, boredom, and sheltering in place potentially increase the risk of use, whereas increased parental monitoring and reduced access to substances and substance-using peers likely decrease the risk. Regardless, the sustained social disruption related to the COVID-19 pandemic will have lasting effects on adolescents. Future research should identify protective factors that decrease use, because these factors might be continued once normal life resumes. Similarly, identifying risk factors associated with increased use could provide targets for treatment. In the meantime, it is likely that partial clinic closures as well as the transition to providing services online uniquely affected the way adolescents engage in treatment. At-risk adolescents may have been particularly affected by these changes. As such, it is important that health care providers consider screening all adolescents for problematic substance use, and regularly monitor adolescents' safety in addition to maintaining treatment gains. Although stay-at-home orders and social distancing guidelines have made certain aspects of substance use disorder treatment more difficult, these restrictions also present a unique opportunity for parents and caregivers, as well as for health care workers. Parents and caregivers can use this time to increase structure in the home and build stronger connections with their children, and health care workers can use lack of access to substances to set up substance cessation goals for their adolescent patients.

CLINICS CARE POINTS

- Telehealth providers should be mindful that adolescents live with a parent or caregiver and because of possible limited privacy within their homes may be less open and honest about their substance use.
- About 1 in 8 adolescents with a substance use disorder lives with at least one parent who is actively using substances; this adolescent may not feel safe engaging in substance use treatment while in their home.
- Pediatricians and primary care providers should screen for substance use during routine checkups and may want to consider administering urine drug screens to concerning patients.
- Treatment providers may want to take advantage of the limited access teens have to cigarettes and vapes during stay-at-home orders and increase motivation to quit; pediatricians may consider prescribing nicotine replacement treatments to help with craving or withdrawal symptoms experienced by adolescents.

DISCLOSURE

Supported by the Lycaki/Young Funds from the State of Michigan.

REFERENCES

1. Eccles JS, Midgley C, Wigfield A, et al. Development during adolescence: the impact of stage-environment fit on young adolescents' experiences in schools and in families. Am Psychol 1993;48:90–101.
2. Richter L. The effects of the COVID-19 pandemic on the risk of youth substance use. Commentary. J Adolesc Health 2020;67:467–8.
3. Brooks SK, Webster RK, Smith LE, et al. The psychological impact of quarantine and how to reduce it: rapid review of the evidence. Lancet 2020;395:912–20.
4. Sarvey D, Welsh JW. Adolescent substance use: challenges and opportunities related to COVID-19. J Subst Abuse Treat 2021;122:108212.
5. Young SE, Corley RP, Stallings MC, et al. Substance use, abuse and dependence in adolescence: prevalence, symptom profiles and correlates. Drug Alcohol Depend 2002;68:309–22.
6. Johnston LD, Miech RA, O'Malley PM, et al. Monitoring the Future national survey results on drug use, 1975-2019: overview, key findings on adolescent drug use. Ann Arbor: Institute for Social Research, The University of Michigan; 2019.
7. Johnston LD, Miech RA, O'Malley PM, et al. Monitoring the Future national survey results on drug use 1975-2020: overview, key findings on adolescent drug use. Ann Arbor: Institute for Social Research, University of Michigan; 2021.
8. As 2020 closes, many questions remain about youth substance use trends. National Institute on Drug Abuse. Available at: https://www.drugabuse.gov/about-nida/noras-blog/2020/12/2020-closes-many-questions-remain-about-youth-substance-use-trends. 2020. Accessed January 26, 2021.
9. Substance Abuse and Mental Health Services Administration. Key substance use and mental health indicators in the United States: results from the 2019 National Survey on Drug Use and Health (HHS publication No. PEP20-07-01-001, NSDUH Series H-55). Rockville, MD: Center for Behavioral Health Statistics and Quality, Substance Abuse and Mental Health Services Administration; 2020. Available at: https://www.samhsa.gov/data/.
10. Substance Abuse and Mental Health Services Administration. Comparing and evaluating youth substance use estimates from the National Survey on Drug Use and Health and other surveys [internet]. Rockville, MD: Substance Abuse and Mental Health Services Administration (US); 2012. Discussion. Available at: https://www.ncbi.nlm.nih.gov/books/NBK533890. Accessed January 8, 2021.
11. Czeisler ME, Lane RI, Petrosky E, et al. Mental health, substance use, and suicidal ideation during the COVID-19 pandemic – United States, June 24-30, 2020. MMWR Mord Mortal Wkly Rep 2020;69:1049–57.
12. Dumas TM, Ellis W, Litt DM. What does adolescent substance use look like during the COVID-19 pandemic? Examining changes in frequency, social contexts, and pandemic-related predictors. J Adolesc Health 2020;67:354–61.
13. Hawke LD, Barbic SP, Voineskos A, et al. Impacts of COVID-19 on youth mental health, substance use, and well-being: a rapid survey of clinical and community samples. The Can J Psychiatry 2020;65:701–9.
14. Gaiha SM, Cheng J, Halpern-Felsher B. Association between youth smoking, electronic cigarette use, and COVID-19. J Adolesc Health 2020;67:519–23.
15. Cooper ML, Kuntsche E, Levitt A, et al. Motivational models of substance use: a review of theory and research on motives for using alcohol, marijuana, and tobacco. In: Sher KJ, editor. The Oxford handbook of substance use disorders, 1. New York, NY: Oxford University Press; 2016.

16. Barnes GM, Hoffman JH, Welte JW, et al. Effects of parental monitoring and peer deviance on substance use and delinquency. J Marriage Fam 2006;68:1084–104.
17. Creswell KG, Chung T, Wright AGC, et al. Personality, negative affect coping, and drinking alone: a structural equation modeling approach to examine correlates of adolescent solitary drinking. Addiction 2015;110:775e83.
18. Bahr SJ, Hoffmann JP, Yang X. Parental and peer influences on the risk of adolescent drug use. J Prim Prev 2005;26(6):529–51.
19. Staff J, Maggs JL. Parents allowing drinking is associated with adolescents' heavy alcohol use. Alcohol Clin Exp Res 2020;44:188e95.
20. Gaiha SM, Lempert LK, Halpern-Fisher B. Underage youth and young adult e-cigarette use and access before and during the coronavirus disease 2019 pandemic. JAMA Netw Open 2020;3(12):1–16, e2027572.
21. Meyers MJ, Delucchi K, Halpern-Felsher B. Access to tobacco among California high school students: the role of family members, peers, and retail venues. J Adolesc Health 2017;61:385–8.
22. Maggs JL. Adolescent life in the early days of the pandemic: less and more substance use. Editorial. J Adolesc Health 2021;67:307–8.
23. Pollard MS, Tucker JS, Green HD. Changes in adult alcohol use and consequences during the COVID-19 pandemic in the US. JAMA Netw Open 2020;3(9):e2022942.
24. Gummin DD, Mowry JB, Beuhler MC, et al. 2019 Annual Report of the American Association of Poison Control Centers' National Poison Data System (NPDS): 37th Annual Report. Clin Toxicol 2020;58(12):1360–541.
25. Mahoney JL, Stattin H. Leisure activities and adolescent antisocial behavior: the role of structure and social context. J Adolesc 2000;23:113e27.
26. Pepper JK, Coats EM, Nonnemaker JM, et al. How do adolescents get their e-cigarettes and other electronic vaping devices? Am J Health Promot 2019;33:420e9.
27. Hawkins J, Catalano R, Miller J. Risk and protective factors for alcohol and other drug problems in adolescent and early adulthood: implications for substance abuse prevention. Psychol Bull 2019;112:64–105.
28. Jordan CJ, Andersen SI. Sensitive periods of substance abuse: early risk for the transition to dependence. Dev Cogn Neurosci 2017;25:29–44.
29. Morales AM, Jones SA, Kliamovich D, et al. Identifying early risk factors for addiction later in life: a review of prospective longitudinal studies. Curr Addict Rep 2020;7:89–98.
30. Davies NG, Klepac P, Liu Y, et al. Age-dependent effects in the transmission and control of COVID-19 epidemics. Nat Med 2020;26:1205–11.
31. COVID-19 questions and answers: for people who use drugs or have substance use disorder. Centers for Disease Control and Prevention Web suite. 2021. Available at: https://www.cdc.gov/coronavirus/2019-ncov/need-extra-precautions/other-at-risk-populations/people-who-use-drugs/QA.html#people-who-use-drugs. Accessed March 2, 2021.
32. Javelle E. Electronic cigarette and vaping should be discouraged during the new coronavirus SARS-CoV-2 pandemic. Arch Toxicol 2020;94:2261–2.
33. Sarkar D, Jung MK, Wang HJ. Alcohol and the immune system. Alcohol Res Curr Rev 2015;37(2):153.
34. McConnell R, Barrington-Trimis JL, Wang K, et al. Electronic cigarette use and respiratory symptoms in adolescents. Am J Respir Crit Care Med 2017;195:1043–9.
35. Ghosh A, Coakley RD, Ghio AJ, et al. Chronic e-cigarette use increases neutrophil elastase and matrix metalloprotease levels in the lung. Am J Respir Crit Care Med 2019;200:1392–401.

36. COVID-19: potential implications for individuals with substance use disorders. National Institute on Drug Abuse; 2020. Available at: https://www.drugabuse.gov/about-nida/noras-blog/2020/04/covid-19-potential-implications-individuals-substance-use-disorders. Accessed February 2, 2021.

37. McKelvey K, Halpern-Felsher B. How and why California young adults are using different brands of pod-type electronic cigarettes in 2019: implications for researchers and regulators. J Adolesc Health 2020;67:46–52.

38. Substance Abuse and Mental Health Services Administration, National Survey of Substance Abuse Treatment Services (N-SSATS): 2019. Data on substance abuse treatment facilities. Rockville, MD: Substance Abuse and Mental Health Services Administration; 2020.

39. NIDA. Evidence-based approaches to treating adolescent substance use disorders. National Institute on Drug Abuse website; 2020. Available at: https://www.drugabuse.gov/publications/principles-adolescent-substance-use-disorder-treatment-research-based-guide/evidence-based-approaches-to-treating-adolescent-substance-use-disorders. Accessed January 18, 2021.

40. APA Presidential Task Force on Evidence-Based Practice. Evidence-based practice in psychology. Am Psychol 2006;6:271–85.

41. Langabeer JR 2nd, Yatsco A, Champagne-Langabeer T. Telehealth sustains patient engagement in OUD treatment during COVID-19. J Subst Abuse Treat 2021;122:108215.

42. McDonnell A, MacNeill C, Chapman B, et al. Leveraging digital tools to support recovery from substance use disorder during the COVID-19 pandemic response. J Subst Abuse Treat 2020. https://doi.org/10.1016/j.sat.2020.108226.

43. Wilens TE, Yule A, Martelon M, et al. Parental history of substance use disorders (SUD) and SUD in offspring: a controlled family study of bipolar disorder. Am J Addict 2014;23(5):440–6.

44. Cohen RIS, Bosk EA. Vulnerable youth and the COVID-19 pandemic. Pediatrics 2020;146:e20201306.

45. Gaither JR, Shabanova V, Leventhal JM. US National Trends in Pediatric Deaths From Prescription and Illicit Opioids, 1999-2016. JAMA Netw Open 2018;1(8):e186558.

46. Slavova S, Rock P, Bush HM, et al. Signal of increased opioid overdose during COVID-19 from emergency medical services data. Drug Alcohol Depend 2020;214:108176.

47. Khatri UG, Pizzicato LN, Viner K, et al. Racial/Ethnic Disparities in Unintentional Fatal and Nonfatal Emergency Medical Services-Attended Opioid Overdoses During the COVID-19 Pandemic in Philadelphia. JAMA Netw Open 2021;4(1):e2034878.

48. Suspected Nonfatal Drug Overdoses During COVID-19. 2021. Centers of Disease Control and Prevention. Available at: https://www.cdc.gov/drugoverdose/data/nonfatal/states/covid-19.html. Accessed March, 2021.

49. Wolfe J. Signs of a substance use issue in teens during COVID-19. Healthy Driven Blogs 2020. Available at: https://www.eehealth.org/blog/2020/04/signs-of-drug-use-in-teens/. Accessed February 18, 2021.

50. Chadi N, Bélanger R. COVID, youth, and substance use: critical messages for youth and families. Canadian Paediatric Society; 2020. Last updated April 20, 2020. Accessed February 17, 2021.

51. Barnes GM, Reifman AS, Farrell MP, et al. The effects of parenting on the development of adolescent alcohol misuse: s six-wave latent growth model. J Marriage Fam 2000;62:175–86.

Child Maltreatment During the COVID-19 Pandemic
A Systematic Rapid Review

Ashley Rapp, MPH[a],*, Gloria Fall, BA[a], Abigail C. Radomsky, BS[b],
Sara Santarossa, PhD[a]

KEYWORDS

- COVID-19 • Pandemic • Child maltreatment • Abuse • Neglect

KEY POINTS

- Findings of the included articles are mixed; 5 articles documented an increase in child maltreatment, 6 articles documented a decrease, and 1 study found no significant difference in child maltreatment rates.
- Of the included articles, rates of child maltreatment reports decreased while hospital cases of child maltreatment increased, calling the accuracy of reporting during the COIVD-19 pandemic into question.
- Most articles (11 of 12) did not include perspectives of children affected by child maltreatment.

It is estimated that each year more than 1 million children worldwide are victims of physical, sexual, or emotional violence. Collectively, this violence has been termed child maltreatment (CM) and defined by the World Health Organization as "the abuse and neglect that occurs to children under 18 years of age."[1] The impacts of CM are multifaceted, having short- and long-term consequences on a child's attitudes and behaviors, as well as their mental and physical well-being.[2–6] Increases in CM have been well-documented in association with increased parental stress,[7] during and after recessions and epidemics, such as the Ebola and AIDS crises.[8–10] Continuing to understand the situations that create, perpetuate, and amplify CM are of the utmost importance to then lower the rates of CM and decrease their impact. Thus, the ongoing coronavirus disease 2019 (COVID-19) pandemic and its subsequent impacts have become an area of interest and concern for linkages to CM.

The ongoing COVID-19 pandemic has permeated daily life and activities, with more than 2.3 million global deaths at the time of this publication.[11] Mass lockdowns, stay-

^a Department of Public Health Sciences, Henry Ford Health System, 1 Ford Place, Detroit, MI 48202, USA; ^b Wayne State University, School of Medicine, 540 E Canfield Street, Detroit, MI 48210, USA
* Corresponding author.
E-mail address: arapp2@hfhs.org

Pediatr Clin N Am 68 (2021) 991–1009
https://doi.org/10.1016/j.pcl.2021.05.006
pediatric.theclinics.com
0031-3955/21/Crown Copyright © 2021 Published by Elsevier Inc. All rights reserved.

at-home orders, shelter-in-place orders, and general encouragement or enforcement to distance from anyone outside of the household have been implemented to mitigate COVID-19 infection rates, hospitalizations, and deaths.[1,12,13] Although the infection and death rates do require drastic isolation measures, there may be negative impacts of such measures as well. The crisis, along with government-implemented isolating measures, have led to economic, psychological, and social hardship for people across the globe.[14–16] These other effects of the pandemic, or the country's response to it, might impact CM.

The pandemic has exacerbated factors that contribute to CM. For parents, quarantines and stay-at-home orders have led to high rates of unemployment, difficulties in relationships, increased rates of depression, and unsurmountable stress.[17–19] Emerging research has suggested that parents experiencing pandemic-related social isolation report an increase in verbal aggression, physical punishment such as spanking or hitting, and neglectful behaviors toward their children.[20] The COVID-19 pandemic has caused significant economic challenges and could have long lasting effects on the global economy.[21,22] Last, more than 80% of children worldwide were affected by school closures during the pandemic.[23] In some countries, educational personnel make up the largest proportion of reporters in cases of CM.[24] Research has shown that because of school closures owing to the COVID-19 pandemic, there is a decrease in CM reports.[25] Routine pediatric medical care has also decreased as a function of the COVID-19 pandemic, leaving fewer opportunities for health care providers to find out about and report a CM case. Although it is clear the COVID-19 pandemic has created a variety of circumstances that are known to be indicative of an increase in CM, the pandemic is still evolving, and currently available studies cannot fully assess the lasting impacts.

The examination of CM during the COVID-19 pandemic has proven to be difficult, with mixed reports of increased, decreased, or varied results in cases of child abuse and neglect.[25] At a time when many victims are isolated within a violent household and are unable to disclose events while separated from the perpetrator,[10] instances of CM are difficult to trace. Thus, a need to better understand and synthesize the existing literature surrounding the COVID-19 pandemic and CM is needed. To the authors' knowledge, this is the first review of its kind to explore the current literature in this field of study and, therefore, this systematic rapid review aims to address (1) the types of study designs used to analyze an ongoing situation, (2) whether CM trends vary by reporting type, and (3) the sources (primary vs secondary) used to gain insight into CM. Synthesizing this information, all published during the pandemic, provides a glimpse into the academic dialogue on this topic in real time.

METHODS
Article Inclusion and Exclusion Criteria

To be included, an article had to (1) include a measure of CM during the COVID-19 pandemic, (2) be published in a peer-reviewed journal, (3) be written in English, and (4) present original empirical findings (eg, no reviews, case studies, or news articles were eligible). Articles were excluded if they were inaccessible to reviewers or if they described the development of a tool or measure. Inaccessible articles are those that did not have a full-text download available or charged a fee.

Search Strategy

The systematic rapid review was conducted in accordance with the 2009 PRISMA statement.[26] Two experienced research librarians independently conducted a literature search on December 28, 2020. Both developed their search strategies in MEDLINE, and translated these searches into Embase, PsycInfo, and CINAHL. The searches were based on a combination of terms related to "maltreatment" (eg, "physical abuse," "sexual abuse," "neglect") AND "child" (eg, "adolescent," "girl," "boy," "young"). It was limited to the COVID-19 pandemic and English language. After their separate searches, the librarians met to compare search results. Duplicate articles between databases and librarians were removed, and the remaining articles were sent to the study team.

Data Extraction

Two independent reviewers (G.F. and A.C.R.) conducted an abstract review of the resulting 234 unique articles. Reviewers indicated whether an article fit or did not fit the inclusion criteria, and each article they disagreed on was discussed among 3 reviewers (G.F., A.C.R., and A.R.) until consensus was reached. A total of 27 articles remained and were retrieved for full-text review and abstraction.

Quality Assessment

Three reviewers (G.F., A.C.R., and A.R.) used the National Institutes of Health National Heart, Lung, and Blood Institute Study Quality Assessment Toolbox[27] to ensure that all of the included articles were free of significant bias.

Ethics

This study was not submitted to an institutional review board because a rapid literature review does not involve human participants.

RESULTS

A total of 234 unique citations were generated from the databases. After the initial abstract screen, 207 articles were removed. Most commonly, articles were removed because they were not original empirical research (n = 131), meaning that they were either a letter to the editor, a viewpoint or debate piece, a review paper, or a news report. Articles were also excluded if they did not include any current child abuse (n = 55), meaning that child abuse was either not mentioned, not included in the statistical analysis, or that child abuse history was only used as a study inclusion factor for adult subjects. Articles that did not include COVID-19 (n = 5) and articles that included neither COVID-19 nor present child abuse (n = 6) were excluded as well. Other reasons for exclusion were that the article was not accessible to reviewers (n = 3 did not have a full-text download available, n = 1 charged a fee to view), only the abstract was published (n = 1), the article was an animal study (n = 1), the article was a program evaluation (n = 1), the research was conducted for development of a clinical tool (n = 1), or the article was a workshop description (n = 1). Each reason for exclusion with only 1 article is categorized as other in **Fig. 1**.

Of the remaining 27 full-text articles that were reviewed, 15 articles were excluded. Articles were removed because they had no current child abuse (n = 6), were not peer reviewed (n = 2), were not original empirical research (n = 5), or did not include COVID-19 (n = 2). A final count of 12 articles were ultimately included in this systematic rapid review, outlined in **Table 1**. Each of these articles were deemed appropriate for inclusion based on the quality assessment measure.[27] Overall, 10 articles received a score of good and 2 received a score of fair. According to the tool, "a 'good' study has the least risk of bias, and results are considered valid, while a 'fair' study is susceptible to some bias deemed not sufficient to invalidate its results."[27] None of the included articles were deemed poor, which would indicate significant bias.

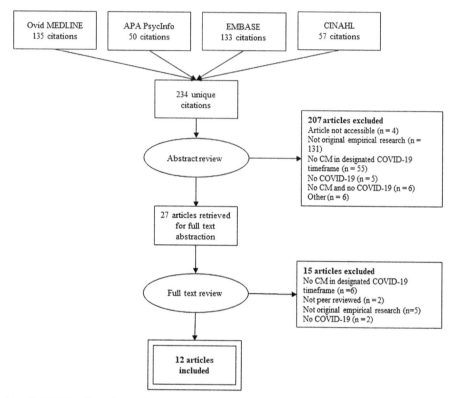

Fig. 1. PRISMA flowchart of the article identification, selection, and abstraction process. APA, American Psychological Association.

Sample Characteristics

Reflective of the global scale of the COVID-19 pandemic, there is geographic diversity among the included articles. Four evaluations took place in the United States,[28–31] and the other 8 are from outside of the United States, including Brazil, the Netherlands, and the UK.[32–39] The articles ranged in sample size, with the smallest sample including 12 children,[38] the median 2 samples including 392 children in one[31] and 414 parents in the other,[32] and the largest sample coming from hospital records of CM for 58,367 children.[33] Of the articles, one was a survey of parents,[32] and one included responses from children.[39] All other articles synthesized information from child abuse reporting or presentation to a hospital. Maltreated children were from all age groups. At the youngest end of the spectrum, Sidpra and associates[38] looked at children from 17 days to 401 days old, with a mean age of 192 days. Conversely, Platt and colleagues[37] included children aged 0 to 19 years, based on the 2002 definition the authors used to define children and adolescents. Three articles did not report a mean age or age range.[30,31,38]

Study Designs

A variety of study designs were used to assess the relationship between the COVID-19 pandemic and CM. The most common study design was retrospective review. Six articles used this method.[29,33–36,38] Two articles use retrospective data to compare

Table 1
Articles assessing CM during the COVID-19 pandemic

Author (Year)	Study Design	Sample Source and Sample Size	Sample Characteristics[a]	Data Time Frame (MM/DD/YY YY)	Child Maltreatment Operational Definition	Findings	NIH NHLBI Study Quality Assessment
Barboza et al,[21] 2020	Negative binomial regression analysis of surveillance data	Los Angeles, CA Reports of CAN to the Los Angeles Police Department Before COVID-19: n = 661 reports COVID-19: n = 614 reports	Before COVID-19: 50% female; 65% Hispanic. 23% Black. 8% White, 1% Asian, 3% other race COVID-19: 49% female: 60% Hispanic, 27% Black, 8% White, 1% Asian, 5% Other race; no age data reported	07/24/2019– 01/20/2020 compared with 01/21/2020– 07/19/2020	Physical abuse and neglect Abuse: Penal Code 273d Neglect: Penal Code 270 Neglect MNBS Parent-Report short version Room for Parents Questionnaire	Compared with the time period immediately preceding it, there was a 7.95% decrease in the number of child abuse and neglect reports during the COVID-19 pandemic	Good
Bérubé et al,[33] 2020	Cross-sectional analysis from a prospective longitudinal cohort	Quebec, Canada MAVIPAN cohort: parents of children aged 0–17 n = 414 parents	85.7% Female; mean age = 40.2; no race data reported	04/29/2020– 05/10/2020	Cognitive and Affective Needs Scale Basic Care Needs Scale	Compared with parents of children aged 0–12, parents of teenaged children were significantly less likely to be able to respond to their child's basic care needs (P<.001)	Fair

(continued on next page)

Table 1
(continued)

Author (Year)	Study Design	Sample Source and Sample Size	Sample Characteristics[a]	Data Time Frame (MM/DD/YY YY)	Child Maltreatment Operational Definition	Findings	NIH NHLBI Study Quality Assessment
Chong et al,[34] 2020	Retrospective review	Singapore Medical records from KK Women's and Children's Hospital, a major pediatric hospital n = 58,367 children	Pre-DORSCON Orange (1): 53% female; mean age = 8.0 y (SD = 4.7); Post-DORSCON Orange: 48% female; mean age = 7.0 y (SD = 4.3); During lockdown (3): 18% female: mean age = 6.9 y (SD = 4.2); After lockdown (4): 44% female: mean age = 7.7 y (SD = 4.4); No race data reported	(1): 01/01/2020– 02/06/2020; (2): 02/07/2020– 04/06/2020; (3) 04/07/2020– 06/01/2020; (4) 06/02/2020– 08/08/2020	Physical abuse SNOMED-CT and ICD codes for child abuse related diagnoses	The hospital saw a greater proportion of child abuse-related emergencies during lockdown (44 children, 0.5% of emergencies) and after lockdown (79%, 0.6%) compared with pre-DORSCON orange (36%, 0.2%) (P<.001)	Good

Degiorgio et al,[35] 2020	Retrospective review	Malta Mater Dei health records and computer databases of all acute pediatric hospital admissions for children aged 0–15 Before COVID: n = 729 admissions; COVID wave I: n = 266 admissions	Before COVID. 2019: 44% female: COVID wave 1: 50% female; No race data reported	Before COVID. 2019: 03/01/2019– 05/09/2019; COVID Wave 1: 03/01/2020– 05/09/2020	Physical abuse EHR	Compared with the same period in 2019, there was a higher percentage of child abuse or social pediatric cases in 2020 (0.14% vs 3.5% of cases) (P<.001)	Good
Garstang et al,[36] 2020	Retrospective review	Birmingham, England CPME referrals for children aged 0–18 at Birmingham Community Healthcare Trust EHR for the children referred 2018: n = 78 referrals 2019: n = 75 referrals 2020: n = 47 referrals	37% Female: median age = 69 mo; no race data reported	Compared 03/2018–6/2018; 03/2019–6/2019; and 03/2020– 6/2020	Physical abuse and neglect Conclusion from CPME History from EHR	Compared with the same period in 2018 and 2019. there was a decrease in CPME referrals in 2020 (39% decrease; 95% CI, (14%–57%).	Good

(continued on next page)

Table 1
(continued)

Author (Year)	Study Design	Sample Source and Sample Size	Sample Characteristics[a]	Data Time Frame (MM/DD/YY YY)	Child Maltreatment Operational Definition	Findings	NIH NHLBI Study Quality Assessment
Kovler et al,[30] 2020	Retrospective review Retrospective population-based study	Maryland, England Cases taken from the trauma registry at a Level 1 pediatric trauma center for children under age 15 2018: n = 60 patients 2019: n = 111 patients 2020: n = 86 patients State of Sergipe, Brazil Official CM registries 2019: n = 70 cases of child abuse 2020: n = 53 cases of child abuse	2018: 0% female: 33% Black, median age = 21 mo; 2019: 50% female; 75% Black, median age = 10 mo; 2020: 62% female; 75% Black; median age = 11.5 mo 2019: 78.6% female; 25.7% aged 0%–11% and 74.3% aged 12%–17%; 24.3% White, 7.1% Black, 60.0% Brown 8.6% missing race data; 2020: 71.7% female; 30.2% aged 0%–11% and 69.8% aged 12%–17%; 15.1% White, 11.3% Black. 62.3% Brown 11.3% missing race data	Compared 3/28/2018–04/27/2018; 3/28/2019–04/27/2019; 3/28/2020–04/27/2020 01/01/2019–06/30/2019 compared with 01/01/2019–06/30/2020	Physical abuse Hospital evaluation Injury pattern Physical abuse Official CM database	Compared with the same period in 2018 and 2019, there was a significantly higher proportion of trauma patients treated for child abuse–related injuries in 2020 (P = .009) Compared with 2019, child physical injury decreased by 24.3% in 2020 Decreasing rates occurred in January, February, March, and May	Good

Mart ins - Filho et al,[37] 2020	Cross-sectional descriptive analysis	State of Santa Catarina, Brazil Notifications of violence against children age 0–19 in the Information System for Notifiable Diseases n = 1851 notifications of interpersonal or self- inflicted violence	Compared 01/01/2020–03/15/2020; 03/16/2020–05/31/2020	Physical abuse, psychological abuse, sexual abuse, neglect Municipality notifications	Compared with the period before the lockdown, there was a decrease of 55.3% in notifications during the isolation period (1192 vs 659 notifications)	Good
Platt et al,[38] 2020	Retrospective analysis using SARIMA modeling	New York City, USA CAN allegations to NYC's Administration for Children's Services Count of NYC CPS investigations warranting child welfare preventative services Stratified CAN allegations data from January 2015 to May 2020 Observed and predicted values generated for March 2019 to February 2020	Created models based on 01/2015–02/2020 Observed actual values from 03/2020–05/2020		Fewer allegations than forecasted from March to May. March: (expected-observed = 1848; 95% CI, 1272–2423, % change = −28.8%) April: (expected-observed = 2976, 95% CI, 2382–3570, % change = −51.5%)	Good

(continued on next page)

Table 1
(continued)

Author (Year)	Study Design	Sample Source and Sample Size	Sample Characteristics[a]	Data Time Frame (MM/DD/YY YY)	Child Maltreatment Operational Definition	Findings	NIH NHLBI Study Quality Assessment
						May: (expected-observed = 2959, 95% CI, 2347–3571, % change = −46.0%)	
Rapoport et al,[31] 2020	Retrospective review	New York City, USA Cases of suspected abusive head trauma at Great Ormond Street Hospital For Children 2017: n = 0 cases; 2018: n = I case; 2019: n = I case; 2020: n = 10 cases	40% Female: mean age = 192 d (range = 17–401 d); no race data reported	Compared 03/23/2020–04/23/2020 with incidence in the previous 3 y (no dates provided)	Physical abuse and neglect Allegations to NYC's Administration for Children's Services Physical abuse Suspected AHT cases at hospital	Compared with the same period in the previous 3 years, there was a 1493% increase in cases of AHT between March 23 and April 23, 2020	Good

| Sidpra et al,[39] 2020 | Mixed methods study: quantitative analysis is longitudinal, qualitative analysis is a substudy | The Netherlands Quantitative: Families that had been reported to CPS for suspected partner violence or child abuse in the Netherlands. Recruited both before and during the pandemic: n = 159 families recruited before COVID and n = 87 families recruited during lockdown Qualitative: these same families and professionals that work with vulnerable families recruited through "contacts with researchers from previous studies" n = 30 parents, n = 9 children, and n = 13 professionals | Parents Before COVID-19: 66% female: 0% aged 18%–24%, 22% aged 25%–34%, 42% aged 35%–44%, 30% aged 45%–55%, and 6% aged 55+ During Lockdown (after 03/16/2020): 63% female, 2% aged 18%–24%, 15% aged 25%–34%, 43% aged 35%–44%, 34% aged 45–55, and 6% aged 55+; No race data reported, no child demographics reported | ~1.5 y before 03/16/2020; 03/16/2020 – ongoing parent study | Physical abuse, psychological abuse, neglect Self-report of parents and teenagers on the CTSPC | No significant difference in number of child abuse and neglect incidents reported by parents or teenagers before the COVID-19 crisis and after 03/16/2020 | Good |

(continued on next page)

Table 1
(continued)

Author (Year)	Study Design	Sample Source and Sample Size	Sample Characteristics[a]	Data Time Frame (MM/DD/YY YY)	Child Maltreatment Operational Definition	Findings	NIH NHLBI Study Quality Assessment
Tierolf et al,[40] 2020	Retrospective analysis using ARIMA modeling	Oklahoma, USA Publicly available court filings from the Oklahoma State Court Network Feb 2020: n = 87 crimes: March 2020: n = 100 crimes; April 2020: n = 83 crimes; May 2020: n = 80 crimes; June 2020: n = 42 crimes	—	Created models based on period starting on 01/01/2010 Observed actual values from 02/01/2020–06/30/2020		25.7% fewer allegations than forecasted from February to June. February: Difference = −21.1, 95% CI, −47.9 to 5.7, % change = −19.5% March: Difference = 0.3, 95% CI, −27.6, to 27.1 % change = 0.3% April: Difference = −23.6, 95% CI, −51.6 to 4.3; % change = −22.2%	Fair

| Whelan et al,[32] 2020 | Physical abuse, sexual abuse, neglect Criminal charges | May: Difference = −29.2, 95% CI, −57.7 to 0.6; % change = −26.7% June: Difference = −63.2, 95% CI, −92.3 to 34.1; % change = −60.1% | Good |

Abbreviations: AHT, abusive head trauma; ARIMA, auto regressive integrated moving average; CAN, child abuse and neglect; CI, confidence interval; COVID -19, coronavirus disease 2019; CPS, Child Protective Services; DORSCON, Disease Outbreak Response System Condition; EHR, electronic health record; ICD, *International Classification of Diseases*; MAVIPAN, "Ma vie et la pandemic au Québec"; MNBS, Multidimensional Neglectful Behavior Scale; NHLBI, National Heart, Lung, and Blood Institute; NIH, National Institutes of Health; SNOMED-CT, Systematized Nomenclature of Medicine – Clinical Terms; SARIMA, seasonal auto regressive integrated moving average.

[a] Indicates that no data is reported.

forecasted trends in CM to actual reports of CM.[30,31] One was a cross-sectional analysis of survey data,[32] and another was a cross-sectional analysis of violence notifications.[37]

Definition of Child Maltreatment

CM was operationalized with some nuance across articles. Some relied solely on diagnostic codes,[33,34] whereas others also considered suspicions or allegations of maltreatment.[29,30,35,37,38] Additionally, the scope of CM varied: 11 of the articles included physical abuse against a child,[28–31,33–39] 7 were inclusive of child neglect,[28,30–32,35,37,39] and 2 included psychological abuse.[37,39]

Qualitative Synthesis of Findings

Overall, 5 articles documented increased CM, 6 articles documented decreased CM, and 1 article found no significant difference in CM trends between the prepandemic period and during the pandemic.

Setting of reports

Four articles discussed incidence of CM in a hospital setting.[29,33,34,38] Six articles discussed incidence of CM from crime reports and Child Protective Services reports.[28,30,31,35–37] Each of the 4 articles that generated reports from a hospital setting found an increased incidence of CM. Contrastingly, each of the 6 articles based on crime and Child Protective Services reports found a decreased incidence of CM.

Forecasted versus actual

Two articles comparing forecasted versus actual trends in CM reports.[30,31] These articles used similar modeling techniques (seasonal autoregressive integrated moving average and autoregressive integrated moving average), in different settings. Rapoport and associates[31] examined New York City, and Whelan and coworkers[32] examined the state of Oklahoma. Both analyses found significantly less allegations during the COVID-19 pandemic than expected. Rapoport and coworkers[31] saw less reports than expected from March to May 2020, and Whelan and colleagues[32] saw less reports than expected in February and April to June 2020.

DISCUSSION

This study used systematic rapid review methodology to explore the impact of the COVID-19 pandemic on CM. The variability in findings across the included articles expose the complexity of this relationship, especially as the situation is developing in real time. The type of study design, the report setting, and the source of the information on the CM were explored and are discussed in detail elsewhere in this article.

The most common study design used was retrospective review, where researchers compared trends in CM from previous time periods with a time period during the lockdown. The lockdown period was defined differently across articles, with one using "COVID Wave One" and the timepoint of interest,[34] another using Disease Outbreak Response System Condition, or DORSCON, stages,[33] and still others defining date ranges of a few months at the height of the lockdown orders.[28,30,31] Thus, data cannot be directly compared owing to differing date ranges.

The rising trends of CM in hospitals and falling trends of CM crime reports during the COVID-19 pandemic is concerning. This trend begets the question of whether reporting is accurate during this time. Access to mandated reporters such as school teachers has been severely limited owing to stay-at-home orders and the transition to virtual schooling, leading to an underreporting of CM.[40] Additionally, during the COVID-19 pandemic, there was an increased hesitancy to visit hospitals and clinics.[41–43] The fear of going to the hospital for issues unrelated to COVID-19 could have different implications: less contact with medical professionals who are mandated reporters or only the most severe cases presenting to the hospital. Telemedicine replaced in-person visits for many medical professionals at the height of the pandemic, and providers may have missed usual warning signs of CM. The hospital-based articles included in the present review, however, reported an increase in CM cases, potentially contradicting this hypothesis.[29,33,34,38]

The articles presented here are predominantly secondary reports. Articles relied on crime reports, health record data, and surveys of parents to understand CM. Just 1 article reported surveying children (aged 3–18 years), but only reported data from the teenagers in the study.[39] It was also unclear whether children were completing surveys away from parental influence. Other reports, like the allegations of abuse documented by Rapoport and associates,[31] also primarily came from adults such as law enforcement, social services, educational personnel, and caregivers. There is absence of information directly from the children affected by CM, despite how useful it could be. Past year incidence data collected directly from young children and adolescents are both reliable and developmentally appropriate, meaning that they have the cognitive capacity to recall and understand instances of CM.[44] The reliance on physical evidence of maltreatment in many of our included articles could result in the underreporting of CM cases, particularly cases where bruises or injuries have healed, where psychological or sexual abuse occurred, or where neglect was involved.[29,33,34,38]

When parents were surveyed,[32] no comparative analyses by sex were completed. Mothers and fathers of children affected by CM were analyzed together as a unit, despite the possibility that parental perspective could vary by gender. It is well-known that parent sex is associated with likelihood of abusing a child and typology of maltreatment committed, although the results are mixed across countries and cultures.[45–48] Sex is also implicated in the relationship between parenting stress and CM potential.[49]

The associations shown here are subject to confounding. One potential confounder in the relationship between the COVID-19 pandemic and CM is parental stress. It is known that parental stress is a major risk factor of CM.[50–52] Parental stress also increased during the COVID-19 pandemic: fear of the virus, job loss, new rules and mandates, and transitions to virtual work and schooling, among other stressors, were rampant during this time.[4,18] Additionally, it is documented that economic hardship is a predictor of child neglect.[53–56] The mass layoffs, financial threats to small businesses, and sometimes minimal relief from governments during the COVID-19 pandemic could all be sources of economic hardship for parents.

The greatest strength of the present study is the rigor with which it was conducted at every stage. A.R. trained G.F. and A.C.R. extensively in data abstraction and article selection using the PRISMA method. Three reviewers took part in the multi-pronged article selection process, and all selected articles were screened for quality assurance using the National Institutes of Health National Heart, Lung, and Blood Institute Study Quality Assessment Toolbox.[27] A limitation of our study is that it was conducted during the ongoing COVID-19 pandemic. Thus, it is likely that additional articles will be published on this topic as the COVID-19 pandemic develops, and of the articles that are included here, some have small sample sizes.[36,38] This factor could impact the potential for generalizability to larger samples or populations.

SUMMARY

The global nature of the COVID-19 pandemic warrants future research conducted by geography. Different countries, states, and even different cities define and handle CM cases differently. This variability could contribute to different rates of reporting and incidence of CM. Policy implications on the accuracy of reports should be explored, as should the efficacy of policy measures on CM prevention.

CLINICS CARE POINTS

- Children are particularly vulnerable during the COVID-19 pandemic because stay-at-home orders, minimized access to mandated reporters, and increased parental stress may be associated with increased CM.
- Providers should take extra care to ask children whether CM is occurring in the home and give examples of the different types of CM. Some children, especially those affected by neglect or psychological violence, may not show visible signs of CM. Other children may not know that what they are experiencing is CM.
- Discourse on school, daycare, church, and other institutional reopenings should include special considerations for children at risk of CM and children with a history of CM victimization.

ACKNOWLEDGMENTS

The authors acknowledge Brianna Andre and Steven Moore from the Sladen Library at Henry Ford Hospital for their assistance with the literature search.

DISCLOSURE

The authors of this publication declare that they have no relevant or material financial interests that relate to the research described in this paper.

REFERENCES

1. WHO Coronavirus Disease Dashboard. Listings of WHO's response to covid-19. World Health Organization. Available at: https://covid19.who.int/. Accessed February 08, 2021.
2. Dube SR, Anda RF, Felitti VJ, et al. Childhood abuse, household dysfunction, and the risk of attempted suicide throughout the life span: findings from the Adverse Childhood Experiences Study. JAMA 2001;286(24):3089–96.
3. Felitti VJ, Anda RF, Nordenberg D, et al. Reprint of: relationship of childhood abuse and household dysfunction to many of the leading causes of death in adults: the adverse childhood experiences (ACE) study. Am J Prev Med 2019; 56(6):774–86.
4. Hailes HP, Yu R, Danese A, et al. Long-term outcomes of childhood sexual abuse: an umbrella review. Lancet Psychiatry 2019;6(10):830–9.
5. Hemmingsson E, Johansson K, Reynisdottir S. Effects of childhood abuse on adult obesity: a systematic review and meta-analysis. Obes Rev 2014;15(11): 882–93.
6. Hughes K, Bellis MA, Hardcastle KA, et al. The effect of multiple adverse childhood experiences on health: a systematic review and meta-analysis. Lancet Public Health 2017;2(8):e356–66.

7. Norman RE, Byambaa M, De R, et al. The long-term health consequences of child physical abuse, emotional abuse, and neglect: a systematic review and meta-analysis. PLoS Med 2012;9(11):e1001349.
8. Crouch JL, Behl LE. Relationships among parental beliefs in corporal punishment, reported stress, and physical child abuse potential. Child Abuse Neglect 2001;25(3):413–9.
9. Kontos M, Moris D, Davakis S, et al. Physical abuse in the era of financial crisis in Greece. Ann Transl Med 2017;5(7):155.
10. Peterman A, Potts A, O'Donnell M, et al. Pandemics and violence against women and children, vol. 528. Washington, DC: Center for Global Development; 2020.
11. Wood JN, French B, Fromkin J, et al. Association of pediatric abusive head trauma rates with macroeconomic indicators. Acad Pediatr 2016;16(3):224–32.
12. Koh D. COVID-19 lockdowns throughout the world. Occup Med 2020;70(5):322.
13. Moris D, Schizas D. Lockdown during COVID-19: the Greek success. In Vivo 2020;34(3 suppl):1695–9.
14. Zhang K, Vilches TN, Tariq M, et al. The impact of mask-wearing and shelter-in-place on COVID-19 outbreaks in the United States. Int J Infect Dis 2020;101:334–41.
15. Tull MT, Edmonds KA, Scamaldo KM, et al. Psychological outcomes associated with stay-at-home orders and the perceived impact of COVID-19 on daily life. Psychiatry Res 2020;289:113098.
16. Wilson JM, Lee J, Fitzgerald HN, et al. Job insecurity and financial concern during the COVID-19 pandemic are associated with worse mental health. J Occup Environ Med 2020;62(9):686–91.
17. Xiong J, Lipsitz O, Nasri F, et al. Impact of COVID-19 pandemic on mental health in the general population: a systematic review. J Affective Disord 2020;277:55–64.
18. Brown SM, Doom JR, Lechuga-Peña S, et al. Stress and parenting during the global COVID-19 pandemic [Article]. Child Abuse Neglect 2020;110(Pt 2):104699.
19. Griffith AK. Parental burnout and child maltreatment during the covid-19 pandemic. J Fam Violence 2020;1–7.
20. Patrick SW, Henkhaus LE, Zickafoose JS, et al. Well-being of parents and children during the COVID-19 pandemic: a national survey. Pediatrics 2020;146(4). e2020016824.
21. Lee SJ, Ward KP, Lee JY, et al. Parental social isolation and child maltreatment risk during the COVID-19 pandemic. J Fam Violence 2020;1–12.
22. Ceylan RF, Ozkan B, Mulazimogullari E. Historical evidence for economic effects of COVID-19. Eur J Health Econ 2020;21(6):817–23.
23. Medel-Herrero A, Shumway M, Smiley-Jewell S, et al. The impact of the Great Recession on California domestic violence events, and related hospitalizations and emergency service visits. Prev Med 2020;139:106186.
24. UNESCO. COVID-19 impact on education. Available at: https://en.unesco.org/covid19/educationrespons. Accessed January 3, 2021.
25. Child Welfare Information Gateway. The role of educators in preventing and responding to child abuse and neglect. Washington, DC: U.S. Department of Health and Human Services, Children's Bureau; 2003.
26. Sharma A, Borah SB. Covid-19 and domestic violence: an indirect path to social and economic crisis. J Fam Violence 2020;1–7.
27. Moher D, Altman DG, Liberati A, et al. PRISMA statement. Epidemiology 2011;22(1):128.

28. Quality assessment tool for observational cohort and cross-sectional studies. National Heart Lung and Blood Institute; 2014. Available at: https://www.nhlbi.nih.gov/node/80102.

29. Barboza GE, Schiamberg LB, Pachl L. A spatiotemporal analysis of the impact of COVID-19 on child abuse and neglect in the city of Los Angeles, California. Child Abuse Neglect 2021;116(Pt 2):104740.

30. Kovler ML, Ziegfeld S, Ryan LM, et al. Increased proportion of physical child abuse injuries at a level I pediatric trauma center during the Covid-19 pandemic. Child Abuse Neglect 2021;116(Pt 2):104756.

31. Rapoport E, Reisert H, Schoeman E, et al. Reporting of child maltreatment during the SARS-CoV-2 pandemic in New York City from March to May 2020. Child Abuse Neglect 2021;116(Pt 2):104719.

32. Whelan J, Hartwell M, Chesher T, et al. Deviations in criminal filings of child abuse and neglect during COVID-19 from forecasted models: an analysis of the state of Oklahoma, USA. Child Abuse Neglect 2021;116(Pt 2):104863.

33. Bérubé A, Clément MÈ, Lafantaisie V, et al. How societal responses to COVID-19 could contribute to child neglect. Child Abuse Neglect 2020;116(Pt 2):104761.

34. Chong SL, Soo JSL, Allen JC, et al. Impact of COVID-19 on pediatric emergencies and hospitalizations in Singapore. BMC Pediatr 2020;20(1):562.

35. Degiorgio S, Grech N, Dimech YM, et al. COVID-19 related acute decline in paediatric admissions in Malta, a population-based study. Early Hum Dev 2020;105251.

36. Garstang J, Debelle G, Anand I, et al. Effect of COVID-19 lockdown on child protection medical assessments: a retrospective observational study in Birmingham, UK. BMJ Open 2020;10(9):e042867.

37. Martins Filho PR, Damascena NP, Lage RCM, et al. Decrease in child abuse notifications during COVID-19 outbreak: a reason for worry or celebration? J Paediatrics Child Health 2020;56(12):1980–1.

38. Platt VB, Guedert JM, Coelho EBS. Violence against children and adolescents: notification and alert in times of pandemic. Rev Paul Pediatr 2020;39:e2020267.

39. Sidpra J, Abomeli D, Hameed B, et al. Rise in the incidence of abusive head trauma during the COVID-19 pandemic [Letter]. Arch Dis Child 2021;106(3):e14.

40. Tierolf B, Geurts E, Steketee M. Domestic violence in families in The Netherlands during the coronavirus crisis: a mixed method study. Child Abuse Neglect 2021;116(Pt 2):104800.

41. Baron EJ, Goldstein EG, Wallace CT. Suffering in silence: how COVID-19 school closures inhibit the reporting of child maltreatment. J Public Econ 2020;190:104258.

42. American Heart Association News. Is it safe to go to the hospital during COVID-19 pandemic? Doctors say yes 2020. Available at: www.heart.org https://www.heart.org/en/news/2020/05/04/is-it-safe-to-go-to-the-hospital-during-covid-19-pandemic-doctors-say-yes.

43. Weiner S. Go to the hospital if you need emergency care, even in the era of COVID-19. Harvard Health Blog 2020. Available at: https://www.health.harvard.edu/blog/go-to-the-hospital-if-you-need-emergency-care-even-in-the-era-of-covid-19-2020050519760.

44. HealthPartners. Is it safe to get health care during COVID-19?: HealthPartners. HealthPartners Blog 2020. Available at: https://www.healthpartners.com/blog/what-were-doing-to-help-you-get-care-safely-during-covid-19/.

45. Mathews B, Pacella R, Dunne MP, et al. Improving measurement of child abuse and neglect: a systematic review and analysis of national prevalence studies. PLoS One 2020;15(1):e0227884.
46. Cui N, Xue J, Connolly CA, et al. Does the gender of parent or child matter in child maltreatment in China? Child Abuse Neglect 2016;54:1–9.
47. Middel F, López ML, Fluke J, et al. The effects of migrant background and parent gender on child protection decision-making: an intersectional analysis. Child Abuse Neglect 2020;104:104479.
48. Romero-Martínez A, Figueiredo B, Moya-Albiol L. Childhood history of abuse and child abuse potential: the role of parent's gender and timing of childhood abuse. Child Abuse Neglect 2014;38(3):510–6.
49. Wolf JP. Parent gender as a moderator: the relationships between social support, collective efficacy, and child physical abuse in a community sample. Child Maltreat 2015;20(2):125.
50. Miragoli S, Balzarotti S, Camisasca E, et al. Parents' perception of child behavior, parenting stress, and child abuse potential: Individual and partner influences. Child Abuse Neglect 2018;84:146–56.
51. Whipple EE, Webster-Stratton C. The role of parental stress in physically abusive families. Child Abuse Neglect 1991;15(3):279–91.
52. Chung G, Lanier P, Wong PYJ. Mediating effects of parental stress on harsh parenting and parent-child relationship during coronavirus (covid-19) pandemic in Singapore. J Fam Violence 2020;1–12.
53. Guterman NB, Lee SJ, Taylor CA, et al. Parental perceptions of neighborhood processes, stress, personal control, and risk for physical child abuse and neglect. Child Abuse Neglect 2009;33(12):897–906.
54. Berger LM, Font SA, Slack KS, et al. Income and child maltreatment in unmarried families: evidence from the earned income tax credit. Rev Econ Household 2017; 15(4):1345–72.
55. Lawson M, Piel MH, Simon M. Child maltreatment during the COVID-19 pandemic: consequences of parental job loss on psychological and physical abuse towards children. Child Abuse Neglect 2020;110(Pt 2):104709.
56. Lefebvre R, Fallon B, Van Wert M, et al. Examining the relationship between economic hardship and child maltreatment using data from the Ontario Incidence Study of Reported Child Abuse and Neglect-2013 (OIS-2013). Behav Sci 2017; 7(1):6.

Pediatric Rheumatologic Effects of COVID-19

Nivine El-Hor, MD[a], Matthew Adams, MD[b],*

KEYWORDS

- COVID-19 • Multisystem inflammatory syndrome in children (MIS-C)
- Kawasaki disease • Intravenous immunoglobulin • Systemic steroids
- Rheumatology

KEY POINTS

- Multisystem inflammatory syndrome is a severe hyperinflammatory post–COVID-19 syndrome sharing characteristics with Kawasaki syndrome, toxic shock syndrome, and hemophagocytic lymphohistiocytosis occurring primarily in children.
- Multisystem inflammatory syndrome in children typically develops 2 to 6 weeks after infection; the usual presenting symptoms are persistent fever, conjunctivitis, peripheral edema, rash, extremity pain, gastrointestinal distress, and advancement to shock.
- Multisystem inflammatory syndrome in children is treated with combinations of systemic steroids, intravenous immunoglobulin, and anti-inflammatory monoclonal antibodies.
- Cardiac sequelae of multisystem inflammatory syndrome in children differ from those of Kawasaki syndrome; specifically coronary artery aneurysms may occur, but are more prominent in Kawasaki.
- Cardiac ventricular dysfunction is more common with multisystem inflammatory syndrome in children, leading to higher troponin levels.

INTRODUCTION

Severe acute respiratory syndrome coronavirus 2 (SARS-CoV-2) was recognized as a novel coronavirus in Wuhan, Hubei Province, China, after several hospitalized patients presented with pneumonia of undetermined origin in December 2019 and January 2020.[1] In March 2020, coronavirus disease 2019 (COVID-19) was declared a pandemic by the World Health Organization.[2] There is now a better understanding of the pathophysiology, disease course, outcomes, and treatment of this virus. It is

[a] Department of Internal Medicine and Pediatrics, Children's Hospital of Michigan, 4201 St. Antoine, UHC 5C, Detroit, MI 48201, USA; [b] Division Chief for Pediatric Rheumatology, Department of Pediatrics, Wayne State University School of Medicine, Wayne Pediatrics, 400 Mack Avenue, Detroit, Michigan 48201, USA
* Corresponding author.
E-mail address: matthew.adams2@wayne.edu

Pediatr Clin N Am 68 (2021) 1011–1027
https://doi.org/10.1016/j.pcl.2021.05.002
0031-3955/21/© 2021 Elsevier Inc. All rights reserved.
pediatric.theclinics.com

recognized that COVID-19 affects adults and children differently, with the virus generally causing milder symptoms of infection in children as compared with adults.[3–5]

In adults, acute respiratory failure accounts for the most common complication from COVID-19.[6] In contrast, healthy children and adolescents may experience a hyperinflammatory syndrome owing to COVID-19 exposure causing a potentially life-threatening response.[6] The hyperinflammatory response seen in the pediatric population is similar in some respects to Kawasaki disease, systemic-onset juvenile idiopathic arthritis, or hemophagocytic lymphohistiocytosis.

MULTISYSTEM INFLAMMATORY SYNDROME IN CHILDREN

Multisystem inflammatory syndrome in children (MIS-C) as a result of SARS-CoV-2 exposure was first reported in April 2020 among 8 healthy children with hyperinflammatory shock over 10 days in the UK.[7] The hyperinflammatory shock was noticed to have comparable characteristics to incomplete Kawasaki disease, Kawasaki disease shock syndrome and toxic shock syndrome.[7] Similarly, between April 27 and May 11, 2020, there were 21 pediatric patients in Paris, France, admitted with Kawasaki-like symptoms associated with SARS-CoV-2.[8] In the United States, cases of MIS-C were noted as early as March 2020.[6] On May 14, 2020, the Centers for Disease Control and Prevention outlined a health advisory that remarked on clinical features of MIS-C and provided a case definition.[9]

Case Definition

The criteria for the proposed case definition of MIS-C are shown in **Table 1**. Per the Centers for Disease Control and Prevention, even if individuals fulfill the criteria for typical or atypical Kawasaki disease, yet meet the criteria for MIS-C, they should be reported.[9] Also, evidence of SARS-CoV-2 infection in any pediatric death should prompt consideration for MIS-C.[9]

PATHOPHYSIOLOGY

In a study of 2135 children (median age, 7 years) diagnosed with COVID-19 in China, the authors noted that SARS-CoV-2 seemed to cause less severe symptoms in children than adults, with more than 90% of children having asymptomatic, mild, or moderate infection.[10] The reasons are unclear, but may in part be owing to age-related nasal epithelium angiotensin-converting enzyme II receptor expression, limiting SARS-CoV-2 host entry via its spike (S) protein.[11,12] Although COVID-19 infection is milder in the pediatric population, a small percentage of the infected or exposed develop MIS-C, a potentially life-threatening condition in children.[6]

MIS-C seems to be temporally associated with COVID-19 infection with clinical symptoms and features (see **Table 1**) developing between 2 and 6 weeks after exposure to the virus.[13–16] Case reports have demonstrated that children admitted for MIS-C most often have positive serum immunoglobulin G (IgG) antibodies against SARS-CoV-2 and are less frequently positive for reverse transcription-polymerase chain reaction (RT-PCR), suggesting that MIS-C is likely a postviral hyperinflammation syndrome rather than an acute COVID-19 infection.[7,8,13–15,17–21]

Gruber and colleagues[13] examined how MIS-C influences the immune system and showed that, compared with pediatric patients with COVID-19, the inflammatory response of MIS-C triggered high levels of cytokines (IL-17A, CD40) and chemokines (CXCL5, CXCL11, CXCL1, CXCL6) that recruit natural killer and T cells. Further, it was noted that patients with MIS-C had increased expression of CD64 on their neutrophils

Table 1
Centers for Disease Control and Prevention case definition of MIS-C—all criteria must be met[9]

Criteria		
1	Age <21 y	
	Fever	≥38°C for ≥24 h or subjective fever ≥24 h
	≥1 elevated marker of inflammation	Including, but not limited to: C-reactive protein, erythrocyte sedimentation rate, fibrinogen, procalcitonin, D-dimer, ferritin, LDH, IL-6, neutrophilia, lymphocytopenia, hypoalbuminemia
	Clinically severe illness necessitating hospitalization	
	Involvement of ≥2 organ systems	Cardiovascular, renal, respiratory, hematologic, gastrointestinal, dermatologic, or neurologic[a]
2	No other reasonable diagnoses	
3	Evidence of SARS-CoV-2 infection or exposure	Positive SARS-CoV-2 infection by RT-PCR, serology or antigen test or COVID-19 exposure within 4 wk before symptom onset

Abbreviations: LDH, lactate dehydrogenase; RT-PCR, reverse transcription-polymerase chain reaction.
  [a] Features of multisystem involvement of ≥2 organ systems may include: cardiovascular (eg, elevated troponin, elevated B-type natriuretic peptide, abnormal echocardiogram, shock, arrhythmia), renal (eg, renal failure, acute kidney injury), respiratory (eg, acute respiratory distress syndrome, pneumonia, pulmonary embolism), hematologic (eg, coagulopathy), gastrointestinal (eg, vomiting/diarrhea, abdominal pain, gastrointestinal bleeding, ileus), dermatologic (eg, rash, mucositis, erythroderma), neurologic (eg, seizure, aseptic meningitis, stroke).
(Table and contents adapted from the Centers for Disease Control and Prevention)[9].

and CD16+ nonclassical monocytes, which are typically seen in autoimmune and autoinflammatory illnesses.[13,22]

Gruber and colleagues[13] hypothesized that MIS-C as a result of SARS-CoV-2 results from the adaptive immune response. They tested MIS-C plasma IgG and immunoglobulin A against a microarray of more than 21,000 human peptides and found 189 peptides that cross-reacted as autoantigens.[13] Interestingly, the tissue expression of these autoantigens was from endothelial, cardiac, and gastrointestinal tract tissue,[13] important sites of clinical involvement. Also noted, plasma IgG from patients with MIS-C reacted with anti-La (seen in systemic lupus erythematosus [SLE] and Sjogren syndrome) and anti–Jo-1 (seen in inflammatory myopathies) antigens.[13] MIS-C pathophysiology may share some mechanisms with these autoimmune diseases[13]; however, further studies need to be conducted to assess whether MIS-C autoantibodies cause an autoimmune pathology.

CLINICAL MANIFESTATIONS

In mid April 2020, the UK began reporting the first cases of 8 previously healthy children (mean age of 8 years) presenting with characteristics similar to incomplete Kawasaki disease or Kawasaki disease shock syndrome.[7] Now recognized as MIS-C, symptoms included persistent fever, conjunctivitis, peripheral edema, rash, extremity pain, and gastrointestinal distress with all the children advancing to distributive shock requiring ionotropic agents.[7] Since these initial reports from the UK, similar cases from other European countries and the United States have emerged.[6,8,13–15,18–20,23]

In the United States, New York City was the first to report 15 cases of MIS-C. Similar to the UK's findings, all of the children (mean age of 12 years) had fever; 87% had gastrointestinal symptoms such as vomiting, abdominal pain, and diarrhea; and less than 50% presented with rash, conjunctivitis, and swollen hands and feet.[18] As in the UK, Riollano-Cruz[18] and colleagues described 87% of children being hypotensive with 60% requiring inotropic agents or vasopressors. In the UK, Riphagen and colleague[7]'s noted that all but 1 child had cardiac involvement, mostly ventricular dysfunction, and in New York City almost 90% of MIS-C cases had severe cardiac pathology with 80% demonstrating abnormal transthoracic echocardiogram results, with 27% showing left ventricular dysfunction.[18]

In another study by Feldstein and colleagues[6] examining 186 pediatric patients with MIS-C (median age of 8.3 years) in 26 US states, the authors noted 92% of children with gastrointestinal involvement, 80% with cardiac involvement with 48% requiring vasopressors owing to cardiogenic shock and 74% with mucocutaneous symptoms,[6] consistent with findings of other case reports.[7,18] After the initial appearance of MIS-C cases in Europe and the United States, numerous other cases have been reported. Fever, abdominal symptoms (pain, emesis, diarrhea), skin rash, oropharyngeal mucosal changes, hypotensive shock, conjunctivitis, cardiac dysfunction, and mucocutaneous findings have been reported as symptoms and signs of MIS-C in the literature.[8,13–15,21,23–26]

LABORATORY TESTS AND IMAGING FINDINGS

Markers of inflammation are prominent in MIS-C and common laboratory studies have been obtained in various case reports with similar reported findings. These include elevations in the erythrocyte sedimentation rate, C-reactive protein, D-dimer, ferritin, fibrinogen, B-type natriuretic peptide, troponin, international normalized ratio, prothrombin time, lactate dehydrogenase, partial thromboplastin time, IL-6, IL-8, and procalcitonin, in addition to anemia, thrombocytopenia, hypoalbuminemia, hyponatremia, leukocytosis with neutrophilia, and lymphopenia.[6,8,13,14,16,18,20,21,23,26–31] These laboratory studies should be considered to help aid in the diagnosis of MIS-C.

In addition to the laboratory testing cited, an electrocardiogram, and echocardiogram should be obtained at baseline for suspected or confirmed patients with MIS-C given arrythmias, cardiac ventricular dysfunction, coronary artery aneurysms, and coronary artery dilation have been observed.[6–8,14,15,20,21,23,25,29] **Table 2** specifies the laboratory and imaging studies that should be considered for a suspected case of MIS-C.

KAWASAKI DISEASE VERSUS MULTISYSTEM INFLAMMATORY DISEASE IN CHILDREN

Kawasaki disease is an acute self-limited systemic small- and medium-sized vessel vasculitis in those typically 6 months to 5 years of age[32–34] with the clinical features presented in **Table 3**. Although the cause remains unknown, it is hypothesized that an infection may trigger the hyperinflammatory response seen in Kawasaki disease,[17] as does SARS-CoV-2 in MIS-C.[13–16] Kawasaki disease can be further distinguished into complete Kawasaki disease, incomplete Kawasaki disease, and Kawasaki disease shock syndrome, with some of their features presenting in MIS-C.[6,8,18,20] For

Table 2
Laboratory testing/imaging for suspected MIS-C[4,6–8,14,15,18,20,21,23,25,29,42,71]

Laboratory testing/Imaging	Values/Features
CMP	Na <135 mmol/L
	Albumin $\leq$ 3 g/dL
CBC with differential	Absolute lymphocyte count <1.0K cell/μL
	Platelets <150,000 cells/μL
	Neutrophilia
Erythrocyte sedimentation rate	$\geq$40 mm/h
C-reactive protein	$\geq$3 mg/dL
BNP or NT-proBNP	>200 pg/mL
Troponin T	Elevated
Procalcitonin	Elevated
Fibrinogen	>400 mg/dL
Ferritin	>600 ng/mL
AST/ALT	At least 2 times the upper limit of normal
Albumin	<3 g/dL
LDH	Elevated
Urinalysis: IL-6/IL-8	Elevated
Coagulation studies	International normalized ratio > 1.1
International normalized ratio	
Prothrombin time	
Partial thromboplastin time	
D-Dimer	>3 mg/L
SARS-CoV-2	RT-PCR positive
	Antigen test positive
	Serology (IgG, immunoglobulin A, IgM)
	positive
Electrocardiogram	Arrythmias
Echocardiogram	Cardiac ventricular dysfunction,
	coronary artery aneurysm,
	coronary artery dilation

Abbreviations: CMP, comprehensive metabolic panel; CBC, complete blood count; NT-proBNP, N-terminal-pro hormone BNP; AST, aspartate aminotransferase; ALT, alanine aminotransferase; IgM, immunoglobulin M; LDH, lactate dehydrogenase.

example, in their study of 186 patients with MIS-C, Feldstein and colleagues[6] report that 40% of patients having Kawasaki disease-like symptoms, and Toubiana and colleagues[8] describe that 52% of patients with MIS-C meeting complete Kawasaki disease criteria, 48% meeting incomplete Kawasaki disease criteria, and 57% developing Kawasaki disease shock syndrome. **Table 3** demonstrates the criteria for complete Kawasaki disease and incomplete Kawasaki disease.

In addition to the features described in **Table 3**, the liver, joints, lungs, central nervous system, and gastrointestinal tract can also be affected in Kawasaki disease.[17] Kawasaki disease shock syndrome includes the features of Kawasaki disease in addition to a 20% systolic blood pressure decrease compared with the patient's age group or signs of hypoperfusion.[35,36] Overlapping features and differences exist between Kawasaki disease and MIS-C. **Table 4** compares and contrasts Kawasaki disease and MIS-C.

Table 3
Complete Kawasaki disease versus incomplete Kawasaki disease[3,6,24,32]

Disease	Features/Criteria

Complete Kawasaki disease	Elevated fever ≥ 5 d
	AND
	At least 4 of 5 of the following:
	  Bilateral nonexudative conjunctivitis
	  Oropharyngeal mucosal changes
	  Cervical lymphadenopathy >1.5 cm
	  Redness and swelling of the hands and feet
	  Erythematous rash

Incomplete Kawasaki disease	Elevated fever ≥5 d
	AND
	  At least 2 of the 5 characteristics in complete
	  Kawasaki disease (see above)
	AND
	  C-reactive protein of ≥3 mg/dL or erythrocyte
	  sedimentation rate of ≥40 mm/h
	AND
	  ≥3 of the following laboratory abnormalities
	  Low hemoglobin for age
	  Platelets of ≥450,000 after fever for 7 d
	  Albumin of ≤3 g/dL
	  White blood count of ≥15,000/mm³
	  ALT of >40 U/L
	OR
	  Cardiac involvement on echocardiogram
	  (eg, coronary artery aneurysms, ventricular dysfunction)

Children with MIS-C and Kawasaki disease shock syndrome tend to have higher C-reactive protein, platelet count, creatinine, N-terminal-pro hormone B-type natriuretic peptide, and troponin levels than those with Kawasaki disease, as well as cardiac ventricular dysfunction.[17] Untreated, 20% to 25% of Kawasaki disease cases will develop coronary artery aneurysms,[32,33] whereas in MIS-C and Kawasaki disease shock syndrome, cardiac ventricular dysfunction is more commonly seen.[7,14,20] In Kawasaki disease, high levels of IL-1 are typically seen, whereas in MIS-C IL-6 and IL-8 are increased, as demonstrated by all 15 MIS-C cases in the study by Riollano-Cruz and associates[18] having high levels of IL-6 and IL-8, and normal IL-1 levels. These findings, in combination with **Table 4**, demonstrate that Kawasaki disease and MIS-C, although sharing similar features, are separate entities.

MULTISYSTEM INFLAMMATORY DISEASE IN CHILDREN TREATMENT

Various treatment options exist for MIS-C (**Table 5**) and many intersect with strategies used for Kawasaki disease. A combination of intravenous immunoglobulin (IVIG) and aspirin are the first-line treatments in the healing process of Kawasaki disease.[32,33] IVIG comprises pooled human IgG antibodies that may work through neutralizing antigens,[37] inhibit proliferation of antigen-specific T cells,[38] prevent the interaction between endothelial and natural killer cells,[39] and induce the secretion of IL-8 and IL-1 receptor antagonist .[40] IVIG has been shown to decrease fever more quickly and decrease the development of coronary artery aneurysms, whereas aspirin aids in decreasing inflammation and inhibiting platelet aggregation in Kawasaki disease.[33]

Table 4
Comparing/contrasting Kawasaki disease and MIS-C[6–8,14–18,20,21,23,25,27,29,31–33,41]

Common similarities	Hyperinflammation Fever, conjunctivitis, oropharyngeal mucosal changes (eg, red cracked lips, strawberry tongue) cervical lymphadenopathy, rash, red and/or swollen hands and feet	
Common differences	Kawasaki Disease	MIS-C
Demographics	Tend to be of East Asian descent, younger (<5 y)	Tend to be Hispanic/Latino, Black/African/Afro-Caribbean descent, Older (around 6–14 y)
Symptoms/signs	Fewer gastrointestinal symptoms	Tend to have more gastrointestinal upset (pain, emesis, diarrhea), hypotension/shock
Laboratory findings	IL-1 > IL-6, leukocytosis with neutrophilia, thrombocytosis	IL-6 > IL-1, lymphopenia, thrombocytopenia, higher: ferritin, C-reactive protein, NT-proBNP, troponin
Cardiac involvement	Tend to have more coronary artery aneurysms	Tend to have more cardiac ventricular dysfunction

Abbreviations: NT-proBNP, N-terminal (NT)-pro hormone BNP.

Owing to the similarities between MIS-C and Kawasaki disease, IVIG and aspirin have been used in the treatment of MIS-C.[7,8,18,20,25] The American College of Rheumatology MIS-C task force recommends using high-dose IVIG (2 g/kg) in patients with MIS-C requiring hospitalization and/or fulfilling the Kawasaki disease criteria, in addition to aspirin if there are no contraindications.[41]

Riollano and colleagues[18] used IVIG and aspirin when Kawasaki disease criteria was met or in those with evidence of cardiac injury. Dufort and colleagues[15] analyzed MIS-C cases in New York state between March and May 2020 and noted that 70% of patients were given IVIG as part of the treatment regimen. Further, Toubiana and colleagues[8] described 21 pediatric patients with MIS-C with gastrointestinal symptoms likely related to bowel vessel vasculitis who all received IVIG with resolution of their symptoms thereafter. Verdoni and colleagues[20] also reported 10 patients between February and April 2020 who all received IVIG in addition to either aspirin or methylprednisolone or both with good response. Corticosteroids tend to be added to the treatment regimen when patients with MIS-C are in shock, if there is an increased risk of developing coronary artery aneurysms, or if the patient is considered high risk, presenting with features similar to incomplete Kawasaki disease.[14,25] Steroids should also be considered when fevers persist for more than 24 hours after IVIG treatment.[42]

Several second -line treatments such as biologics and antiviral analogs are used for MIS-C.[18,23] Remdesivir, an antiviral nucleoside analog, is given to those who meet compassionate use criteria, especially in those who have a positive PCR or presentation typical of COVID-19 infection.[18,23,27] Markedly, biologic agents tocilizumab, an anti–IL-6 receptor monoclonal antibody (anti–IL-6R), and anakinra, a recombinant human IL-1 receptor antagonist, have been used for refractory MIS-C not responding to IVIG,[18,42] just as anakinra has been used in IVIG-resistant Kawasaki disease[43,44] and tocilizumab for juvenile idiopathic arthritis.[45] Guidelines from the Inova health system recommend that anakinra be given for refractory MIS-C when fevers persist for more than 24 hours after IVIG or steroids and ferritin levels are greater than 1000 ng/mL or for worsening echocardiogram findings, whereas tocilizumab should be given for MIS-C refractory to anakinra.[42]

In their study, Riollano and colleagues[18] report tocilizumab and anakinra use for patients with MIS-C with hemodynamic instability and rapid clinical deterioration. Some patients with MIS-C received anakinra for unresolving severe inflammation, respiratory distress, persistent fevers, thrombocytopenia, or unresolving cardiac dysfunction.[14,29,31] Further, some received tocilizumab for high IL-6 levels, which play a part in the cytokine storm and the subsequent myocardial injury seen in MIS-C.[23] In a series of 9 patients with MIS-C in New York City between April and June 2020, all were treated with either IVIG or tocilizumab within 1 day of admission with resolution of their symptoms leading to favorable outcomes and a median 6-day admission.[13]

Waltuch and colleagues[46] describe case reports in children with MIS-C treated with IVIG and biologic agents. In 1 case, a 13-year-old patient presented with features of atypical Kawasaki disease, toxic shock syndrome, and COVID-19 cytokine storm with elevated IL-6 levels for which he was treated with IVIG, anakinra, and tocilizumab.[46] In another case, a 10-year-old boy with elevated IL-6 levels was treated with IVIG and tocilizumab for atypical Kawasaki disease and cytokine storm, respectively.[46] Balasubramanian and colleagues[47] report a case of an 8-year-old boy with MIS-C presenting with features of toxic shock syndrome and Kawasaki disease who was initially treated with IVIG and then tocilizumab 72 hours later owing to continued high-grade fevers and elevated C-reactive protein. At 12 hours after receiving 8 mg/kg IV tocilizumab infused over 2 hours, his fevers improved and his markers of inflammation normalized. Alongside other case reports and studies, the authors demonstrate that tocilizumab seems successful in decreasing the hyperinflammatory response in IVIG refractory MIS-C.[47]

In addition to using anakinra and tocilizumab as treatments for MIS-C, in a case series Whittaker and colleagues report that 8 of 58 patients with MIS-C received infliximab, a tumor necrosis factor (TNF)-alpha antagonist.[21] Similarly, Dolinger and colleagues[48] describe a 14-year-old boy presenting with active Crohn's disease and MIS-C with high levels of IL-6, IL-8, and TNF-alpha levels with a deteriorating clinical course including hypotension, tachycardia and persistent fevers. To treat both the Crohn's disease and the MIS-C in the setting of elevated TNF-alpha levels, 10 mg/kg infliximab was given with resolution of the fevers, hypotension, and tachycardia within hours, normalization of TNF-alpha levels, and a decrease in other cytokine levels.[48] In another study by Abdel-Haq and coworkers,[49] infliximab was used as a second-line therapy in 12 of 22 critically ill patients with MIS-C (median age of 7 years) with myocardial dysfunction refractory to IVIG, or persistent inflammation/fever with consequent improvement after treatment. These studies suggest that infliximab may be another beneficial treatment for MIS-C in those presenting with worsening systemic signs and high cytokine levels.

In a cohort of 185 patients with MIS-C, Feldstein and colleagues[6] reported that 77% of patients received IVIG, 49% received steroids, 8% received tocilizumab or siltuximab (anti–IL-6R), and 13% received anakinra. Similar studies examining patients with MIS-C used treatments that also included a combination of IVIG, aspirin, steroids, and/or IL-6 and IL-1 inhibitors.[14,18,20,23,25] Similarly, an 11-year-old girl with MIS-C and elevated IL-6 levels significantly improved within 24 hours after combination treatment with tocilizumab, convalescent plasma, remdesivir, steroids, and IVIG with resolution of fevers, tachycardia, and discontinuation of pressor support.[50]

Table 5
Treatment strategies to be considered in MIS-C[4,7,8,13,14,18,20,23,25,27,29,41,42]

Therapy	Dosage/Duration	Indication
IVIG (neutralizes autoantibodies)	Single 2 g/kg/d infusion ×1 over 10–12 h. Refrain from giving a second dose for refractory MIS-C owing to potential volume overload and hemolytic anemia risk	KD-like illness. Cardiac involvement. Severe hyperinflammation (ferritin of >700 ng/mL, C-reactive protein of >30 g/dL). Multisystem organ failure
Aspirin[a]	3–5 mg/kg/d for at least 4–6 wk until inflammatory markers, platelet count and echocardiogram findings have normalized	
Steroids	1–2 mg/kg/d prednisolone or methylprednisolone for 5 d followed by a 2-wk taper. Consider high dose methylprednisolone 10–30 mg/kg/d (max 1 g) IV for 3 d with taper in those with shock	Adjunct to IVIG in those with severe disease/high risk. Infants, C-reactive protein of >130 g/dL, echocardiogram Z score of >2.5 or aneurysms, shock. Refractory disease
Biologics		
Tocilizumab (anti–IL-6R)[c]	Weight < 30 kg = 12 mg/kg/dose ×1. Weight ≥ 30 kg = 8 mg/kg/dose (max 800 mg) ×1. Repeat 12 h later if needed	Refractory to IVIG and steroids or contraindication to IVIG/steroids. Hemodynamic instability or acute clinical decompensation. Persistent hyperinflammation
Anakinra (anti–IL-1R)	2–4 mg/kg/d IV or SQ (max 100 mg/dose)	
Infliximab (TNF-alpha antagonist)	10 mg/kg IV	
Remdesivir (antiviral nucleoside analog)	5 mg/kg load IV once (max dose 200 mg) on day 1, then 2.5 mg/kg (100 mg max dose) IV daily for 9 d	Presentation consistent with SARS-CoV-2 infection AND/OR Positive RT-PCR for COVID-19
Anticoagulation	Consult hematology for appropriate dosing. Continue for at least 2 wk after discharge	Consider for moderate to severe LV dysfunction (LVEF of <35%). Coronary artery aneurysm z-score of ≥10[b]. Thrombosis. Critically ill patients

Abbreviations: anti–IL-1R, interleukin-1 receptor antagonist; IVIG, intravenous immunoglobulin; KD, Kawasaki disease; LV, left ventricular; LVEF, left ventricular ejection fraction; SQ, subcutaneous; TNF, tumor necrosis factor.

[a] Platelet count should be ≥80,0000 cells/μL to give aspirin and it should be avoided in active bleeding or in those with high bleeding risk. For the acute phase of illness, some institutions recommend aspirin 30 to 80 mg/kg/d divided 4 times a day and 3 to 5 mg/kg/d for at least 4 wk once afebrile for 24 to 72 h.

[b] Continue lifelong therapy for coronary artery aneurysm z-score of ≥10.

[c] American College of Rheumatology MIS-C task force does not recommend tocilizumab for most COVID-19 pediatric patients based on randomized control adult studies in those with COVID-19 pneumonia that show this medication does not decrease mortality at 28 d and instead prefer Anakinra.

Interestingly, in the United States 5% of patients who present with Kawasaki disease require vasoactive support for cardiogenic shock, whereas Feldstein and colleagues[6] report almost 50% of their patients with MIS-C needing such agents, highlighting that MIS-C tends to cause more shock than Kawasaki disease. Vasopressors and ionotropic agents were widely used in those having shock with MIS-C in other case reports.[14,15,18,19,24] Further, anticoagulation, most notably enoxaparin, has been used in the treatment of patients with MIS-C as either prophylaxis or in those with high D-dimer, fibrinogen, electrocardiogram changes, left ventricular dysfunction, or coronary artery abnormalities.[18,23,25]

RHEUMATOLOGIC MANIFESTATIONS OF SARS-CoV-2

COVID-19 has been shown to cause a hyperinflammatory response in children (MIS-C),[7] similar to how rheumatologic disorders such as juvenile idiopathic arthritis and SLE may induce a hyperinflammatory state like in macrophage activation syndrome (MAS).[51] SARS-CoV-2 enters cells via the host angiotensin-converting enzyme II receptor that, in addition to the respiratory tract, can be found in skeletal muscle, smooth muscle, synovial fluids, small vessel endothelium, and bowel tissue causing symptoms such as fatigue, myalgia, and arthralgias, which are also seen in rheumatologic pathology.[52] Viral infections can trigger rheumatologic diseases,[52] and case reports have demonstrated that SARS-CoV-2 infection may trigger rheumatologic entities in children and adolescents such as SLE, arthritis, MAS, chilblains, and antiphospholipid syndrome.[20,53–55] Understanding that COVID-19 may present with or potentially precipitate rheumatologic manifestations aides in improving patient care by expanding the differential diagnosis to enhance treatment plans and to consider COVID-19 infection as part of the work-up in an individual presenting with new-onset rheumatologic disease in correlation with the clinical picture.

COVID-19 AND MACROPHAGE ACTIVATION SYNDROME

MAS is characterized by high serum ferritin levels and cytokines causing hyperinflammation leading to multiorgan failure, similar to what is seen in MIS-C.[20,56] In their case series, Verdoni and colleagues[20] describe a group of children diagnosed with Kawasaki-like disease in which 50% also met MAS criteria in the setting of SARS-CoV-2 exposure (80% with positive IgG serology). SARS-CoV-2 infection induces a hyperinflammatory syndrome as seen in MIS-C, which has similar features to MAS, a hyperferritinemic syndrome where macrophage activation allows for high levels of ferritin release (ferritin of >300 ng/mL).[51,56] MAS, commonly treated by rheumatologists, already has established treatment methods (such as steroids, anakinra and tocilizumab)[27] and understanding the overlapping clinical features and pathogenesis between MAS and MIS-C will likely aid in the treatment strategies for this new inflammatory entity.

COVID-19 AND NEW-ONSET SYSTEMIC LUPUS ERYTHEMATOUS

Systemic lupus erythematous is a relapsing and remitting chronic multisystemic autoimmune disorder resulting from autoantibodies against host cytoplasmic and nuclear antigens that can be triggered by viral infections.[53,57] Mantovani and colleagues[53] described the first case of an 18-year-old Hispanic girl with a positive COVID-19 PCR result with a past medical history of autism and panic disorder presenting with new-onset SLE and probable antiphospholipid syndrome. The patient presented with shortness of breath, productive cough, fevers, upper respiratory symptoms, pericardial effusion, and fatigue with consequent hemodynamic instability leading to cardiac arrest with ROSC.[53] RT-PCR for SARS-CoV-2 was negative twice and, owing to continued high clinical suspicion for COVID-19 infection, she was retested a third time with RT-PCR resulting positive.[53] During her hospital course, she developed kidney failure and had lymphopenia, anemia, proteinuria, and hematuria.[53] Also, she was found to have positive serology for antinuclear antibodies (1:2560), anti–double stranded DNA, low complement (C3 and C4) levels, leading to a diagnosis of SLE based on the American College of Rheumatology/European League Against Rheumatism 2019 criteria.[53] Further, she was treated for possible antiphospholipid syndrome in the setting of multiple deep venous thromboses and thrombocytopenia in the setting of anticardiolipin antibodies and positive lupus anticoagulant.[53]

Adaptive immunity in SLE does not function as well as in healthy individuals and thus may be further weakened by COVID-19.[53] SLE decrease the T helper cell type 1 response by impairing the production of cytokines such as IL-1, IL-2, and TNF-alpha.[53] This process causes a less effective T helper cell type 2 response to evade viruses owing to SLE causing increased autoantibodies and heightened autoreactivity of helper, cytotoxic T cells, and B-cell differentiation.[53] This concept of changing from a T helper cell type 1 response to a T helper cell type 2 response owing to autoreactivity and autoantibodies altering cytokine profiles has been seen in HIV and may explain the autoimmune phenomena seen in COVID-19.[53]

COVID-19 AND NEW-ONSET CUTANEOUS LESIONS

Chilblain-like lesions have been described as vaso-occlusive erythematous to purpuric, violaceous-edematous lesions with cyanotic areas on the toes, hands, and fingers measuring between 5 and 20 mm in diameter.[54,58–63] Outbreaks of chilblain-like lesions, also known as pseudo-chilblain, pernio-like, acute acro-ischemia, or COVID toes have been increasingly documented in the setting of the SARS-CoV-2 pandemic,[54,58–60,64] associating a potential relationship between the lesions and the virus. To further demonstrate this correlation, in a study by Colmenero and colleagues,[65] skin biopsies from 7 children showed lymphocytic vasculitis and immunohistochemistry demonstrated SARS-CoV-2 in the endothelial and epithelial cells of eccrine glands. Moreover, in a case series of 19 adolescents (mean age 14 years) with chilblain-like lesions, El Hachem and colleagues[66] report positive immunoglobulin A serology for the S1 domain of the COVID-19 spike protein.

Chilblains tend to be more common in adults than children resulting from an inflammatory vascular response.[54] Cold, nonfreezing temperatures typically induce primary chilblains, whereas secondary chilblains can be due to autoimmune disorders and viral infections.[54,58] The term chilblain-like has been used given these lesions do not seem to be precipitated by cold and there is typically no prior personal history of these cutaneous manifestations, even though they look similar to chilblains.[54,58,67] In Italy, Piccolo and colleagues[58] reported 63 healthy patients (median age of 14 years) with erythematous–edematous chilblain-like lesions mostly affecting the toes and soles (85.7%), but also observed on the hands. Although 25.4% of the lesions were asymptomatic, there was pain and pruritis in more than 50% of cases.[58] In the study, it was difficult to attain COVID-19 status for all cases; however, some patients had either positive serology or PCR or both, although others in the study had individuals they lived with that were positive for SARS-CoV-2.[58] In another case report, Locatelli and colleagues[67] describe a 16-year-old boy who tested positive by RT-PCR for SARS-CoV-2 with erythematous–edematous macules and plaques on the fingers and toes with histology consistent with chilblains.

COVID-19 can cause a type I interferon response that in turn causes microvascular injury as seen in chilblains and retinal vasculitis. Interestingly, Quintana-Castanedo and coworkers[63] report the first case of an otherwise healthy asymptomatic 11-year-old boy presenting with a 2-week history of chilblains on his dorsal toes bilaterally and retinal vasculitis in the setting of positive IgG serology to SARS-CoV-2. An eye examination was performed as routine owing to possible thromboembolic events owing to COVID-19.[63] Further, in a case series during the highest COVID peak in northern Spain where 85.2% of cases were less than 21 years of age (median age of 14 years) with no history of rheumatic disease, Gómez-Fernández and associates[68] reported chilblain-like lesions with positive cryofibrinogen proteins in 68.2% of patients between the ages of 0 and 20 years. This finding could potentially suggest that cryofibrinogenemia may play a role in the pathogenesis of chilblains owing to COVID-19.[68]

Gallizzi and colleagues[69] report 9 cases of chilblain-like lesions during the COVID-19 outbreak in Italy in children aged 5 to 15 years old with more than 50% experiencing systemic symptoms around 2 weeks before developing the lesions. Antinuclear antibodies and antiphospholipid antibodies were positive in 4 children.[69] One child with a history of Raynaud phenomenon a few years prior was noted to be positive for extractable nuclear antigens autoantibodies SS-A and rheumatoid factor, in addition to antinuclear antibodies (1:5120), leading the authors to diagnose him with a connective tissue disorder and, although it is hard to say, COVID-19 could have potentially been the trigger given the timing of the onset of events.[69]

Piccolo and colleagues[58] reported only 6 of 63 patients with an autoimmune disorder, and other case reports reported similar findings,[54,60,67] suggesting that chilblain-like lesions are likely not due to an underlying rheumatic disease, but rather exposure to SAR-CoV-2 infection. Chilblain-like lesions seemed to manifest after systemic symptoms, such as gastrointestinal and respiratory distress, headache, and fever,[54,58,59,62,67] and can present with itchiness and pain.[54,59,62] Typically, these patients were negative for COVID-19 PCR or serology; however, there were patients in case reports who had coinhabitants with confirmed COVID-19 infection, upper respiratory tract symptoms, or potential COVID-19 exposure from family that worked closely with these patients.[54,58,59,61,62] Further, in a case series of 20 pediatric patients with Chilblain-like lesions, RT-PCR and serology were negative for COVID-19.[70] PCR and serology seem to be negative in those presenting with Chilblain-like lesions, and this observation seems to indicate that the lesions are a late manifestation of COVID-19.[54,62,68] Observing chilblain-like lesions in a pediatric patient may prompt an investigation of previous COVID-19 infection and help to mitigate efforts for surveillance and screening of this virus.

COVID-19 AND NEW-ONSET ARTHRITIS

Reactive arthritis tends to occur in men between the ages of 20 to 50 years.[55] It is also a postinfectious arthritis with sterile synovial fluid mostly occurring secondary to sexually transmitted or gastrointestinal infections and less commonly from viral infections.[55] Houshmand and colleagues[55] describe a case of a 10-year-old boy with positive SARS-CoV-2 RT-PCR presenting with a 1-week of history of fever and urticaria and 5 days of swelling and pain in his bilateral knees and right elbow. Other than morning stiffness and pain with movement, he had no other systemic symptoms.[55] On physical examination, he had warmth, tenderness, swelling, and decreased range of motion of affected joints.[55] His rheumatoid factor and antinuclear antibodies were normal and knee joint aspiration did not reveal any fluid.[55] He improved with supportive treatment and antihistamines.[55] Although difficult to discern whether SARS-CoV-2 infection induces reactive arthritis, this case describes potential postviral arthritis, likely owing to COVID-19 in the setting of positive serology.[55]

SUMMARY

SARS-CoV-2 continues to spread widely around the world. The more we learn about COVID-19, including its presentation and pathophysiology, the better its features become recognized to diagnose and treat its manifestations. In children, the Kawasaki-like disease, multisystem inflammatory syndrome, causes severe life-threatening symptoms. Although not common, several case reports have documented new-onset rheumatologic disease in children concerning SARS-CoV-2 infection, such as SLE, arthritis, and MAS. Rheumatologists commonly treat hyperinflammation syndromes and these same therapies have been used to direct treatment for the severe hyperinflammation seen in COVID-19. As reviewed in this article, the literature documents rheumatologic manifestations owing to prior SAR-CoV-2 infection in children. Although it is difficult to pinpoint definitively whether the virus triggered these rheumatologic presentations, these cases raise awareness that there could be a link between COVID-19 and new-onset rheumatologic diseases, which will help to guide future research efforts to further understand this correlation, establish diagnoses, and initiate treatment plans.

CLINICS CARE POINTS

- Children with COVID-19 infection generally have asymptomatic or mild disease.
- MIS-C is a severe post–COVID-19 syndrome similar to Kawasaki disease, but differing in several ways.
- COVID-19 can cause an inflammatory vascular response leading to chilblains in children.
- Flares of existing or new onset of rheumatologic diseases have been reported in children with COVID-19.

DISCLOSURE

The authors declare no conflict of interest.

UNCITED REFERENCE

72.

REFERENCES

1. Zhu N, Zhang D, Wang W, et al. A novel coronavirus from patients with pneumonia in China, 2019. N Engl J Med 2020;382(8):727–33.
2. Cucinotta D, Vanelli M. WHO declares COVID-19 a pandemic. Acta Biomed 2020;91(1):157–60.
3. Lu X, Zhang L, Du H, et al. SARS-CoV-2 infection in children. N Engl J Med 2020; 382(17):1663–5.
4. Ludvigsson JF. Systematic review of COVID-19 in children shows milder cases and a better prognosis than adults. Acta Paediatr 2020;109(6):1088–95.

5. Castagnoli R, Votto M, Licari A, et al. Severe acute respiratory syndrome corona-virus 2 (SARS-CoV-2) infection in children and adolescents: a systematic review. JAMA Pediatr 2020;174(9):882–9.

6. Feldstein LR, Rose EB, Horwitz SM, et al. Multisystem inflammatory syndrome in U.S. children and adolescents. N Engl J Med 2020;383(4):334–46.

7. Riphagen S, Gomez X, Gonzalez-Martinez C, et al. Hyperinflammatory shock in children during COVID-19 pandemic. The Lancet 2020;395(10237):1607–8.

8. Toubiana J, Poirault C, Corsia A, et al. Kawasaki-like multisystem inflammatory syndrome in children during the covid-19 pandemic in Paris, France: prospective observational study. BMJ 2020;369:m2094.

9. Centers for Disease Control and Prevention Health Alert Network (HAN). Multi-system inflammatory syndrome in children (MIS-C) associated with coronavirus disease 2019 (COVID-19) 2020. Available at: https://emergency.cdc.gov/han/2020/han00432.asp. Accessed March 20, 2021.

10. Dong Y, Mo X, Hu Y, et al. Epidemiology of COVID-19 Among Children in China. Pediatrics 2020;145(6):e20200702.

11. Zhou P, Yang XL, Wang XG, et al. A pneumonia outbreak associated with a new coronavirus of probable bat origin. Nature 2020;579(7798):270–3.

12. Bunyavanich S, Do A, Vicencio A. Nasal gene expression of angiotensin-converting enzyme 2 in children and adults. J Am Med Assoc 2020;323(23):2427–9.

13. Gruber CN, Patel RS, Trachtman R, et al. Mapping systemic inflammation and antibody responses in multisystem inflammatory syndrome in children (MIS-C). Cell 2020;183(4):982–95.e14.

14. Belhadjer Z, Méot M, Bajolle F, et al. Acute heart failure in multisystem inflamma-tory syndrome in children in the context of global SARS-CoV-2 pandemic. Circu-lation 2020;142(5):429–36.

15. Dufort EM, Koumans EH, Chow EJ, et al. Multisystem inflammatory syndrome in children in New York State. N Engl J Med 2020;383(4):347–58.

16. Levin M. Childhood multisystem inflammatory syndrome - a new challenge in the pandemic. N Engl J Med 2020;383(4):393–5.

17. Nakra NA, Blumberg DA, Herrera-Guerra A, et al. Multi-system inflammatory syn-drome in children (MIS-C) following SARS-CoV-2 infection: review of clinical pre-sentation, hypothetical pathogenesis, and proposed management. Children (Basel) 2020;7(7):69.

18. Riollano-Cruz M, Akkoyun E, Briceno-Brito E, et al. Multisystem inflammatory syn-drome in children related to COVID-19: a New York City experience [published online ahead of print, 2020 Jun 25]. J Med Virol 2020;93:424–33. https://doi.org/10.1002/jmv.26224.

19. Belot A, Antona D, Renolleau S, et al. SARS-CoV-2-related paediatric inflamma-tory multisystem syndrome, an epidemiological study, France, 1 March to 17 May 2020. Euro Surveill 2020;25(22):2001010.

20. Verdoni L, Mazza A, Gervasoni A, et al. An outbreak of severe Kawasaki-like dis-ease at the Italian epicentre of the SARS-CoV-2 epidemic: an observational cohort study. Lancet 2020;395(10239):1771–8.

21. Whittaker E, Bamford A, Kenny J, et al. Clinical characteristics of 58 children with a pediatric inflammatory multisystem syndrome temporally associated with SARS-CoV-2. J Am Med Assoc 2020;324(3):259–69.

22. Li Y, Lee PY, Sobel ES, et al. Increased expression of FcgammaRI/CD64 on circu-lating monocytes parallels ongoing inflammation and nephritis in lupus. Arthritis Res Ther 2009;11(1):R6.

23. Kaushik S, Aydin SI, Derespina KR, et al. Multisystem inflammatory syndrome in children associated with severe acute respiratory syndrome coronavirus 2 infection (MIS-C): a multi-institutional study from New York City. J Pediatr 2020; 224:24–9.
24. Godfred-Cato S, Bryant B, Leung J, et al. COVID-19-associated multisystem inflammatory syndrome in children - United States, March-July 2020. MMWR Morb Mortal Wkly Rep 2020;69(32):1074–80.
25. Capone CA, Subramony A, Sweberg T, et al. Characteristics, cardiac involvement, and outcomes of multisystem inflammatory syndrome of childhood associated with severe acute respiratory syndrome coronavirus 2 infection. J Pediatr 2020;224:141–5.
26. Miller J, Cantor A, Zachariah P, et al. Gastrointestinal symptoms as a major presentation component of a novel multisystem inflammatory syndrome in children that is related to coronavirus disease 2019: a single center experience of 44 cases. Gastroenterology 2020;159(4):1571–4.e2.
27. Hennon TR, Penque MD, Abdul-Aziz R, et al. COVID-19 associated multisystem inflammatory syndrome in children (MIS-C) guidelines; a Western New York approach [published online ahead of print, 2020 May 23]. Prog Pediatr Cardiol 2020;101232.
28. Davies P, Evans C, Kanthimathinathan HK, et al. Intensive care admissions of children with paediatric inflammatory multisystem syndrome temporally associated with SARS-CoV-2 (PIMS-TS) in the UK: a multicentre observational study [published correction appears in Lancet Child Adolesc Health. 2020 Jul 17]. Lancet Child Adolesc Health 2020;4(9):669–77.
29. Pouletty M, Borocco C, Ouldali N, et al. Paediatric multisystem inflammatory syndrome temporally associated with SARS-CoV-2 mimicking Kawasaki disease (Kawa-COVID-19): a multicentre cohort. Ann Rheum Dis 2020;79(8):999–1006.
30. Licciardi F, Pruccoli G, Denina M, et al. SARS-CoV-2-induced Kawasaki-like hyperinflammatory syndrome: a novel COVID phenotype in children. Pediatrics 2020;146(2):e20201711.
31. Chiotos K, Bassiri H, Behrens EM, et al. Multisystem inflammatory syndrome in children during the coronavirus 2019 pandemic: a case series. J Pediatr Infect Dis Soc 2020;9(3):393–8.
32. Kawasaki T. Kawasaki disease. Proc Jpn Acad Ser B Phys Biol Sci 2006;82(2): 59–71.
33. Burns JC, Glodé MP. Kawasaki syndrome. The Lancet 2004;364(9433):533–44.
34. Elakabawi K, Lin J, Jiao F, et al. Kawasaki disease: global burden and genetic background. Cardiol Res 2020;11(1):9–14.
35. Zhang MM, Shi L, Li XH, et al. Clinical analysis of Kawasaki disease shock syndrome. Chin Med J (Engl) 2017;130(23):2891–2.
36. Gatterre P, Oualha M, Dupic L, et al. Kawasaki disease: an unexpected etiology of shock and multiple organ dysfunction syndrome. Intensive Care Med 2012; 38(5):872–8.
37. Jolles S, Sewell WA, Misbah SA. Clinical uses of intravenous immunoglobulin. Clin Exp Immunol 2005;142(1):1–11.
38. Aktas O, Waiczies S, Grieger U, et al. Polyspecific immunoglobulins (IVIg) suppress proliferation of human (auto)antigen-specific T cells without inducing apoptosis. J Neuroimmunol 2001;114(1–2):160–7.
39. Finberg RW, Newburger JW, Mikati MA, et al. Effect of high doses of intravenously administered immune globulin on natural killer cell activity in peripheral blood. J Pediatr 1992;120(3):376–80.

40. Ruiz de Souza V, Carreno MP, Kaveri SV, et al. Selective induction of interleukin-1 receptor antagonist and interleukin-8 in human monocytes by normal polyspecific IgG (intravenous immunoglobulin). Eur J Immunol 1995;25(5):1267–73.

41. Henderson LA, Canna SW, Friedman KG, et al. American College of Rheumatology clinical guidance for pediatric patients with multisystem inflammatory syndrome in children (MIS-C) associated with SARS-CoV-2 and hyperinflammation in COVID-19. version 2. Arthritis Rheum 2021;72(11):1791–805.

42. Developed by pediatric infectious diseases, critical care, cardiology, rheumatology, and pharmacy providers. Guideline: evaluation and management of COVID-19 multisystem inflammatory syndrome in children (MIS-C). Falls Church (VA): Inova Health System; 2020.

43. Kone-Paut I, Cimaz R, Herberg J, et al. The use of interleukin 1 receptor antagonist (anakinra) in Kawasaki disease: a retrospective cases series. Autoimmun Rev 2018;17(8):768–74.

44. Blonz G, Lacroix S, Benbrik N, et al. Severe late-onset Kawasaki Disease successfully treated with anakinra. J Clin Rheumatol 2020;26(2):e42–3.

45. Brunner HI, Ruperto N, Zuber Z, et al. Efficacy and safety of tocilizumab for polyarticular-course juvenile idiopathic arthritis in the open-label 2-year extension of a phase 3 trial [published online ahead of print, 2020 Sep 20]. Arthritis Rheum 2015;74:1110–7.

46. Waltuch T, Gill P, Zinns LE, et al. Features of COVID-19 post-infectious cytokine release syndrome in children presenting to the emergency department. Am J Emerg Med 2020;38(10):2246.e3–6.

47. Balasubramanian S, Nagendran TM, Ramachandran B, et al. Hyper-inflammatory syndrome in a child with COVID-19 treated successfully with intravenous immunoglobulin and tocilizumab. Indian Pediatr 2020;57(7):681–3.

48. Dolinger MT, Person H, Smith R, et al. Pediatric Crohn disease and multisystem inflammatory syndrome in children (MIS-C) and COVID-19 treated with infliximab. J Pediatr Gastroenterol Nutr 2020;71(2):153–5.

49. Abdel-Haq N, Asmar BI, Deza Leon MP, et al. SARS-CoV-2-associated multisystem inflammatory syndrome in children: clinical manifestations and the role of infliximab treatment [published online ahead of print, 2021 Jan 16]. Eur J Pediatr 2021;180(5):1–11.

50. Greene AG, Saleh M, Roseman E, et al. Toxic shock-like syndrome and COVID-19: multisystem inflammatory syndrome in children (MIS-C). Am J Emerg Med 2020;38(11):2492.e5–6.

51. Cron RQ, Chatham WW. The rheumatologist's role in COVID-19. J Rheumatol 2020;47(5):639–42.

52. Ciaffi J, Meliconi R, Ruscitti P, et al. Rheumatic manifestations of COVID-19: a systematic review and meta-analysis. BMC Rheumatol 2020;4:65.

53. Mantovani Cardoso E, Hundal J, Feterman D, et al. Concomitant new diagnosis of systemic lupus erythematosus and COVID-19 with possible antiphospholipid syndrome. Just a coincidence? A case report and review of intertwining pathophysiology. Clin Rheumatol 2020;39(9):2811–5.

54. Andina D, Noguera-Morel L, Bascuas-Arribas M, et al. Chilblains in children in the setting of COVID-19 pandemic. Pediatr Dermatol 2020;37(3):406–11.

55. Houshmand H, Abounoori M, Ghaemi R, et al. Ten-year-old boy with atypical COVID-19 symptom presentation: a case report [published online ahead of print, 2020 Nov 16]. Clin Case Rep 2021;9(1):304–8.

56. Colafrancesco S, Alessandri C, Conti F, et al. COVID-19 gone bad: a new character in the spectrum of the hyperferritinemic syndrome? Autoimmun Rev 2020; 19(7):102573.

57. Fortuna G, Brennan MT. Systemic lupus erythematosus: epidemiology, pathophysiology, manifestations, and management. Dent Clin North Am 2013;57(4): 631–55.

58. Piccolo V, Neri I, Filippeschi C, et al. Chilblain-like lesions during COVID-19 epidemic: a preliminary study on 63 patients. J Eur Acad Dermatol Venereol 2020;34(7):e291–3.

59. Colonna C, Monzani NA, Rocchi A, et al. Chilblain-like lesions in children following suspected COVID-19 infection. Pediatr Dermatol 2020;37(3):437–40.

60. Mazzotta F, Troccoli T, Bonifazi E. A new vasculitis at the time of COVID-19. Eur J Pediat Dermatol 2020;30(2):75–8.

61. Landa N, Mendieta-Eckert M, Fonda-Pascual P, et al. Chilblain-like lesions on feet and hands during the COVID-19 Pandemic. Int J Dermatol 2020;59(6):739–43.

62. Cordoro KM, Reynolds SD, Wattier R, et al. Clustered cases of acral perniosis: clinical features, histopathology, and relationship to COVID-19. Pediatr Dermatol 2020;37(3):419–23.

63. Quintana-Castanedo L, Feito-Rodríguez M, Fernández-Alcalde C, et al. Concurrent chilblains and retinal vasculitis in a child with COVID-19. J Eur Acad Dermatol Venereol 2020;34(12):e764–6.

64. Hernandez C, Bruckner AL. Focus on "COVID Toes". JAMA Dermatol 2020; 156(9):1003.

65. Colmenero I, Santonja C, Alonso-Riaño M, et al. SARS-CoV-2 endothelial infection causes COVID-19 chilblains: histopathological, immunohistochemical and ultrastructural study of seven paediatric cases. Br J Dermatol 2020;183(4):729–37.

66. El Hachem M, Diociaiuti A, Concato C, et al. A clinical, histopathological and laboratory study of 19 consecutive Italian paediatric patients with chilblain-like lesions: lights and shadows on the relationship with COVID-19 infection. J Eur Acad Dermatol Venereol 2020;34(11):2620–9.

67. Locatelli AG, Robustelli Test E, Vezzoli P, et al. Histologic features of long-lasting chilblain-like lesions in a paediatric COVID-19 patient. J Eur Acad Dermatol Venereol 2020;34(8):e365–8.

68. Gómez-Fernández C, López-Sundh AE, González-Vela C, et al. High prevalence of cryofibrinogenemia in patients with chilblains during the COVID-19 outbreak. Int J Dermatol 2020;59(12):1475–84.

69. Gallizzi R, Sutera D, Spagnolo A, et al. Management of pernio-like cutaneous manifestations in children during the outbreak of COVID-19 [published online ahead of print, 2020 Sep 19]. Dermatol Ther 2020;33(6):e14312. https://doi.org/ 10.1111/dth.14312.

70. Roca-Ginés J, Torres-Navarro I, Sánchez-Arráez J, et al. Assessment of acute acral lesions in a case series of children and adolescents during the COVID-19 pandemic. JAMA Dermatol 2020;156(9):992–7.

71. Centers for Disease Control and Prevention. Information for healthcare provides about multisystem inflammatory syndrome in children (MIS-C). Available at: https://www.cdc.gov/mis-c/hcp/. Accessed August 28, 2020; National Center for Immunization and Respiratory Diseases (NCIRD).

72. Rowley AH. Understanding SARS-CoV-2-related multisystem inflammatory syndrome in children. Nat Rev Immunol 2020;20(8):453–4.

Impact of COVID-19 on Pediatric Immunocompromised Patients

James A. Connelly, MD[a], Hey Chong, MD, PhD[b],
Adam J. Esbenshade, MD, MSCI[c], David Frame, PharmD[d],
Christopher Failing, MD[e], Elizabeth Secord, MD[f],
Kelly Walkovich, MD[g],*

KEYWORDS

- Immunocompromised • Immunodeficiency • SARS-CoV-2 • COVID-19 • Pediatric
- HIV • Cancer • Autoimmune

KEY POINTS

- Children and adolescents with primary or secondary immune deficiencies have not generally had increased incidence or severity of COVID-19 infection as was initially feared.
- Decreased access to care has led to delayed diagnosis and increased morbidity in some groups of immunocompromised patients, especially those with malignancies and rheumatologic disease.
- The current vaccines available for COVID-19 are not live vaccines and should be able to be safely used in immunocompromised children and adolescents, but the efficacy will have to be monitored carefully for each immune defect.
- The COVID-19 pandemic has normalized some infection-control procedures that are routine for immunocompromised children and adolescents and may bring more tolerance for their needs.

[a] Pediatric Hematology/Oncology, Monroe Carell Jr Children's Hospital, Vanderbilt University, 2220 Pierce Avenue, 389 PRB, Nashville, TN 37232, USA; [b] Pediatric Allergy & Immunology, UPMC Children's Hospital of Pittsburgh, One Children's Hospital Drive, 4401 Penn Avenue, Pittsburgh, PA 15224, USA; [c] Pediatric Hematology/Oncology, Monroe Carell Jr Children's Hospital, Vanderbilt University, 2220 Pierce Avenue, 388 PRB, Nashville, TN 37232, USA; [d] School of Pharmacy, University of Michigan, 1500 East Medical Center Drive, Ann Arbor, MI 48109, USA; [e] Pediatric Rheumatology, Essentia Health, 1702 South University Drive, Fargo, ND 58103, USA; [f] Pediatric Allergy & Immunology, Wayne State University, Wayne Pediatrics, 400 Mack Avenue, Detroit, MI 48201, USA; [g] Pediatric Hematology/Oncology, C.S. Mott Children's Hospital, University of Michigan, 1540 East Medical Center Drive, Ann Arbor, MI 48109, USA
* Corresponding author.
E-mail address: kwalkovi@med.umich.edu

Pediatr Clin N Am 68 (2021) 1029–1054
https://doi.org/10.1016/j.pcl.2021.05.007
0031-3955/21/© 2021 Elsevier Inc. All rights reserved.

INTRODUCTION

The severe acute respiratory syndrome coronavirus-2 (SARS-CoV-2) has caused critical coronavirus disease 2019 (COVID-19) most often in the elderly and individuals with comorbid medical conditions. Although growing evidence supports the importance of an intact innate immune response at the onset of viral infection, mortality caused by dysregulated immune responses, particularly in adults, has shown a spotlight on the delicate balance of a robust, but coordinated and controlled, immune activity against infection.[1] The pathologic role of the immune system has also been emphasized by the new multisystem inflammatory syndrome in children (MIS-C), which currently is believed to be a result of an aberrant adaptive immune response to SARS-CoV-2 infection.[2] The necessity of this immune equilibrium has manifested in the clinical care of severe COVID-19 and MIS-C with administration of immune suppressants to offset inappropriate immune activation.

This complex network of infection, immune response, and inflammation with SARS-CoV-2 has created concerns, questions, and challenges for immunocompromised children beyond fear of death from contracting SARS-CoV-2. This review examines how adaptations by health care systems to reduce SARS-CoV-2 transmission and treat the surge of COVID-19 patients impacted immunocompromised pediatric patients. While expansion of some services, such as telemedicine, provided a new safe venue to provide care for some patients, contraction of other services or parental anxiety to present to medical care units resulted in impaired access for other patients. We will also examine how the perceived danger of severe infection early in the pandemic triggered modifications of immune suppression, with negative ramifications in some patients, and the impact of prolonged quarantine-intensified psychosocial concerns in children and adolescents.

In addition, this publication will examine questions commonly faced among health care providers including how to test for SARS-CoV-2 with high sensitivity, how to treat active SARS-CoV-2 infection in immunocompromised youth, how to consider the safety and efficacy of COVID vaccine for the immunocompromised, and how to provide medical and psychosocial support while reducing infectious exposure in immunocompromised children. The outcomes of SARS-CoV-2 in immunocompromised patients to date are also reviewed. Lessons learned caring for immunocompromised children during the pandemic, including some unforeseen benefits of the lockdown, are presented as valuable education for providers caring for both healthy and sick children.

Testing for SARS-CoV-2 Infection in Immunocompromised Patients

Despite the potential for an altered immune response to SARS-CoV-2, asymptomatic presentations are common in pediatric immunocompromised patients (13%–62% in published cohorts; **Table 1**), emphasizing that the lack of signs and symptoms does not rule out infection. However, identifying SARS-CoV-2 infection is especially important in patients with immune deficits, where decisions on admission, treatment, and procedures may be dependent on ruling out acute infection. In addition, given that many immunocompromised children receive care in proximity to other immunocompromised patients in infusion centers or inpatient wards, using high-sensitivity testing is critical to curb exposures.

To that end, the Infectious Disease Society of America (IDSA), in recommendations from January 2021,[3] specifically recommends SARS-CoV-2 RNA testing in asymptomatic immunocompromised patients being admitted to the hospital and before hematopoietic stem cell (HSCT) or solid organ transplant (SOT) regardless of COVID-19

Table 1
Summary of published studies on pediatric immunocompromised patients and COVID-19

Cancer and hematopoietic stem cell transplant

Country and Study Period	Study Design	Testing Strategy (%) and Detection (% Positive)	Patients Characteristics (%)	Clinical Course (%)	Treatment (%)	Outcomes (%)
Czech Republic[105] Up to 3/16/20	Care provider survey; 32 centers	>200 tested patients; 8 positive cases	8 patients: 7 ST, 1 ALL	All patients asymptomatic or had mild symptoms	2 HCQ, 2 AZI, 1 LPV/r	No deaths or ICU admissions
US (NY)[106] 3/10/20–4/6/20	Retrospective cohort; 2 centers	Asymptomatic (before admission, before procedure, before chemotherapy, contact, transfer), symptomatic (84); NP PCR; positive cases (11)	19 patients: Leukemia/lymphoma (32), ST (42), nonmalignant hematology (16), HSCT (11)	Asymptomatic (16), MV (2), ICU (26)	HCQ + AZI (16); Cancer-directed therapy delayed in oncology patients (64)	No deaths in oncology patients; 1 sickle cell patient died
Spain[107] Up to 4/15/20	Retrospective cohort in Madrid	NP PCR	15 patients: ALL (53), AML/MDS (13), lymphoma (7), NBL (7), ST (20)	Asymptomatic (13), mild/moderate (87)	HCQ (73); chemotherapy delayed (40)	No deaths or ICU admission at time of report
Italy[60] 2/20/20–4/15/20	Retrospective cohort in Lombardia; 6 centers	Asymptomatic (74): screening (65) or close contact (9); positive cases (7)	21 patients: leukemia (48), lymphoma (10), CNS (5), ST (38)	Severe (10)	Cancer treatment modified (48)	No deaths
France[108] Up to 4/16/20	Physician survey; 30 centers	NP PCR or CT; 33 cases identified and only reporting 5 severe cases	5 patients: 3 ALL, 1 allo-HSCT, 1 CNS	All 5 patients admitted to ICU	N/A	No deaths at time of reporting

(continued on next page)

Table 1
(continued)

Country and Study Period	Study Design	Testing Strategy (%) and Detection (% Positive)	Patients Characteristics (%)	Clinical Course (%)	Treatment (%)	Outcomes (%)
Italy[35] 2/23/20–4/24/20	Registry study; 13 centers	Asymptomatic (before chemotherapy or procedure) or symptomatic; NP PCR or bronchoalveolar lavage	29 patients: ALL (48), AML (7), lymphoma (10), CNS (3), ST (28), histiocytosis (3); 3 patients also had HSCT (10)	Asymptomatic (62), mild (24), moderate (14), severe/critical (0)	HCQ (31), AZI (31), LPV/r (10), GC (3); treatment suspended (55) or reduced/ delayed (7)	No deaths or ICU admissions; 1 lymphoma patient had progression after chemotherapy withdrawal due to COVID
United States (NY, NJ)[12] 1/15/20–4/27/20	Retrospective cohort; 13 centers	Asymptomatic (before procedure, treatment) and symptomatic; NP PCR; 578 tested, 98 positive cases (17)	98 patients: ALL (53), AML (9), lymphoma (3), CNS (9), NBL (5), ST (16), auto-HSCT (5), allo-HSCT (3); obese (22)	Asymptomatic (25), mild (45), moderate (11), severe (17), ICU (23), MV (8)	HCQ (15), AZI (15), TCZ (5), RDV (4), CVP (2), ANR + GC (1); interruptions to chemotherapy (67)	Died (4) – none solely due to COVID
France[52] Up to 5/28/20	Retrospective and prospective cohort; multicenter	NP PCR (92), serology (5), clinical + radiological diagnosis (3)	37 patients; ALL (27), AML (3), CML (3), NHL (3), CNS (19), ST (30), NBL (3); HSCT (11); 1 patient each for aplastic anemia, sickle cell, EBV-MAS, familial septic granulomatosis	Asymptomatic (24), ICU (15), MV (5)	HCQ (5), RDV (3), TCZ (5); treatment delayed in oncology patients (48) for a mean of 14 d	1 Patient with ALL died (3) from severe macrophage activation syndrome with COVID

Turkey[51] 3/11/20–5/31/20	Physician survey; 66 centers	Asymptomatic (contact history, before HSCT, before surgery) and symptomatic; NP PCR or symptomatic + chest CT findings/contact history	51 patients: leukemia (51), lymphomas, and LCH/HLH (10), CNS (10), NBL (8), ST (22); 6 had undergone HSCT (12)	Asymptomatic/mild (49), moderate/severe (33), critical (18), ICU (18), MV (6)	No treatment (20), AZI (20), HCQ (8), HCQ + AZI (27), AZI + antivirals (2), HCQ + AZI + antivirals (6), CVP (2); interruption/delay in chemotherapy (63)	1 HSCT patient died (2) from COVID and also had concurrent recurrent leukemia and fungal infection
Egypt[47] mid-April to mid-June 2020	Prospective, non-intervention	NP PCR conducted on all admitted pediatric oncology patients	15 patients: ALL (67), AML (7), lymphoma (13), SOT (13)	Asymptomatic (33), mild (67)	HCQ, AZI, ceftriaxone, enoxaparin used per hospital guidelines; chemotherapy revised on individual basis	Died (13) – not related to COVID; 1 new oncology diagnosis patient died from treatment delay related to COVID
Mexico[11] 3/20/20–6/20/20	Retrospective cohort; 1 center	Only symptomatic tested; PCR; positive cases (58)	14 patients: leukemia (63), lymphoma (7), ST (21), CNS (7)	Oxygen required (80), no ICU or MV	Cancer treatment delayed until negative PCR	1 patient died with pulmonary metastases and pulmonary hemorrhage
Peru[109] 3/6/20–7/7/20	Retrospective cohort; 9 centers	PCR (49), serology (33), not reported (18)	69 patients: ALL (52), AML (4), lymphoma (7), CNS (5), ST (14), other (17)	Asymptomatic (54), ICU (4), but 2 patients who died did not have ICU beds available	AZI/IVM/GC (13); chemotherapy stopped (100)	Died due to COVID (4), died not related to COVID (6)
United Kingdom[110] 3/12/20–7/31/20	Retrospective + prospective registry study; 20 centers	Asymptomatic (before admission) and symptomatic; NP PCR	54 patients: ALL (44), AML (7), lymphoma (4), CNS (9), NBL (11), ST (19), other (6)	Asymptomatic (28), mild (63), moderate (2), severe (2), critical (6)	N/A	Died (2) – not related to COVID

(continued on next page)

Table 1
(continued)

Country and Study Period	Study Design	Testing Strategy (%) and Detection (% Positive)	Patients Characteristics (%)	Clinical Course (%)	Treatment (%)	Outcomes (%)
Mexico[111] 3/12/20– 9/25/20	Retrospective cohort; 1 center	Asymptomatic (before procedure, before admission); NP PCR	38 patients: ALL (55), AML (8), histiocytosis (8), CNS (5), ST (21), NBL (3)	Asymptomatic (18), mild (71), ICU (5), MV (5)	Treatment delay (68)	Deaths (8) – not related to COVID
United States Pediatric Oncology COVID-19 Case Report[53] As of 1/21/21	Registry study; 93 centers	Asymptomatic and symptomatic	657 patients: HM (64), ST (36); in addition, a proportion of patients had an allo-HSCT (6) or auto-HSCT (3)	Asymptomatic: HM (33), ST (41); intubation: HM (4), ST (4); ICU: HM (13), ST (8); MIS-C: HM (2), ST (2)	Change in oncology therapy: HM (47), ST (37)	Died (2)
Global Global Registry of COVID-19 in Childhood Cancer[54] As of 2/10/21	Registry study; 48 countries	Asymptomatic and symptomatic; testing included NP (80.5), nasal (18.0), oropharyngeal swab (8.4), and blood serology (5.2)	1557 patients: ALL (49.1), ST (24.5), CNS (8.1), other HM (17.9), after HSCT for nonmalignant disorders (0.39); in addition, a proportion of cancer patients had an HSCT (5.16)	Asymptomatic (34.9), mild (36.1), moderate (9.3), severe (12.1), critical (17.6); ICU (9.1), MV (4.4)	No treatment (70.3), AZI (20.2), GC (14.7), RDV (4.8), IVIG (4.4), HCQ (4.0), LPV/r (2.0), CP (0.7), TZM (0.4), FPV (0.1); chemotherapy reduced (5.9) or withheld (37.6)	Died from COVID-19 (3.44), died from other causes (2.19)
Solid organ transplant						
United States (TX, CA, FL, CO)[50] 4/1/20–7/20/20	Retrospective cohort; 5 centers	NP PCR	26 SOT patients: liver (38), kidney (31), heart (23), lung (8); median time to COVID-19 from transplant 1246 d (range 12–6574 d)	Asymptomatic (23), hospitalized (20) for COVID-19 for median of 3 d, none required supplemental oxygen	No change in IST (92); 1 patient developed acute cellular rejection (kidney) 7 d after IST reduction for COVID	No deaths or ICU admissions

Europe[62]	Care provider survey; 18 centers	N/A	5 SOT patients: 2 kidney, 3 liver; 3 HSCT patients	All SOT had mild symptoms; HSCT: 1 mild, 2 moderate/severe	No change in IST for all patients	No deaths or ICU admissions
Rheumatologic disorders						
Turkey[112] 3/11/20–4/15/20	Parent survey	23 patients with suspicion for COVID-19 tested with NP PCR (30% positive)	7 patients: 7 FMF (all on colchicine), 1 PFAPA	2 asymptomatic, 4 outpatient therapy, 1 hospitalized for 5 d	5 HCQ, 3 AZI, 4 OTV, 2 none	No deaths or ICU admissions
Spain[113] Up to 6/30/20	Registry study; 49 hospitals	N/A	8 patients: 3 JIA, 1 JDM, 1 cytoplasmic-ANCA vasculitis, 1 PFAPA, 1 polyarteritis nodosa, 1 phospholipid antibody syndrome	3 required oxygen, 1 with central line associated thrombosis, 1 with venous thrombosis and adrenal hemorrhage	5 HCQ, 1 RDV, 1 LPV/r, 1 TCZ, 1 enoxaparin; 1 reduction in IST	1 death in JDM from rapidly progressive interstitial lung disease before COVID
Chronic kidney disease on immunosuppressive therapy						
Spain[114] 3/1/20–4/15/20	Physician survey; 43 hospitals	PCR	16 patients: NS (31), renal dysplasia (31), uropathy (13), IgA nephropathy (6), vasculitis (6), scarring nephropathy (6), cortical necrosis (6); 9 patients (56) on IST and 3 patients had a kidney transplant (19)	Asymptomatic (19), no patients required oxygen	HCQ (38), LPLV/r (6); azathioprine stopped in vasculitis patient; MMF decreased in 2 of 3 and tacrolimus decreased in 1 of 3 transplant patients	No deaths or ICU admissions
Global[115] 3/15/20–End of April 2020	Retrospective survey; 16 centers	N/A	18 patients: kidney transplant (61), NS (17), ANCA-vasculitis (11), aHUS (6), ESKD with IBD (6)	Outpatient (39), oxygen support (17)	N/A	No deaths or ICU admissions

(continued on next page)

Table 1
(continued)

Country and Study Period	Study Design	Testing Strategy (%) and Detection (% Positive)	Patients Characteristics (%)	Clinical Course (%)	Treatment (%)	Outcomes (%)
Global[116] 3/15/20–7/5/20	Registry study; 30 countries	113 cases (104 by PCR or antibody testing, 9 clinically suspected)	113 patients: kidney transplant (47), NS (27), SLE (10), glomerulonephritis/vasculitis (6), other (11); all on IST	Asymptomatic (21), admitted but no respiratory support (38), admitted with respiratory support (17), MV (4)	N/A	Died (4)
Inflammatory bowel disease						
Global[78] Before 3/26/20	Registry study; 102 sites	6 by NP PCR or 2 with symptoms + positive first degree relative	8 patients: 5 Crohn's disease, 2 Ulcerative colitis, 1 unclassified	All 8 with mild disease and no admissions	No suspension of IBD-related medications	No deaths or ICU admissions
Global[45] Before May 2020	Registry study; 33 countries	NP PCR	29 patients	Hospitalized (10)	N/A	No deaths or ICU admissions
Italy[65] 3/9/20–5/4/20	Retrospective cohort; 21 centers	6 COVID-19 cases identified out of 2291 patients (0.2%) by NP test	6 patients: 4 Crohn's disease, 2 ulcerative colitis	1 asymptomatic, 4 mild, 1 hospitalized for 7 d	No suspension of IBD-related medications	No deaths
Global[16] Before 10/1/20	Registry study; 23 countries	N/A	209 patients: Crohn's disease (66), ulcerative colitis (29), unclassified (5)	Hospitalized (7), MV (1); of the 2 patients on MV, 1 patient had MIS and 1 patient had secondary infection	N/A	No deaths

Inborn errors of immunity

Global[41] 3/16/20– 6/30/20	Physician survey	Asymptomatic, symptomatic; PCR or serology	32 pediatric patients: CID (28, CVID or antibody deficiency (13), CGD (9), AGS (9), ALPS (9), WAS (6), XLA (3), CTLA4 deficiency (3), CMC with recurrent sepsis (3), MSMD (3), STAT1 GOF (3), GATA2 haploinsufficiency (3), XIAP deficiency (3), BMF (3); 2 had received HSCT, 1 gene therapy	Asymptomatic (25), ICU admission (28), MIS-C in patient with MSMD (*IFNGR2*)	Antibiotics (31), GC (16), immunoglobulin (16), RDV (9), LPV/r (3), CP (6), TCZ (3), chloroquine (3), aspirin (3), enoxaparin (3)	Deaths (6): 1 child with CGD and *Burkholderia* sepsis and HLH; 1 child following HSCT for XIAP deficiency, severe gut GVHD, septic shock, HLH
Israel[40] Mid-February to Mid-September 2020	Care provider survey; 10 centers	Contact tracing (27), symptomatic (73); NP PCR	11 pediatric patients: 3 Hyper-IgM, 2 X-linked agammaglobulinemia, 3 CID (*RELB* mutation), 2 CGD, 1 22q11.2 deletion syndrome	None hospitalized, asymptomatic (46), mild (54)	Additional dose of IVIG (9); no change in treatment for immune disorder	No deaths or ICU admissions
Iran[55]	Prospective study; 38 centers	Symptomatic only; PCR; incidence of 1 in 144 PID patients	16 pediatric patients: SCID (19), Omenn's syndrome (6), CID (13), CGD (13), IGF syndrome (13), WAS (6), AT (6), hyper-IgM (6), specific IgA deficiency (6), Griscelli syndrome type 2 (6), DIRA (6)	ICU (50)	AZI (69), IVIG (63), HCQ (50), other antibiotics (44), GC (6)	Death (50): 4 of 4 SCID/ Omenn's syndrome, STK4 deficiency, 1 of 2 IGF syndrome, Griscelli syndrome type 2, DIRA

(continued on next page)

Table 1
(continued)

Country and Study Period	Study Design	Testing Strategy (%) and Detection (% Positive)	Patients Characteristics (%)	Clinical Course (%)	Treatment (%)	Outcomes (%)
Other immunocompromised cohorts						
Spain[117] 3/1/20–3/31/20	Retrospective cohort; 1 center	NP PCR	8 patients: 5 HO (3 after HSCT), 2 SOT (1 liver, 1 kidney), 1 CKD	1 required oxygen, 1 HLH-like syndrome	5 Anti-viral treatment, 1 GC, 1 TCZ, 6 IST decreased or withdrawn	No deaths or ICU admissions
United Arab Emirates[118]	Retrospective cohort; 1 center	Contact tracing or symptomatic; NP PCR	5 patients: 1 CVID, 1 ST, 1 after splenectomy, 1 CKD, 1 SLE	3 asymptomatic, 2 mild	3 HCQ, 1 RDV, 1 FPV	No deaths or ICU admissions

Table includes only studies with at least 5 pediatric (age < 21 y) immunocompromised patients.

Abbreviations: AGS, Aicardi-Goutieres syndrome; aHUS, atypical hemolytic uremic syndrome; ALL, acute lymphoblastic leukemia; Allo-HSCT, allogeneic hematopoietic stem cell transplant; AML, acute myelogenous leukemia; ANCA, antineutrophil cytoplasmic antibody; ANR, anakinra; AT, ataxia telangiectasia; Auto-HSCT, autologous hematopoietic stem cell transplant; AZI, azithromycin; BMF, bone marrow failure; CID, combined immunodeficiency; CGD, chronic granulomatous disease; CKD, chronic kidney disease; CMC, chronic mucocutaneous candidiasis; CNS, central nervous tumor; CT, computed tomography; CVP, convalescent plasma; DIRA, deficiency of IL-1 receptor antagonist; EBV-MAS, EBV-induced macrophage activation syndrome; ESKD, End-stage kidney disease; FMF, familial mediterranean fever; FPV, favipiravir; GC, glucocorticosteroids; GOF, gain-of-function; HCQ, hydroxychloroquine; HM, hematologic malignancy; HO, Hematologic-oncologic; HSCT, hematopoietic stem cell transplant; IBD, inflammatory bowel disease; ICU, intensive care unit; IGF, immunodeficiency; centromere instability, facial anomalies; IST, immunosuppressive therapy; IVIG, intravenous immunoglobulin; IVM, ivermectin; JDM, juvenile dermatomyositis; JIA, juvenile idiopathic arthritis; LPV/r, Lopinavir-ritonavir; MIS, multisystem inflammatory syndrome; MIS-C, multisystem inflammatory syndrome in children; MSMD, mendelian susceptibility to mycobacterial diseases; MV, mechanical ventilation; N/A, not available; NBL, neuroblastoma; NP, nasopharyngeal; NS, nephrotic syndrome; OTV, oseltamivir; PCR, polymerase chain reaction; PFAPA, periodic fever-aphthous stomatitis-pharyngitis-adenitis; RDV, remdesivir; SCID, severe combined immunodeficiency; SLE, systemic lupus erythematosus; SOT, solid organ transplant; ST, solid tumor; TCZ, tocilizumab; WAS, Wiskott-Aldrich syndrome; XLA, X-linked agammaglobulinemia; MDS, myelodysplastic syndrome; CML, chronic myeloid leukemia; NHL, non-Hodgkin lymphoma; LCH Langerhan cell histiocytosis; HLH, hemophagocytosis lymphohistiocytosis; TZM, temozolamide; CVID, common variable immunodeficiency; ALPS, autoimmune lymphoproliferative syndrome; CTLA4, cytotoxic T-lymphocyte-associated protein 4; STAT1, signal transducer and activator of transcription 1; XIAP, X-linked inhibitor of apoptosis protein; GVHD, graft versus host disease; PID, primary immunodeficiency.

exposure history or community SARS-CoV-2 infection rate.[4-6] This recommendation was based on the presumed risk of nosocomial transmission, although data are limited.[7] Of note, the IDSA guidelines specifically include cytotoxic chemotherapy, biologic or cellular therapy, high-dose steroids, and SOT or HSCT. There is no inclusion of patients with primary immunodeficiency, immune dysregulatory disorders, or HIV under the "immunocompromised patients," but biologically their immune deficits are similar. For asymptomatic outpatients receiving chemotherapy or other immunosuppressive medications for autoimmune disease, the IDSA recommends that the decision for testing before therapy be individualized as there remains a significant evidence gap to reliably guide practice.

It is important to note that numerous tests to detect the SARS-CoV-2 virus have emergency use authorization (EUA) and that their sensitivities and turn-around times are not uniform.[3,8] These assays detect parts of the virus via RNA or antigen testing, and molecular analysis can be completed via rapid reverse transcription polymerase chain reaction (sensitivity 98%, specificity 97%, 45–60 minutes for test completion), standard laboratory-based nucleic acid amplification testing (NAAT) (sensitivity 98%, specificity 97%), or rapid isothermal NAAT (sensitivity 81%, specificity 99%, 5–15 minutes for test completion) testing.[3] Thus, providers should appreciate the potential for false negative testing from rapid bedside testing, which may be less sensitive and miss asymptomatic patients as they are frequently completed via rapid isothermal NAAT. Beyond assay limitations, specimen inadequacy (eg, tentatively swabbing the nasopharynx of patients with thrombocytopenia) and timing of collection relative to the onset of symptoms can contribute to false negative tests.[8]

Serology testing is also available to detect past SARS-CoV-2 infection, but the utility of the test is unknown in patients with humoral immune defects who may fail to seroconvert as the assays rely on detection of anti-SARS-CoV-2 IgG, IgM, IgA, or total antibody. In addition, as immunoglobulin replacement products begin to include anti-SARS-CoV-2 IgG, the value of serologic detection will be unclear for patients on replacement therapy. Standard IDSA approaches for the use of serologic testing for SARS-CoV-2 infection should be followed for immunocompromised pediatric patients.[9]

Prevalence of SARS-CoV-2 Infection in Pediatric Immunocompromised Patients

Understanding the infectivity rate of SARS-CoV-2 has been a huge epidemiologic undertaking. In theory, immunocompromised children may be less likely to contract SARS-CoV-2 secondary to already ingrained infection prevention techniques, for example, hand washing and social isolation. However, interaction with the health care system may raise the risk of a positive contact as demonstrated in a Madrid study in which 4 of 15 cases (27%) of SARS-CoV-2 infections in pediatric oncology patients were traced to nosocomial exposure.[10] Comparison of infectivity rates with healthy children is difficult secondary to discrepancies in testing practices in immunocompromised patients who are more likely to undergo testing over concerns of developing severe COVID-19 or as a screen before hospital admissions, surgical procedures, or receiving chemotherapy. Therefore, immunocompromised children are more likely to be screened when asymptomatic, theoretically falsely raising the relative prevalence of SARS-CoV-2 in this population compared with immunocompetent children.

In review of the current 13 articles that detailed their testing strategy for pediatric oncology patients, just one cohort limited SARS-CoV-2 testing to symptomatic patients only.[11] Interestingly, this strategy was adopted in Mexico where resources for broad testing are limited, indicating that studies in poorly resourced countries may also underestimate the prevalence secondary to less aggressive screening. Among pediatric oncology hospitals in New York and New Jersey, the positivity rate at the height of the pandemic was 16.95% with 32.7% of the cases being identified in asymptomatic patients.[12] Symptomatic patients were also more likely to be tested early in the pandemic as demonstrated in a single-center study at the UPMC Children's Hospital of Pittsburgh where immunocompromised pediatric patients with fever or respiratory symptoms were 3-times (58.0% vs 19.5%) as likely to be tested for SARS-CoV-2 in comparison to immunocompetent patients.[10] It is important to note that testing strategies continue to evolve as changes in disease prevalence and access to test supplies have fluctuated, and these early reports may not reflect current screening practices.

Another strategy to evaluate the burden of SARS-CoV-2 is to assess seroprevalence in pediatric cohorts. The UPMC Children's Hospital of Pittsburgh tested for the presence of SARS-CoV-2 IgG in convenience blood samples from immunocompromised and general pediatric patients.[10] In 485 immunocompromised patients, 1% were found to have IgG antibodies to SARS-CoV-2 spike protein, which was similar to the immunocompetent cohort (0.6%). Seroprevalence was highest in rheumatology (4.3%) and SOT (1.9%), with no detection of antibodies in HSCT, primary immunodeficiency, or inflammatory bowel disease (IBD) patients, although these data may underestimate the true prevalence given the possibility of poor humoral response to SARS-CoV-2 in some immunocompromised patients.

As of March 1, 2021, 2617 patients have met the case definition of MIS-C in the United States.[13] Estimating the prevalence of MIS-C in immunocompromised patients may prove more difficult as unlike SARS-CoV-2, MIS-C does not have specific testing but requires a constellation of symptoms and laboratory evidence of inflammation for diagnosis that may overlap with the underlying disorder, especially in rheumatology patients. MIS-C has been diagnosed in patients with underlying IBD, but presenting features including fever, gastrointestinal disease, mouth ulcers, and elevation of inflammatory markers are common manifestations of both conditions.[14–16] MIS-C, therefore, has the potential to be both underdiagnosed and overdiagnosed in immunocompromised patients and may require more specific findings such as Kawasaki-like features to confirm a MIS-C diagnosis.

Treatment of SARS-CoV-2 in Pediatric Immunocompromised Patients

Despite a large number of therapeutic studies related to COVID-19 being carried out over the past year, most participants are immunocompetent adults.[17,18] As such, treatment of immunocompromised patients mirrors that of immunocompetent patients. At the time of this publication, remdesivir, a nucleoside analog that when incorporated into RNA inhibits the replication of SARS-CoV-2 by causing delayed chain termination, is the only agent with Food and Drug Administration (FDA) approval for COVID-19 treatment. Remdesivir is approved for hospitalized patients (aged $\geq$12 years and weighing $\geq$40 kg) requiring supplemental oxygen[17,19,20] and through an EUA for hospitalized children weighing $\geq$3.5 kg. Currently there are insufficient data for use in nonhospitalized mild to moderate cases or for non–oxygen-requiring hospitalized patients, with the argument that remdesivir should be considered in these situations for immunocompromised patients. For hospitalized adult patients, dexamethasone afforded a survival benefit in patients receiving respiratory support and led to increased ventilator-free days in mechanically ventilated patients.[21,22] Dexamethasone in combination with remdesivir may be considered for immunocompromised patients with severe or critical COVID-19 requiring respiratory support but must be balanced with the risk for inadequate viral control and secondary infections.

Immunocompromised patients who have decreased ability or inability to make antibodies may be at risk for prolonged illness with decreased capacity to clear the virus.[23] While no specific trials have been reported in this population, two therapies that could be considered are anti-SARS-CoV-2 monoclonal antibodies and convalescent plasma. Currently, the FDA has issued an EUA for the anti-SARS-CoV-2 monoclonal antibodies bamlanivimab,[24] bamlanivimab plus etesevimab,[25] and casirivimab plus imdevimab[26] for nonhospitalized adult and pediatric patients ($\geq$12 years and weighing $\geq$40 kg), who are at high risk for disease progression or hospitalization, including those with immunosuppressive disorders or those receiving immunosuppressive treatment. Convalescent plasma from recovered COVID-19 donors also received an EUA from the FDA for hospitalized patients early in the course of disease and those hospitalized with impaired humoral immunity.[27,28] This recommendation, however, is not fully supported by pediatric subspecialist groups who have advocated against routine administration of monoclonal antibodies for COVID-19 treatment because of the lack of evidence for safety and efficacy in children.[29]

As demonstrated in **Table 1**, although multiple additional therapies have been used in immunocompromised patients, there are no robust data to demonstrate the benefits or harm in this population. Until more data are available, immunocompromised pediatric patients should be followed up very closely, and therapeutic intervention considered on an individual basis.

Patients on immunosuppressive treatment for their underlying disorder present additional quandaries as there are limited studies that provide guidance regarding management of chronic immunosuppressant therapies in patients with COVID-19.[30] Concerns in pediatric immunocompromised patients with SARS-CoV-2 infection that must be balanced in the decision to maintain or modify chronic immune suppression include poor viral control, dysregulated immune responses, flare of underlying disorders, and acquisition of secondary infections. Universal guidelines are difficult if not impossible to develop given the diversity of disease and underlying risks of modifying immune suppression, as well as the knowledge that some immunosuppressant therapies (eg, cyclosporine A, thiopurine metabolites, mycophenolic acid)[31,32] have antiviral properties while others (eg, tocilizumab, dexamethasone)[21,33] have been attempted to control dysregulated immune responses in severe COVID-19. This dilemma has led physicians to perform an individualized risk-benefit evaluation to weigh the risk of reducing immunosuppression against the risk of disease flare or worsening disease activity which potentially could have both devastating short- and long-term consequences.[34] Thankfully, guidance in pediatric immunocompromised patient care is developing as our experience in COVID-19 expands. For example, the current recommendation for pediatric cancer patients with SARS-CoV-2 infections is to avoid major alterations in underlying therapy unless there is evidence of severe COVID-19 infection.[35]

Outcomes of SARS-CoV-2 in Pediatric Immunocompromised Patients

At the onset of the COVID-19 pandemic, it was assumed that poor antiviral immunity in immunocompromised patients would place them at high risk for complications as seen for other respiratory viruses including influenza, respiratory syncytial virus, and common strains of human coronavirus (OC43, NL63, HKU1, and 229E).[36–38] However, immunocompromised status and poor outcomes have not been reported during the SARS-CoV-1 and Middle East respiratory syndrome coronavirus (MERS-CoV) epidemics.[1] This somewhat paradoxic observation may stem from the unique immune pathology induced by SARS-CoV-2. The usual immune response to SARS-CoV-2 is an initial innate immune response through type I interferons followed by an adaptive humoral and cellular immune response.[39] Although adequate immune function is necessary to control SARS-CoV-2 infection, significant toxicity and death are often a sequelae of inappropriate and dysregulated immune responses and not a direct consequence of viral invasion and replication.[40] This has raised the intriguing possibility that patients with primary or secondary immune defects may not be at increased risk of death from COVID-19 but also that certain subsets of patients may be protected from severe disease by their inability to mount a pathologic immune response to SARS-CoV-2.[41]

Initial studies in adults, however, have demonstrated that oncology and SOT patients are at higher risk for severe outcomes including intubation and death from COVID-19.[42–44] In contrast, IBD and rheumatology adult patients taking biologics and Janus kinase inhibitors displayed no increased incidence of severe disease.[45,46] The difference in outcomes may be related to the type and degree of immune suppression, but comorbidities such as hypertension, heart disease, diabetes, and chronic kidney disease were also highly prevalent in adult cancer and SOT patients with severe COVID-19.[42]

Clinical outcomes in immunocompetent children with COVID-19 are superior to adults, and several mechanisms including lower angiotensin-converting enzyme (ACE)-2 expression, enhanced immune tolerance, and fewer comorbidities have been proposed as reasons for the discrepant outcomes.[47] These protective features may be minimized in some immunocompromised populations as ACE-2 can be overexpressed in some patients with IBD and systemic lupus erythematous (SLE).[48,49] In addition, immune tolerance mechanisms may be disrupted by inborn errors of immunity such as pathogenic variants in *FOXP3* or *CTLA4*, and comorbidities exist because of the underlying genetic defect or toxicities related to treatment or prior infection.[49] Children may also be on relatively higher doses of immune suppression than adults for some conditions such as SOT, and therefore, COVID-19 outcome trends seen in immunosuppressed adults may not be translatable to pediatrics.[50]

A summary of currently published studies on pediatric immunocompromised cohorts is provided in **Table 1**, permitting some interesting early observations. First, in pediatric oncology patients, the risk of death is less than that in adults but appears to be higher than that of the general pediatric population and may be worse when compounded by certain high-risk demographics, for example, male, obese, and older age, or in patients with hematologic malignancies.[12,51–54] In contrast to oncology patients, published cohorts of pediatric rheumatology patients, SOT, chronic kidney disease on immune suppression, and IBD reported low rates of severe complications, but the literature is less extensive in these diseases.

COVID-19 severity in patients with inborn errors of immunity is dependent on the underlying defect. Although there is potential for reporter bias, complete absence of adaptive immunity appears lethal with mortality from COVID-19 in all reported severe combined immunodeficiency (SCID) patients not yet transplanted in an Iranian case series that included 3 patients with SCID and 1 patient with Omenn syndrome.[55] However, pediatric patients with nonsevere defects in adaptive immunity presented with asymptomatic or mild COVID-19 disease in a global (14 patients) and Israeli (9 patients) survey of medical providers.[40,41] Despite the concern for excessive immune activation in autoinflammatory disorders, severe disease has not been frequently reported and may be a misguided concern or the inflammation is well attenuated by preventive immunosuppression in these patients.[41] A similar concern is whether MIS-C will be more prevalent or severe in patients with autoinflammatory disorders, but it is too early to speculate as only a few anecdotal cases of MIS-C in patients with immune disorders are published to date.[14–16,41]

Overall, the clinical course in immunocompromised patients with SARS-CoV-2 is favorable, but some caution is warranted in caring for these patients. First, based on recent data demonstrating the importance of type I interferons in initial SARS-

CoV-2 control, patients who have severely deficient type I interferon signaling or immune disorders, for example, secondary to Toll-like receptor 3 or interferon regulatory factor 7 defects, or those that predispose to autoantibodies against type I interferons may be at risk for critical disease.[40,56,57] Second, some cases of death have been attributed to concurrent infections or an underlying primary disorder, highlighting the need for continued monitoring for additional infections, disease progression, and immune-related adverse events that may be independent or indirectly related to SARS-CoV-2 infection.[41] Third, changing therapy and supportive care measures against COVID-19 and evolution of new SARS-CoV-2 strains may alter outcomes in immunocompromised patients. Finally, atypical manifestations of SARS-CoV-2, such as hemophagocytic lymphohistiocytosis and cytopenias, have been infrequently reported, and providers need to remain vigilant for these and other new complications of COVID-19.

Impact to Access of Clinical Care for Immunocompromised Patients

The COVID-19 pandemic impacted access to care for non–SARS-CoV-2-infected patients as hospital systems scrambled to accommodate the surge of infected patients and limit transmission of infection among staff and patients. Unfortunately, the need to implement social distancing protocols, mobilization of SARS-CoV-2 testing, redeployment of providers and reduction in staff, use of critical care beds for severe COVID-19 patients, and parental and patient anxiety of traveling to medical centers all contributed to delayed access and untoward consequences for some immunocompromised patients. For example, surveyed pediatric rheumatologists indicated one-third of patients suffered a delayed diagnosis or joint injections due to lack of access for evaluation, and 21.9% had patients who experienced a flare due to delayed appointments.[58] A parental survey of children with rheumatic disease reported 14.3% had a treatment interruption with social restrictions and anxiety over new health center arrangements listed as the primary barrier to medical care access.[59]

In pediatric oncology, a significant drop in new diagnoses, including a decrease of 45% of expected new acute lymphoblastic leukemia diagnoses in Lombardia, Italy, and a gap of 35 days between new leukemia patients at the Children's Hospital of Philadelphia, where the historic mean gap between new diagnoses is 2.96 days, occurred early in the pandemic.[60,61] Although these reports have yet to describe a rebound of cancer diagnoses, extreme sickness in new cancer patients is documented, and these presentation delays to oncology centers have been attributed to parental reluctance to seek medical care, decreased referrals to major medical centers, limitations of telemedicine, and a diagnostic bias toward COVID-19 for presenting signs of a malignancy.[61] A survey of SOT and HSCT centers in Europe reported that two-third of centers reduced their transplant activity.[62] However, pediatric kidney transplants in the United States has largely returned to baseline after the initial surge of COVID-19.[63] In the United Kingdom, restrictions on endoscopy procedures resulted in most pediatric patients being diagnosed with "presumed IBD" without histologic confirmation.[64] IBD admissions for new diagnoses and endoscopic re-evaluation were also significantly reduced during the lock down in Italy.[65]

In attempts to maintain access to care while minimizing infectious exposure and conserving personal protective equipment, subspecialty providers pivoted toward telemedicine.[66] Expansion of telemedicine services was greatly aided by changes in reimbursement policies during the COVID-19 pandemic.[67] While not all clinical situations are amenable to virtual visits, subspecialists quickly adapted care for telemedicine including devising standardized virtual joint examinations and facilitating "care in place" with local laboratory evaluation and primary care collaboration for vital signs, weight checks, and key examination findings as needed. The reduced risk of inadvertent infectious exposure as well as the historical advantages of increased flexibility of access and decreased financial burden (eg, travel, days of missed work, childcare) contributed to telemedicine appeal among immunocompromised patients. For example, 38 childhood cancer survivors or their proxies surveyed about their long-term follow-up virtual visits were highly satisfied with their visits (with 86% and 95%, "completely/very satisfied," respectively) with 82% preferring video visits to remain an option after the pandemic.[68] Further study of parental preferences is needed to optimize the telehealth care models.

In addition to medical care, continuation of psychosocial services to immunocompromised children and adolescents during this pandemic is vitally important. Patients with immunodeficiency, even before the pandemic, had lower health-related quality of life (HRQoL) than healthy peers and those with other chronic conditions.[69] With the onset of COVID-19, a nationwide pediatric healthy cohort of 1586 families from Germany reported lower HRQoL (measured by KIDSCREEN-10), more mental health problems (measured by SDQ), and increased anxiety (measured by SCARED) than before the pandemic.[70] While not yet formally assessed, it is anticipated that similar trends exist in immunocompromised patients.

Immunocompromised children and parents seeking trustworthy information and peer support have historically relied on philanthropic foundations, for example, Immune Deficiency Foundation, Race for Immunology, Alex's Lemonade Stand, and resources such as the Ryan White HIV/AIDS Program. Providers, similarly, have turned to prepandemic psychosocial service models such as those used for people with HIV that have historically used home visits, telemedicine and adherence programs inclusive of directly observed therapy, motivational interviewing sessions, and social work check-ins.[71-73] Home delivery of medication was already occurring for many high-risk patients, and continuation of this service has minimized treatment gaps for some patients. Unfortunately, the same services have not been available in many resource-poor areas of the United States and abroad, and services to those with HIV have suffered interruptions of heath care.[74-76] The same service interruptions may be inferred for other high-risk immune-deficient patients in poor-resource areas.

Changes to Management in Immunocompromised Patient in the COVID-19 Era

At the onset of the pandemic, uncertainty over the risk of severe COVID-19, drug shortages for medications used for both immunocompromised patients and SARS-CoV-2, and reallocation of resources to COVID-19 patient care and research led to numerous changes in management of immunocompromised children. Early in the pandemic, pediatric oncologists regularly delayed chemotherapy (48%–100% in published cohorts; see **Table 1**), and reports of patient deaths secondary to disease progression while delaying induction or pausing chemotherapy during SARS-CoV-2 infection have been reported. Pediatric oncology clinical trial enrollment decreased as resources were diverted to COVID-19 research, restrictions on research were made in an effort to curb SARS-CoV-2 transmission, and research staff furloughed to limit the negative institutional financial impact of COVID-19. As such, some pediatric oncology patients, particularly those with relapsed/refractory disease, had less options for therapy because of delays in opening new studies.[77]

In China and South Korea, 20% of pediatric IBD patients suffered disease exacerbation when infliximab infusions were delayed.[78] In the UK, standard treatment with a Tumor necrosis factor inhibitor was replaced with exclusive enteral nutrition for new IBD patients as diagnosis could not be confirmed secondary to reduction in endoscopy procedures.[64] Early guidance in pediatric rheumatology patients stressed continuing current immune suppression to avoid disease flare.[79] However, concerns over SARS-CoV-2 also led to hesitancy to starting new immune suppression with worsening disease[58] despite that control of disease activity may also help reduce risk of severe infection in certain systemic disorders as demonstrated in adult patients with rheumatoid arthritis.[80,81]

In addition, drug shortages forced changes in management and mandated strategic planning to preserve doses for critical care.[82] In pediatric and adult rheumatology, many patients receiving IV tocilizumab were switched to the subcutaneous (SQ) form as the supply of IV tocilizumab was consumed for treatment of severe COVID-19. This switch to SQ tocilizumab resulted in patient/parent anxiety of the risk of disease flare or worsening disease activity even though switching to SQ route has been found to be an effective alternative for children with juvenile idiopathic arthritis.[83] Other drugs, for example, hydroxychloroquine, demonstrated a huge surge in prescriptions early in the pandemic presumably attributed to off-label use for COVID-19 treatment raising concern for decreased availability of the drug for SLE or other autoimmune indications.[84–86]

With concerns for nosocomial exposure, providers prioritized home-administered therapeutic options when possible, particularly for immunocompromised patients. The National Institute for Health and Care Excellence published COVID-19 rapid guidelines specifically recommending clinicians to consider switching IV medications to SQ form to minimize exposure of SARS-CoV-2. Anecdotally, children receiving IgG replacement were transitioned from IV IgG in-hospital infusion areas to either SQ or at-home IV IgG and when feasible, and outpatient chemotherapy regimens were favored, for example, SQ cytarabine versus IV vinblastine with prednisone for children with Langerhans cell histiocytosis given the success of cytarabine monotherapy in refractory disease.[87]

Considerations for COVID-19 Vaccination in Immunocompromised Patients

In December of 2020, Pfizer-BioNTech and Moderna both received EUAs for their COVID-19 vaccines from the FDA,[88,89] with the Janssen Biotech COVID-19 vaccine receiving an EUA in February 2021.[90] With the exception of HIV, patients with immune deficiency were largely excluded from the clinical trials.[91–93] Despite the current lack of safety and efficacy data in patients with compromised immune systems, there is general consensus among physicians that these nonlive vaccines should be administered to the vast majority of immunosuppressed patients.[94] The Centers for Disease Control and Prevention (CDC) also suggests that immunocompromised individuals receive the COVID-19 vaccine, with counseling on unknown safety profile and efficacy in this population.[95] Timing of vaccination in relation to immunosuppressive therapies is not completely understood, but adult patients with rheumatoid arthritis receiving the seasonal influenza vaccination demonstrated improved response if methotrexate was not given for at least 2 weeks after HCT.[96] It was also noted that flares were more common in patients with 4-week pauses of their methotrexate around the time of vaccination.[97] But the effects of immune suppression on COVID-19 vaccine response are not yet determined, and consideration to hold immunosuppressants after vaccination need to be considered on a case-by-case basis and ideally studied in clinical trials.[98] The CDC at the time of publication does not recommend revaccination of those who may have received the vaccine during chemotherapy or while on immunosuppressive medications and does not suggest antibody testing to assess for immunity after vaccination.[95]

Safety of vaccines in the immune compromised is different compared with that in immune-competent individuals. Live attenuated vaccines can cause disease in immunocompromised patients because of the inability to control the replication of the pathogen even in its weakened state. The Pfizer-BioNTech and Moderna COVID-19 vaccines are not live, nor do they contain any actual virus to cause disease, and instead contain mRNA encoding the spike protein of SARS-CoV-2. The Janssen COVID-19 vaccine uses a recombinant, replication-incompetent adenovirus vector containing the full-length SARS-CoV-2 spike protein gene.[93] The vector shuttles the gene into the nucleus of the cell where it is transcribed and translated into the spike protein, but the genetic material does not integrate into host DNA, and because the vector does not replicate, it cannot cause human disease.[99] Therefore, as all 3 vaccines cannot result in infection, they are likely safe for patients with immunodeficiency. However, live attenuated COVID-19 vaccines are in development or clinical trials, so in the future, it will be important to know which vaccine is being offered with the live attenuated vaccines being avoided until workup and discussion with an immunologist.[100] Another theoretic concern is administration of vaccines in patients with autoimmune and autoinflammatory disorders with excessive production of inflammatory cytokines in response to viral products. However, given the risk of SARS-CoV-2 infection in these disorders, the immunology community has provided cautious support for vaccination in these patients and recommended it ideally should be administered during periods of low disease activity.[101]

In addition to safety concerns, efficacy of these vaccines is unclear and likely variable depending on the immune defect. Classically, antibody production is used as a measure of the protection offered from immunization, but vaccines may generate T-cell responses as well, which could be of benefit in those with humoral defects. Studies examining patients recovered from COVID-19 have found the presence of SARS-CoV-2-specific CD4+ and CD8+ T cells in circulation, and studies of the Pfizer-BioNTech vaccine found that two doses elicit T-cell responses against the SARS-CoV-2 spike protein.[102,103]

SUMMARY

While the COVID-19 pandemic triggered numerous clinical practice changes and resulted in severe consequences either directly or indirectly for select pediatric patients, important lessons were learned, and there are silver linings for immunocompromised children evident among the chaos. At a minimum, the pandemic raised global awareness of infection risk, viral transmissibility, and the immune system. Handwashing, comprehensive disinfection practices of shared surfaces, and mask wearing are more normalized. School shutdowns during the COVID-19 pandemic not only kept children from exposure to SARS-CoV-2 but also decreased the incidence of pneumonia, otitis media, streptococcal pharyngitis, urinary tract infections, croup, gastrointestinal infections, and asthma.[104] Strategies to mitigate SARS-CoV-2 infection including ventilation upgrades and cohorting methods are likely to help attenuate infectious exposures as students return to the classroom. In addition, the broad acceptance of virtual learning and incorporation of virtual learners in a hybrid classroom are practices expected to be of value to immunodeficient patients. Beyond schooling, the creative transition of other activities, for example, dance, karate, and enrichment opportunities, for example, art classes and streaming concerts, has allowed immunocompromised children to participate with their peers. As risk of SARS-CoV-2 transmission lessens, immunocompetent children will return to school and other in-person activities; the expanded services offered during the pandemic need to be continued for children with weakened immune systems.

From a health care perspective, the massive uptake of telemedicine provided an alternative strategy for patients with compromised immune systems to maintain access to care with increased convenience and decreased cost. Given that immunocompromised patients are likely to benefit from continued telehealth options after the pandemic, it is imperative that action be taken to preserve the expansion of compensated telehealth options, while also appreciating that in-person visits are vital for some patients to diagnose new or progressive disease. In addition, strategies to mitigate barriers for telehealth uptake to improve equity of access as well as parental/patient preferences for care received in-person versus virtually must be explored.

Although global efforts have accelerated our understanding and care of SARS-CoV-2 patients, our knowledge of clinical outcomes and treatment in immunocompromised patients is limited, particularly in inborn errors of immunity and pediatric HIV. Challenges remaining for pediatricians include sustained, global collaboration to consolidate knowledge in these rare patient groups, continued adaptation of knowledge gained from immunocompetent patients to immunocompromised cohorts, and further study on the safety and efficacy of current and developing vaccines. Persistent advocacy for rare diseases is even more critical as the clinical, scientific, and philanthropic communities remain focused on COVID-19 care and research.

Finally, a comment that immunocompromised parents hear is, "I finally understand what it is like to live like you. I am afraid to get an infection. I cannot just go anywhere I want to go anymore". Although the COVID-19 pandemic has been difficult for everyone on a personal and professional level, the anxiety of infection and social isolation will persist for immunocompromised families even as the risk of SARS-CoV-2 transmission subsides. It is imperative that we leverage knowledge gained from this pandemic to improve the health and quality of life of immunocompromised children so that they may live without fear.

REFERENCES

1. D'Antiga L. Coronaviruses and Immunosuppressed Patients: The Facts During the Third Epidemic. Liver transplantation : official publication of the American Association for the Study of Liver Diseases and the. Int Liver Transplant Soc 2020;26(6):832–4.

2. Kabeerdoss J, Pilania RK, Karkhele R, et al. Severe COVID-19, multisystem inflammatory syndrome in children, and Kawasaki disease: immunological mechanisms, clinical manifestations and management. Rheumatol Int 2021;41(1): 19–32.

3. Hanson KE, Caliendo AM, Arias CA, et al. The Infectious Diseases Society of America Guidelines on the Diagnosis of COVID-19: Molecular Diagnostic Testing. Clin Infect Dis 2021. https://doi.org/10.1093/cid/ciab048.

4. Waghmare A, Abidi MZ, Boeckh M, et al. Guidelines for COVID-19 Management in Hematopoietic Cell Transplantation and Cellular Therapy Recipients. Biol Blood Marrow Transplant 2020;26(11):1983–94.

5. Ljungman P, Mikulska M, de la Camara R, et al. The challenge of COVID-19 and hematopoietic cell transplantation; EBMT recommendations for management of hematopoietic cell transplant recipients, their donors, and patients undergoing CAR T-cell therapy. Bone Marrow Transplant 2020;55(11):2071–6.

6. Ritschl PV, Nevermann N, Wiering L, et al. Solid organ transplantation programs facing lack of empiric evidence in the COVID-19 pandemic: A By-proxy Society Recommendation Consensus approach. Am J Transplant 2020;20(7):1826–36.

7. Abbas S, Raybould JE, Sastry S, et al. Respiratory viruses in transplant recipients: more than just a cold. Clinical syndromes and infection prevention principles. Int J Infect Dis 2017;62:86–93.

8. Ravi N, Cortade DL, Ng E, et al. Diagnostics for SARS-CoV-2 detection: A comprehensive review of the FDA-EUA COVID-19 testing landscape. Biosens Bioelectron 2020;165:112454.

9. Hanson KE, Caliendo AM, Arias CA, et al. Infectious diseases Society of America guidelines on the diagnosis of COVID-19:serologic testing. Clin Infect Dis 2020. https://doi.org/10.1093/cid/ciaa1343.

10. Freeman MC, Rapsinski GJ, Zilla ML, et al. Immunocompromised Seroprevalence and Course of Illness of SARS-CoV-2 in One Pediatric Quaternary Care Center. J Pediatr Infect Dis Soc 2020. https://doi.org/10.1093/jpids/piaa123.

11. López-Aguilar E, Cárdenas-Navarrete R, Simental-Toba A, et al. Children with cancer during COVID-19 pandemic: Early experience in Mexico. Pediatr Blood Cancer 2021;68(2):e28660.

12. Madhusoodhan PP, Pierro J, Musante J, et al. Characterization of COVID-19 disease in pediatric oncology patients: The New York-New Jersey regional experience. Pediatr Blood Cancer 2021;68(3):e28843.

13. Center for Disease Control and Prevention. Health Department-reported Cases of Multisystem Inflammatory Syndrome in Children (MIS-C) in the United States. Available at: https://www.cdc.gov/mis-c/cases/index.html. Accessed March 1, 2021.

14. Meredith J, Khedim CA, Henderson P, et al. Paediatric Inflammatory Multisystem Syndrome temporally associated with SARS-CoV-2 (PIMS-TS) in a patient receiving Infliximab therapy for Inflammatory Bowel Disease. J Crohn's Colitis 2020. https://doi.org/10.1093/ecco-jcc/jjaa201.

15. Dolinger MT, Person H, Smith R, et al. Pediatric Crohn Disease and Multisystem Inflammatory Syndrome in Children (MIS-C) and COVID-19 Treated With Infliximab. J Pediatr Gastroenterol Nutr 2020;71(2):153–5.

16. Brenner EJ, Pigneur B, Focht G, et al. Benign Evolution of SARS-Cov2 Infections in Children With Inflammatory Bowel Disease: Results From Two International Databases. Clin Gastroenterol Hepatol 2021;19(2):394–6.e5.

17. Wang Y, Zhang D, Du G, et al. Remdesivir in adults with severe COVID-19: a randomised, double-blind, placebo-controlled, multicentre trial. Lancet (London, England) 2020;395(10236):1569–78.

18. Kalil AC, Patterson TF, Mehta AK, et al. Baricitinib plus Remdesivir for Hospitalized Adults with Covid-19. N Engl J Med 2021;384(9):795–807.

19. Beigel JH, Tomashek KM, Dodd LE, et al. Remdesivir for the Treatment of Covid-19 - Final Report. N Engl J Med 2020;383(19):1813–26.

20. Spinner CD, Gottlieb RL, Criner GJ, et al. Effect of Remdesivir vs Standard Care on Clinical Status at 11 Days in Patients With Moderate COVID-19: A Randomized Clinical Trial. JAMA 2020;324(11):1048–57.

21. Horby P, Lim WS, Emberson JR, et al. Dexamethasone in Hospitalized Patients with Covid-19. N Engl J Med 2021;384(8):693–704.

22. Tomazini BM, Maia IS, Cavalcanti AB, et al. Effect of Dexamethasone on Days Alive and Ventilator-Free in Patients With Moderate or Severe Acute Respiratory Distress Syndrome and COVID-19: The CoDEX Randomized Clinical Trial. JAMA 2020;324(13):1307–16.

23. Focosi D, Franchini M. COVID-19 neutralizing antibody-based therapies in humoral immune deficiencies: A narrative review. Transfus Apheresis Sci 2021;103071. https://doi.org/10.1016/j.transci.2021.103071.

24. Food and Drug Administration. Bamlanivimab EUA Letter of Authorization. Available at: https://www.fda.gov/media/143602/download. Accessed March 2, 2021.

25. Food and Drug Administration. Bamlanivimab and etesevimab EUA Letter of Authorization. Available at: https://www.fda.gov/media/145801/download. Accessed February 25, 2021.
26. Food and Drug Administration. Casirivimab plus imdevimab EUA Letter of Authorization. Available at: https://www.fda.gov/media/145610/download. Accessed February 25, 2021.
27. Joyner MJ, Bruno KA, Klassen SA, et al. Safety Update: COVID-19 Convalescent Plasma in 20,000 Hospitalized Patients. Mayo Clin Proc 2020;95(9): 1888–97.
28. Food and Drug Administration. Convalescent plasma EUA Letter of Authorization. Available at: https://www.fda.gov/media/141477/download. Accessed February 23, 2021.
29. Wolf J, Abzug MJ, Wattier RL, et al. Initial Guidance on Use of Monoclonal Antibody Therapy for Treatment of COVID-19 in Children and Adolescents. J Pediatr Infect Dis Soc 2021. https://doi.org/10.1093/jpids/piaa175.
30. Ladani AP, Loganathan M, Danve A. Managing rheumatic diseases during COVID-19. Clin Rheumatol 2020;39(11):3245–54.
31. Cheng KW, Cheng SC, Chen WY, et al. Thiopurine analogs and mycophenolic acid synergistically inhibit the papain-like protease of Middle East respiratory syndrome coronavirus. Antiviral Res 2015;115:9–16.
32. Pfefferle S, Schöpf J, Kögl M, et al. The SARS-coronavirus-host interactome: identification of cyclophilins as target for pan-coronavirus inhibitors. PLoS Pathog 2011;7(10):e1002331.
33. Rosas IO, Bräu N, Waters M, et al. Tocilizumab in Hospitalized Patients with Severe Covid-19 Pneumonia. N Engl J Med 2021. https://doi.org/10.1056/NEJMoa2028700.
34. Warraich R, Amani L, Mediwake R, et al. Immunosuppression drug advice and COVID-19: are we doing more harm than good? Br J Hosp Med (London, Engl: 2005) 2020;81(6):1–3.
35. Bisogno G, Provenzi M, Zama D, et al. Clinical Characteristics and Outcome of Severe Acute Respiratory Syndrome Coronavirus 2 Infection in Italian Pediatric Oncology Patients: A Study From the Infectious Diseases Working Group of the Associazione Italiana di Oncologia e Ematologia Pediatrica. J Pediatr Infect Dis Soc 2020;9(5):530–4.
36. Memoli MJ, Athota R, Reed S, et al. The natural history of influenza infection in the severely immunocompromised vs nonimmunocompromised hosts. Clin Infect Dis 2014;58(2):214–24.
37. Asner S, Stephens D, Pedulla P, et al. Risk factors and outcomes for respiratory syncytial virus-related infections in immunocompromised children. Pediatr Infect Dis J 2013;32(10):1073–6.
38. Ogimi C, Englund JA, Bradford MC, et al. Characteristics and Outcomes of Coronavirus Infection in Children: The Role of Viral Factors and an Immunocompromised State. J Pediatr Infect Dis Soc 2019;8(1):21–8.
39. Batu ED, Özen S. Implications of COVID-19 in pediatric rheumatology. Rheumatol Int 2020;40(8):1193–213.
40. Marcus N, Frizinsky S, Hagin D, et al. Minor Clinical Impact of COVID-19 Pandemic on Patients With Primary Immunodeficiency in Israel. Front Immunol 2020;11:614086.
41. Meyts I, Bucciol G, Quinti I, et al. Coronavirus disease 2019 in patients with inborn errors of immunity: An international study. J Allergy Clin Immunol 2021; 147(2):520–31.

42. Fung M, Babik JM. COVID-19 in Immunocompromised Hosts: What We Know So Far. Clin Infect Dis 2020. https://doi.org/10.1093/cid/ciaa863.

43. Kuderer NM, Choueiri TK, Shah DP, et al. Clinical impact of COVID-19 on patients with cancer (CCC19): a cohort study. Lancet (London, England) 2020; 395(10241):1907–18.

44. Akalin E, Azzi Y, Bartash R, et al. Covid-19 and Kidney Transplantation. N Engl J Med 2020;382(25):2475–7.

45. Brenner EJ, Ungaro RC, Gearry RB, et al. Corticosteroids, But Not TNF Antagonists, Are Associated With Adverse COVID-19 Outcomes in Patients With Inflammatory Bowel Diseases: Results From an International Registry. Gastroenterology 2020;159(2):481–91.e3.

46. Gianfrancesco M, Hyrich KL, Al-Adely S, et al. Characteristics associated with hospitalisation for COVID-19 in people with rheumatic disease: data from the COVID-19 Global Rheumatology Alliance physician-reported registry. Ann Rheum Dis 2020;79(7):859–66.

47. Ebeid FSE, Ragab IA, Elsherif NHK, et al. COVID-19 in Children With Cancer: A Single Low-Middle Income Center Experience. J Pediatr hematology/oncology 2020. https://doi.org/10.1097/mph.0000000000002025.

48. Garg M, Burrell LM, Velkoska E, et al. Upregulation of circulating components of the alternative renin-angiotensin system in inflammatory bowel disease: A pilot study. J Renin-Angiotensin-Aldosterone Syst 2015;16(3):559–69.

49. Sawalha AH, Zhao M, Coit P, et al. Epigenetic dysregulation of ACE2 and interferon-regulated genes might suggest increased COVID-19 susceptibility and severity in lupus patients. Clin Immunol (Orlando, FL) 2020;215:108410.

50. Goss MB, Galván NTN, Ruan W, et al. The pediatric solid organ transplant experience with COVID-19: An initial multi-center, multi-organ case series. Pediatr Transplant 2020;e13868. https://doi.org/10.1111/petr.13868.

51. Kebudi R, Kurucu N, Tuğcu D, et al. COVID-19 infection in children with cancer and stem cell transplant recipients in Turkey: A nationwide study. Pediatr Blood Cancer 2021;e28915. https://doi.org/10.1002/pbc.28915.

52. Rouger-Gaudichon J, Thébault E, Félix A, et al. Impact of the First Wave of COVID-19 on Pediatric Oncology and Hematology: A Report from the French Society of Pediatric Oncology. Cancers 2020;12(11). https://doi.org/10.3390/cancers12113398.

53. The Pediatric COVID-10 Cancer Case Report. POCC Rep as January 20, 2021. Available at: https://www.uab.edu/medicine/icos/icos-research/the-pocc-report/reports-updates. Accessed February 10, 2021.

54. COVID-19 and Childhood Cancer Registry. Available at: https://global.stjude.org/en-us/global-covid-19-observatory-and-resource-center-for-childhood-cancer/registry.html. Accessed February 10, 2021.

55. Delavari S, Abolhassani H, Abolnezhadian F, et al. Impact of SARS-CoV-2 Pandemic on Patients with Primary Immunodeficiency. J Clin Immunol 2021; 41(2):345–55.

56. Zhang Q, Bastard P, Liu Z, et al. Inborn errors of type I IFN immunity in patients with life-threatening COVID-19, 370. New York: Science; 2020. p. 6515.

57. Bastard P, Rosen LB, Zhang Q, et al. Autoantibodies against type I IFNs in patients with life-threatening COVID-19, 370. New York: Science; 2020. p. 6515.

58. Batu ED, Lamot L, Sag E, et al. How the COVID-19 pandemic has influenced pediatric rheumatology practice: Results of a global, cross-sectional, online survey. Semin Arthritis Rheum 2020;50(6):1262–8.

59. Koker O, Demirkan FG, Kayaalp G, et al. Does immunosuppressive treatment entail an additional risk for children with rheumatic diseases? A survey-based study in the era of COVID-19. Rheumatol Int 2020;40(10):1613–23.
60. Ferrari A, Zecca M, Rizzari C, et al. Children with cancer in the time of COVID-19: An 8-week report from the six pediatric onco-hematology centers in Lombardia, Italy. Pediatr Blood Cancer 2020;67(8):e28410.
61. Ding YY, Ramakrishna S, Long AH, et al. Delayed cancer diagnoses and high mortality in children during the COVID-19 pandemic. Pediatr Blood Cancer 2020;67(9):e28427.
62. Doná D, Torres Canizales J, Benetti E, et al. Pediatric transplantation in Europe during the COVID-19 pandemic: Early impact on activity and healthcare. Clin Transplant 2020;34(10):e14063.
63. Charnaya O, Chiang TP, Wang R, et al. Effects of COVID-19 pandemic on pediatric kidney transplant in the United States. Pediatr Nephrol (Berlin, Germany) 2021;36(1):143–51.
64. Ashton JJ, Kammermeier J, Spray C, et al. Impact of COVID-19 on diagnosis and management of paediatric inflammatory bowel disease during lockdown: a UK nationwide study. Arch Dis Child 2020;105(12):1186–91.
65. Arrigo S, Alvisi P, Banzato C, et al. Impact of COVID-19 pandemic on the management of paediatric inflammatory bowel disease: An Italian multicentre study on behalf of the SIGENP IBD Group. Dig Liver Dis : official J Ital Soc Gastroenterol Ital Assoc Study Liver 2021;53(3):283–8.
66. Hare N, Bansal P, Bajowala SS, et al. Work Group Report: COVID-19: Unmasking Telemedicine. J Allergy Clin Immunol In Pract 2020;8(8):2461–73.e3.
67. Kircher SM, Mulcahy M, Kalyan A, et al. Telemedicine in Oncology and Reimbursement Policy During COVID-19 and Beyond. J Natl Compr Cancer Netw 2020;1–7. https://doi.org/10.6004/jnccn.2020.7639.
68. Kenney LB, Vrooman LM, Lind ED, et al. Virtual visits as long-term follow-up care for childhood cancer survivors: Patient and provider satisfaction during the COVID-19 pandemic. Pediatr Blood Cancer 2021;e28927. https://doi.org/10.1002/pbc.28927.
69. Peshko D, Kulbachinskaya E, Korsunskiy I, et al. Health-Related Quality of Life in Children and Adults with Primary Immunodeficiencies: A Systematic Review and Meta-Analysis. J Allergy Clin Immunol In Pract 2019;7(6):1929–57.e5.
70. Ravens-Sieberer U, Kaman A, Erhart M, et al. Impact of the COVID-19 pandemic on quality of life and mental health in children and adolescents in Germany. Eur Child Adolesc Psychiatry 2021;1–11. https://doi.org/10.1007/s00787-021-01726-5.
71. Glikman D, Walsh L, Valkenburg J, et al. Hospital-based directly observed therapy for HIV-infected children and adolescents to assess adherence to antiretroviral medications. Pediatrics 2007;119(5):e1142–8.
72. Parsons GN, Siberry GK, Parsons JK, et al. Multidisciplinary, inpatient directly observed therapy for HIV-1-infected children and adolescents failing HAART: A retrospective study. AIDS Patient Care and STDs 2006;20(4):275–84.
73. Saberi P, Siedle-Khan R, Sheon N, et al. The Use of Mobile Health Applications Among Youth and Young Adults Living with HIV: Focus Group Findings. AIDS patient care and STDs 2016;30(6):254–60.
74. Ponticiello M, Mwanga-Amumpaire J, Tushemereirwe P, et al. Everything is a Mess": How COVID-19 is Impacting Engagement with HIV Testing Services in Rural Southwestern Uganda. AIDS Behav 2020;24(11):3006–9.

75. Lodge W 2nd, Kuchukhidze S. COVID-19, HIV, and Migrant Workers: The Double Burden of the Two Viruses. AIDS Patient Care and STDs 2020;34(6):249–50.

76. Shiau S, Krause KD, Valera P, et al. The Burden of COVID-19 in People Living with HIV: A Syndemic Perspective. AIDS Behav 2020;24(8):2244–9.

77. Auletta JJ, Adamson PC, Agin JE, et al. Pediatric cancer research: Surviving COVID-19. Pediatr Blood Cancer 2020;67(9):e28435.

78. Turner D, Huang Y, Martín-de-Carpi J, et al. Corona Virus Disease 2019 and Paediatric Inflammatory Bowel Diseases: Global Experience and Provisional Guidance (March 2020) from the Paediatric IBD Porto Group of European Society of Paediatric Gastroenterology, Hepatology, and Nutrition. J Pediatr Gastroenterol Nutr 2020;70(6):727–33.

79. Licciardi F, Giani T, Baldini L, et al. COVID-19 and what pediatric rheumatologists should know: a review from a highly affected country. Pediatr Rheumatol Online J 2020;18(1):35.

80. Accortt NA, Lesperance T, Liu M, et al. Impact of Sustained Remission on the Risk of Serious Infection in Patients With Rheumatoid Arthritis. Arthritis Care Res 2018;70(5):679–84.

81. Au K, Reed G, Curtis JR, et al. High disease activity is associated with an increased risk of infection in patients with rheumatoid arthritis. Ann Rheum Dis 2011;70(5):785–91.

82. Moss JD, Schwenk HT, Chen M, et al. Drug Shortage and Critical Medication Inventory Management at a Children's Hospital During the COVID-19 Pandemic. J Pediatr Pharmacol Ther 2021;26(1):21–5.

83. Ayaz NA, Karadağ Ş G, Koç R, et al. Patient satisfaction and clinical effectiveness of switching from intravenous tocilizumab to subcutaneous tocilizumab in patients with juvenile idiopathic arthritis: an observational study. Rheumatol Int 2020;40(7):1111–6.

84. Vaduganathan M, van Meijgaard J, Mehra MR, et al. Prescription Fill Patterns for Commonly Used Drugs During the COVID-19 Pandemic in the United States. JAMA 2020;323(24):2524–6.

85. Mendel A, Bernatsky S, Thorne JC, et al. Hydroxychloroquine shortages during the COVID-19 pandemic. Ann Rheum Dis 2020. https://doi.org/10.1136/annrheumdis-2020-217835.

86. Plüß M, Chehab G, Korsten P. Concerns and needs of patients with systemic lupus erythematosus regarding hydroxychloroquine supplies during the COVID-19 pandemic: results from a patient-centred survey. Ann Rheum Dis 2020. https://doi.org/10.1136/annrheumdis-2020-217967.

87. Simko SJ, McClain KL, Allen CE. Up-front therapy for LCH: is it time to test an alternative to vinblastine/prednisone? Br J Haematol 2015;169(2):299–301.

88. Food and Drug Administration. Pfizer COVID-19 Vaccine EUA Letter of Authorization. Available at: https://www.fda.gov/media/144412/download. Accessed February 25, 2021.

89. Food and Drug Administration. Moderna COVID-19 Vaccine EUA Letter of Authorization. Available at: https://www.fda.gov/media/144636/download. Accessed February 25, 2021.

90. Food and Drug Administration. Janssen Biotech COVID-19 Vaccine EUA Letter of Authorization. Available at: https://www.fda.gov/media/146303/download. Accessed February 27, 2021.

91. Polack FP, Thomas SJ, Kitchin N, et al. Safety and Efficacy of the BNT162b2 mRNA Covid-19 Vaccine. N Engl J Med 2020;383(27):2603–15.

92. Baden LR, El Sahly HM, Essink B, et al. Efficacy and Safety of the mRNA-1273 SARS-CoV-2 Vaccine. N Engl J Med 2021;384(5):403–16.
93. Sadoff J, Le Gars M, Shukarev G, et al. Interim Results of a Phase 1-2a Trial of Ad26.COV2.S Covid-19 Vaccine. N Engl J Med 2021. https://doi.org/10.1056/NEJMoa2034201.
94. D'Amico F, Rabaud C, Peyrin-Biroulet L, et al. SARS-CoV-2 vaccination in IBD: more pros than cons. Nat Rev Gastroenterol Hepatol 2021;1–3. https://doi.org/10.1038/s41575-021-00420-w.
95. Centers for Disease Control and Prevention. Interim Clinical Considerations for Use of COVID-19 Vaccines Currently Authorized in the United States. Available at: https://www.cdc.gov/vaccines/covid-19/info-by-product/clinical-considerations.html. Accessed March 3, 2021.
96. Park JK, Choi Y, Winthrop KL, et al. Optimal time between the last methotrexate administration and seasonal influenza vaccination in rheumatoid arthritis: post hoc analysis of a randomised clinical trial. Ann Rheum Dis 2019;78(9):1283–4.
97. Park JK, Lee MA, Lee EY, et al. Effect of methotrexate discontinuation on efficacy of seasonal influenza vaccination in patients with rheumatoid arthritis: a randomised clinical trial. Ann Rheum Dis 2017;76(9):1559–65.
98. Sonani B, Aslam F, Goyal A, et al. COVID-19 vaccination in immunocompromised patients. Clin Rheumatol 2021;40(2):797–8.
99. Livingston EH, Malani PN, Creech CB. The Johnson & Johnson Vaccine for COVID-19. JAMA 2021. https://doi.org/10.1001/jama.2021.2927.
100. Zhao J, Zhao S, Ou J, et al. COVID-19: Coronavirus Vaccine Development Updates. Front Immunol 2020;11:602256.
101. Velikova T, Georgiev T. SARS-CoV-2 vaccines and autoimmune diseases amidst the COVID-19 crisis. Rheumatol Int 2021;41(3):509–18.
102. Sahin U, Muik A, Derhovanessian E, et al. COVID-19 vaccine BNT162b1 elicits human antibody and T(H)1 T cell responses. Nature 2020;586(7830):594–9.
103. Anderson EJ, Rouphael NG, Widge AT, et al. Safety and Immunogenicity of SARS-CoV-2 mRNA-1273 Vaccine in Older Adults. N Engl J Med 2020;383(25):2427–38.
104. Hatoun J, Correa ET, Donahue SMA, et al. Social Distancing for COVID-19 and Diagnoses of Other Infectious Diseases in Children. Pediatrics 2020;146(4). https://doi.org/10.1542/peds.2020-006460.
105. Hrusak O, Kalina T, Wolf J, et al. Flash survey on severe acute respiratory syndrome coronavirus-2 infections in paediatric patients on anticancer treatment. Eur J Cancer 2020;132:11–6.
106. Gampel B, Troullioud Lucas AG, Broglie L, et al. COVID-19 disease in New York City pediatric hematology and oncology patients. Pediatr Blood Cancer 2020;67(9):e28420.
107. de Rojas T, Pérez-Martínez A, Cela E, et al. COVID-19 infection in children and adolescents with cancer in Madrid. Pediatr Blood Cancer 2020;67(7):e28397.
108. André N, Rouger-Gaudichon J, Brethon B, et al. COVID-19 in pediatric oncology from French pediatric oncology and hematology centers: High risk of severe forms? Pediatr Blood Cancer 2020;67(7):e28392.
109. Montoya J, Ugaz C, Alarcon S, et al. COVID-19 in pediatric cancer patients in a resource-limited setting: National data from Peru. Pediatr Blood Cancer 2021;68(2):e28610.
110. Millen GC, Arnold R, Cazier JB, et al. Severity of COVID-19 in children with cancer: Report from the United Kingdom Paediatric Coronavirus Cancer Monitoring Project. Br J Cancer 2021;124(4):754–9.

111. Palomo-Collí M, Fuentes-Lugo AD, Cobo-Ovando SR, et al. COVID-19 in Children and Adolescents With Cancer From a Single Center in Mexico City. J Pediatr Hematol Oncol 2020. https://doi.org/10.1097/MPH.0000000000002040.

112. Haslak F, Yildiz M, Adrovic A, et al. Management of childhood-onset autoinflammatory diseases during the COVID-19 pandemic. Rheumatol Int 2020;40(9): 1423–31.

113. Calvo C, Udaondo C, Group tRDE-AW. COVID-19 in Children With Rheumatic Diseases in the Spanish National Cohort EPICO-AEP. J Rheumatol 2021. https://doi.org/10.3899/jrheum.201548.

114. Melgosa M, Madrid A, Alvárez O, et al. SARS-CoV-2 infection in Spanish children with chronic kidney pathologies. Pediatr Nephrol 2020;35(8):1521–4.

115. Marlais M, Wlodkowski T, Vivarelli M, et al. The severity of COVID-19 in children on immunosuppressive medication. Lancet Child Adolesc Health 2020;4(7): e17–8.

116. Marlais M, Wlodkowski T, Al-Akash S, et al. COVID-19 in children treated with immunosuppressive medication for kidney diseases. Arch Dis Child 2020. https://doi.org/10.1136/archdischild-2020-320616.

117. Pérez-Martinez A, Guerra-García P, Melgosa M, et al. Clinical outcome of SARS-CoV-2 infection in immunosuppressed children in Spain. Eur J Pediatr 2021; 180(3):967–71.

118. El Dannan H, Al Hassani M, Ramsi M. Clinical course of COVID-19 among immunocompromised children: a clinical case series. BMJ Case Rep 2020; 13(10). https://doi.org/10.1136/bcr-2020-237804.

Changes in Clinical Care of the Newborn During COVID-19 Pandemic

From the Womb to First Newborn Visit

Pezad N. Doctor, MBBS[a],*, Deepak Kamat, MD, PhD[b],
Beena G. Sood, MD, MS[c]

KEYWORDS

- SARS-CoV-2 • Newborn • Perinatal transmission • Pandemic

KEY POINTS

- Perinatal transmission of SARS-CoV-2 is mainly horizontal, necessitating strict control measures for preventing spread of infection to newborns.
- Universal screening for SARS-CoV-2 for all pregnant women is necessary to guide delivery room preparation and postdelivery care of newborns and mothers.
- Newborns infected with SARS-CoV-2 are usually asymptomatic or have mild clinical disease; therefore, other causes need to be investigated in case of severe illness.
- Breast feeding and bonding between newborn and SARS-CoV-2 infected mother can be encouraged with proper education and infection control measures.
- All newborns should have routine newborn care irrespective of their SARS-CoV-2 status as early discharge has not shown to reduce the spread of infection.

INTRODUCTION

Coronavirus disease 2019 (COVID-19), caused by severe acute respiratory syndrome coronavirus 2 (SARS-CoV-2), which was first reported in the Wuhan region of China in December in 2019 has struck the world, affecting humans across all age groups.[1] Initially, it was thought to affect mainly the respiratory system causing a "pneumonia of unknown etiology,"[2] but it was soon discovered that it affects multiple organ systems with significant morbidity and mortality. SARS-CoV-2 has been demonstrated to be transmitted by respiratory droplets, contact, and fomites.[3–5] SARS-CoV-2 has

[a] Department of Pediatrics, Children's Hospital of Michigan, 3901, Beaubien Boulevard, Detroit, MI 48201, USA; [b] Department of Pediatrics, UT Health Science Center, UT Health San Antonio, San Antonio, TX 78229, USA; [c] Department of Pediatrics, Wayne State University School of Medicine, 540E Canfield Street, Detroit, Michigan 48201, USA
* Corresponding author. Office of Pediatric education, 3901 Beaubien, Detroit, MI 48201.
E-mail address: pezaddoctor@gmail.com

Pediatr Clin N Am 68 (2021) 1055–1070
https://doi.org/10.1016/j.pcl.2021.05.008
0031-3955/21/© 2021 Elsevier Inc. All rights reserved.

proven to be highly contagious with a reproduction number of 2.2 to 5.7, which means that 1 person with SARS-CoV-2 infection can infect on an average 2 to 5 people around him or her if no precautions are followed.[6] SARS-CoV-2 gains entry into the lungs and gut by binding to the angiotensin-converting enzyme receptor 2 present abundantly on the type 2 pneumocytes and gastrointestinal epithelium. There is controversy regarding in utero transmission of SARS-CoV-2. However, there is increasing evidence of horizontal transmission from mother to neonate. There is a scarcity of data regarding pregnant women affected with COVID-19, and its implications during pregnancy: prenatal visits, antenatal scans, testing, and management of symptomatic women, and delivery, as well as delivery room preparedness, logistics, and postnatal care of newborns.[7–10] In this review, we highlight major changes in clinical practice implemented during delivery and postnatal care of newborns born to mothers with confirmed or suspected SARS-CoV-2 infection during the pandemic, based on various expert opinions and evolving evidence.

SARS-CoV-2 INFECTION IN PREGNANCY

Early speculations regarding SARS-CoV-2 infection in pregnancy were concerning owing to changes in cellular immunity during pregnancy along with an array of physiologic changes in the cardiovascular, respiratory, and coagulation systems. Few studies have investigated whether SARS-CoV-2 infection poses additional risk during pregnancy.[11] Studies so far have shown similar COVID-19 symptoms in pregnant and nonpregnant women.[12,13] Surveillance data from the Centers for Disease Control and Prevention (CDC) including 91,412 women of reproductive age group (15–45 years of age) with laboratory-confirmed SARS-CoV-2 infection showed no difference between pregnant (8207) and nonpregnant women (83,205) in terms of cough and shortness of breath.[14] Headache, fever, chills, diarrhea, and muscle aches were in fact less frequently noted in pregnant women compared with nonpregnant women. Initial studies from New York showed a significant asymptomatic carrier rate ($\leq$33%) in pregnant women.[15,16] Therefore, universal screening for SARS-CoV-2 infection in all pregnant women during hospitalization or at the time of delivery was proposed and soon became the standard of care. In a series of 54 pregnant women with confirmed (n = 38) and suspected (n = 16) SARS-CoV-2 infections reported by Sentilhes and colleagues,[17] oxygen supplementation was required in 24.1%, intensive care unit admission in 9.3%, and severe illness was observed in those over the age of 35 years or those with comorbidities, such as asthma and obesity. A recent report by the CDC's Coronavirus Disease 19-Associated Hospitalization Surveillance Network surveillance team found that, of the 598 pregnant women hospitalized in 13 states across the country with COVID-19 between March 1 and August 22, 2020, the majority of them (55%) were asymptomatic.[18] However, severe illness was observed in symptomatic women that included intensive care admission in 16%, mechanical ventilation in 8%, and mortality in 1%.[18] In an analysis of approximately 400,000 women aged 15 to 44 years with symptomatic COVID-19 by the CDC's Surveillance for Emerging Threats to Mothers and Babies Network (SET-NET), intensive care unit admission, invasive ventilation, extracorporeal membrane oxygenation, and death were more likely in pregnant women than in nonpregnant women.[19] In a 35-year-old woman infected with COVID-19, placental pathology showed inflammation and the presence of SARS-CoV-2 by immunohistochemistry at 22 weeks gestation, possibly contributing to the development of early-onset preeclampsia, hypertension, and disseminated coagulopathy.[20] Hence, a multidisciplinary team of maternal and fetal medicine specialists and neonatologists is essential in the care of pregnant women with SARS-CoV-2 infection and their infants.

IMPACT ON ROUTINE ANTENATAL VISIT AND SCANS

Since the declaration of SARS-CoV-2 as a pandemic by World health Organization (WHO), the American College of Obstetrics and Gynecology (ACOG) has proposed various modifications in the existing guidelines of antenatal visits and ultrasounds. These modifications were primarily made to decrease the amount contact between the pregnant women and health care facilities as well as to decrease the transmission of SARS-CoV-2 throughout the general population.[21] Minimal data are available on the impact on maternal and fetal health after these guideline changes. In a 28-year-old pregnant woman with gestational diabetes mellitus and chronic hypertension who was found to be COVID-19 positive at 34 weeks gestation, her routine nonstress testing and amniotic fluid index testing were delayed owing to her COVID-19–positive status. Ultimately, her nonstress testing revealed category 2 tracing persistently, requiring urgent cesarean section.[22] This case highlights that the frequency of antenatal visits and testing should be decided on an individualized basis, especially for high-risk pregnancies.

TRANSMISSION FROM MOTHER TO NEWBORN

The first case of SARS-CoV-2 infection in a neonate was reported in February 2020. The infant presented at 17 days of age with a fever, cough, runny nose, and vomiting.[23] This presentation led to suspicion of vertical transmission in utero because the mother of the newborn had tested positive for SARS-CoV-2. Early studies conducted in China were unable to isolate SARS-CoV-2 from amniotic fluid, vaginal mucus, cord blood, placenta, urine, feces, or breast milk. Similarly, Silva and colleagues did not find SARS-CoV-2 by reverse transcriptase polymerase chain reaction (RT-PCR) in 18 samples of amniotic fluid, umbilical cord, and placenta obtained from COVID-19–positive mothers.[24] Therefore, the risk of vertical transmission was considered highly unlikely.[25–29] However, in a retrospective cohort study of 3497 respiratory, urine, stool, and serum samples from adults analyzed for SARS-CoV-2 viral load, the median duration of the virus in stools (22 days; interquartile range [IQR], 17–31 days) was significantly longer than in respiratory (18 days; IQR, 13–29 days; $P = .02$) and serum samples (16 days; IQR, 11–21 days; $P < .001$).[30] In a study by Zeng and colleagues,[9] 3 of the 33 neonates born to COVID-19–positive mothers tested positive by RT-PCR from nasopharyngeal and anal swabs by 2 days of age despite strict isolation of the newborn soon after delivery. Two of the 3 neonates were born at full term with mild symptoms such as fever, vomiting, and lethargy; the third neonate was born at 31 weeks of gestation and developed respiratory distress syndrome and pneumonia, along with leukocytosis and thrombocytopenia requiring noninvasive positive pressure ventilation and antibiotics because his blood culture was positive for *Enterobacter* spp. Hence, the contribution of SARS-CoV-2 in causing symptoms in the third neonate was dubious. However, in a case reported by Dong and colleagues[31] of a neonate born to a SARS-CoV-2–positive mother was found to have high levels of SARS-CoV-2–specific IgM antibodies at 2 hours of age despite negative pressure room delivery and strict adherence to precautions. Her PCR results were negative on 5 consecutive samples during the first 16 days of life. Her IgM and IgG levels were still elevated at 16 days of life, but were trending down. Because IgM antibodies are elevated only after 3 to 7 days after the infection, high IgM levels in the infant only at the 2 hours of age strongly suggested an intrauterine infection. In a review of 217 neonates born to SARS-CoV-2–infected mothers, only 7 (3%) tested positive.[32] Of the 7, 3 had positive serum IgM and IgG levels with negative PCR and the remaining 4 had a positive PCR from nasopharyngeal or anal swabs. In the national registry of perinatal

COVID-19 infection established by the American Academy of Pediatrics Section on Neonatal Perinatal Medicine (AAP SONPM NPC-19 registry), which includes 295 centers, 139 of 6229 infants (2.2%) born to COVID-19–positive mothers tested positive as of February 20, 2021.[33] More than one-third (2888) of these newborns had contact, droplet, and air-borne isolation, 2303 (28%) had contact and droplet isolation, 1677 (20%) had contact, droplet, air-borne, and negative pressure isolation, 466(6%) had unspecified form of isolation, and 873 (11%) had no isolation.[33] Because the evidence for vertical transmission is weak, newborns are most likely infected via horizontal transmission after delivery from mother or other caregivers. Therefore, implementing strict infection control measures during and after delivery, quarantine of infected mothers, and close monitoring of neonates in the perinatal period was essential in decreasing horizontal transmission. The CDC's SET-NET had information of 2869 newborns delivered from 13 jurisdictions between March 29 and October 14, 2020. They reported 610 infants (21.3%) who were tested and 16 (2.6%) of them were positive for SARS-CoV-2. They were primarily those born to women with infection at delivery.[34] This result led to the development and implementation of essential delivery preparedness strategies across various birthing centers to curb the spread of SARS-CoV-2.

COVID-19 VACCINATION DURING PREGNANCY

The US Food and Drug Administration recently approved 2 vaccines against SARS-CoV-2 (Pfizer-BioNtech mRNA vaccine and Moderna mRNA-1273 vaccine) under the context of an Emergency Use Authorization in high-risk priority groups. The CDC's Advisory Committee on Immunization Practices and the ACOG have recommended their use in pregnant and lactating women.[35,36] However, the data are lacking regarding the benefits (to the mother and transplacental passage of passive immunity to the fetus) and side effects of these vaccines in this subset of patients because pregnant women were not involved in the studies during vaccine development.[37] In a study by Flannery and colleagues[38] involving 1714 mothers who delivered from April to August 2020 in the northeastern United States, 83 (6%) had detectable IgG and/or IgM antibodies at delivery. However, the majority of infants born to these seropositive mothers (72/83) had detectable IgG levels at birth, suggesting transplacental transfer during pregnancy. For Moderna mRNA-1273 vaccine, the WHO revised the recommendation on January 29, 2021, stating that "pregnant women at high risk of exposure to SARS CoV-2 (e.g. health workers) or who have comorbidities which add to their risk of severe disease, may be vaccinated in consultation with their health care provider."[39] Although immunization may be the best available options for pregnant and lactating mothers to protect themselves and their infants, longitudinal clinical studies are necessary to implement safe vaccination guidelines.

DELIVERY ROOM AND NEWBORN RESUSCITATION PRACTICES

Much of delivery room preparedness recommendations depended on the COVID-19 status of the mother. Therefore, a short turnaround time of the test was crucial for optimal preparedness during delivery. If resources were available, all mothers were tested for SARS-CoV-2 at delivery, regardless of their clinical profile, to prevent nosocomial spread to other patients and health care workers.[40] All mothers whose COVID-19 status was unknown either owing to a lack of resources, testing refusal, or in whom the test results were not back by the time they delivered were considered positive owing to the high asymptomatic carrier state.[15] Important aspects of delivery room preparedness included the availability of KN95 masks, appropriate personal protective equipment, medical professionals experienced in neonatal resuscitation to minimize aerosolization during newborn resuscitation, and separation of the mother from the newborn.[15,40] Discussion and planning between the obstetric and neonatal teams guided maternal and newborn care, such as the use of maternal steroids (dexamethasone for COVID-19–related lung injury in mother vs betamethasone for fetal lung maturity), magnesium sulfate for preterm delivery, unfractionated heparin for thromboembolism prophylaxis, and the use of remdesvir.[41] Positive pressure ventilation using bag and mask, endotracheal intubations, and high-flow nasal cannula have the potential to aerosolize the respiratory droplets, allowing SARS-CoV-2 to remain in air for more than 3 hours and propagate for more than 2 months.[42] Pregnant women who are COVID-19 positive or unknown should deliver preferably in a negative pressure room, if available, with an adjoining room for neonatal resuscitation.[40,43,44] If not available, a single room with minimal entry and exit of essential caregivers from the room is paramount.[43,44] Earlier, delayed cord clamping was deferred owing to the unknown risk of vertical transmission.[8] However, according to recent recommendations from the ACOG and the AAP SONPM, delayed cord clamping can be practiced in suspected or confirmed COVID-19–positive mothers because there is no strong evidence to suggest transplacental viral transmission at this time.[43,45]

Mode of Delivery

Varied speculations have been made on the mode of delivery in pregnant women with SARS-CoV-2.[46–49] Cesarean section was performed for routine obstetric indications or worsening respiratory distress and exhaustion owing to COVID-19.[40] Some centers also preferred cesarean section for decreasing the total hospital stay of the mother and to minimize cross-infection.[40,47] However, in a case reported by Iqbal and colleagues,[48] a full-term female infant who was born by vaginal delivery to a SARS-CoV-2–infected mother was asymptomatic and discharged home on the 6th day of life. A retrospective cohort study among adults found that SARS-CoV-2 was present in stool samples for a longer duration compared with serum and respiratory mucosa.[30] Therefore, caution should be taken in mothers with diarrhea during vaginal delivery. In a systematic review by Khan and colleagues49 that which included 8 studies, comprising a total of 100 women with COVID-19, cesarean section was noted in 85%, premature deliveries in 29%, and low birthweight infants in 16%. However, there is a shift in this trend; recent data from the AAP SONPM NPC-19 registry showed that of 7486 suspected or confirmed COVID-19–positive pregnant women, 4872 (65%) delivered vaginally and the remaining 2614 (35%) underwent cesarean section as of February 20, 2021.[33]

BREAST MILK AND BREASTFEEDING

The AAP, along with other academic organizations such as the Academy of Breast Feeding, the CDC, and the WHO recommend breastfeeding in mothers with confirmed or suspected COVID-19 while taking the necessary precautions.[45,50–53] Mothers can either pump breast milk or directly nurse the baby while wearing a face mask and performing breast and hand hygiene.[52] The mother can either wash her hands with soap and water or use sanitizer with at least 60% alcohol before touching the baby. Preferably, expressed breast milk should be fed by an uninfected healthy caregiver not at risk of developing severe illness from SARS-CoV-2.[54] Earlier studies were unable to detect SARS-CoV-2 in breast milk.[13,25,27,55,56] However, in few studies SARS-CoV-2 was detected in breast milk.[57,58] A case was reported of a 32-week gestational age preterm baby who was breastfed SARS-CoV-2–positive breast milk but did not become infected. The baby was inadvertently fed expressed breast milk from the mother who later tested positive for SARS-CoV-2. Her expressed milk also tested positive by RT-PCR despite using a face mask and standard personal protective equipment while expressing the milk. However, the newborn tested negative for SARS-CoV-2 nasopharyngeal swab as well as for antibodies at 30 days after the exposure.[59] Similarly, in a series of 14 infants breast fed by SARS-CoV-2–positive mothers, breast milk tested positive in only 1 case. Four of the 14 infants (including the one fed the infected breast milk) tested positive for SARS-CoV-2, but the clinical course of all the infants was uneventful. The repeat testing of these 4 infants was negative for SARS-CoV-2 at 6 weeks.[60] Although there is no clear evidence that infants fed breast milk from COVID-19–positive mothers are protected from SARS-CoV-2 infection, breast milk may contain antibodies against SARS-CoV-2 providing passive immunity and protecting the baby. The Human Milk Banking Association of North America milk banks provide heat-treated pasteurized donor breast milk that has been shown to inactivate viruses similar to SARS-CoV-2.[61] Hence, human donor milk could be used in preterm and term neonates admitted to the nursery and neonatal intensive care unit (NICU) for longer durations.

MOTHER AND NEWBORN SEPARATION

Owing to the unknown infective properties of the virus, the Chinese Neonatal 2019-nCoV expert working Group published its first consensus statement in February 2020 soon after the first case of SARS-CoV-2 was reported in a neonate.[8] They recommended separation of mother and child based on a systematic review of the adult literature on SARS-CoV-2 as well as previous reports of Middle East respiratory syndrome-related coronavirus and severe acute SARS-CoV infections.[8] As more cases were reported from China and around the world affecting newborns as early as few hours, separation of the mother with suspected or confirmed SARS-CoV-2 from newborn was strongly recommended by other health organizations such as the AAP, ACOG, and CDC.[43,45,62] However, separation may not be always feasible owing to the lack of infrastructure and resources available in other parts of the world. Recent amendments to the CDCs guidelines allow a case-by-case approach and takes into account decision made between the health care provider and mother, the clinical condition of the mother and infant, availability of testing, staffing, space, personal protective equipment, and test results of the newborn.[62] As of August 3, 2020, the CDC recommends mothers to remain separated for at least 10 days after the occurrence of first symptoms (20 days if critically ill or the mother is immunocompromised), and at least 24 hours after the last fever without use of antipyretics and improvement in other symptoms.[62] If the newborn is tested COVID-19 positive, there is no need for separation. If the mother refuses separation, the newborn and mother should be placed in a negative pressure room with 6 feet or more distance between the two. In addition, the newborn should be placed in a temperature-regulated isolette to minimize droplet spread from mother. The Italian Society of Neonatology guidelines endorsed by the Union of European Neonatal and Perinatal Societies suggest that rooming-in of mother and newborn is workable if a mother is SARS-CoV-2 positive, or is a person under investigation, or is asymptomatic, or has minimal symptoms at delivery, but with strict infection control measures.[63] Ample research-based evidence has concluded that early maternal–newborn bonding positively impacts the growth and development in term and preterm neonates.[64,65] Early separation may negatively affect the bonding, breast milk production, and mental health of the mother during the hospital stay and after discharge with uncertain short- and long-term implications. In a recent study of 45 newborns born to SARS-CoV-2–positive mothers, 33 (73%) roomed-in with the mother. Thirty-one of the 33 newborns were breastfed within the 1 hour of birth. All 33 newborns tested negative for SARS-CoV-2, did not require NICU admission, and remained asymptomatic at their 2-week telemedicine follow-up visit.[66]

CLINICAL FEATURES OF SARS-CoV-2 INFECTION IN NEONATES

Various clinical studies have concluded that newborns and infants are less susceptible to SARS-CoV-2 infection and have a fairly mild clinical course with lower mortality compared with adults. A few theories have been proposed explaining this difference in clinical susceptibility. These include immature angiotensin-converting enzyme receptor 2 in neonates, which may prevent or decrease binding of the virus to the epithelial cells and naïve immune system of newborn mounting a poor inflammatory response.[67,68] However, the exact pathogenesis of COVID-19 is still being investigated. Neonates and children are usually asymptomatic or develop mild symptoms such as respiratory distress and feeding difficulties. A clinical finding of COVID-19 specific to newborns has not been recognized. The first few case series from China reported that the majority of newborns born to SARS-CoV-2–confirmed positive mothers were unaffected.[25,26] Later, a few publications reported varied presentations such as respiratory distress, shock, tachycardia, sepsis, thrombocytopenia, and occasionally death in neonates.[8,9,32,69] Other presenting symptoms include temperature instability, poor feeding, diarrhea, vomiting, and abdominal distension. Associated risk factors such as prematurity, prolonged rupture of membranes, and sepsis were also present in these neonates. In another case series of 4 neonates ranging between 30 hours and 17 days of age with a confirmed SARS-CoV-2 positive result by nucleic acid testing, 2 had fever, 1 developed respiratory distress, 1 had cough, and 1 had no symptoms.[69] Recently, another case of a SARS-CoV-2–positive neonate was reported who developed cyanosis and hypoxemia with respiratory distress at 48 hours of life. His chest radiograph showed ground glass opacity and he improved on high-flow nasal cannula with a 30% Fio_2.[70] Aghdam and colleagues[71] reported a 15-day-old neonate who presented with fever, tachycardia, and respiratory distress who improved quickly and was discharged 6 days later. In China, a greater proportion of infants less than 1 year of age had severe or critical disease compared with older children (10.6% vs 4.8%).[72] Owing to the high incidence of asymptomatic cases, other causes should be investigated in newborns with confirmed SARS-CoV-2 infection who demonstrate clinical deterioration. However, in a recent review of 18 PubMed articles that included 25 SARS-CoV-2–positive confirmed newborns less than 28 days of age, with a mean age of 8.2 ± 8.5 days, a gestational age of 37.4 ± 4.0 weeks, and a birth weight of 3041.6 ± 866.0 grams, the clinical features included fever in 28%, vomiting in 16%, cough or shortness of breath in 12%, diarrhea, lethargy or respiratory difficulty in 8% or cyanosis, feeding intolerance, hyperpnea, mild intercostal retractions, mottling, sneezing, nasal stuffiness, and paroxysmal episodes in 4%; only 16% of these newborns were completely asymptomatic.[73] Deaths were not reported in any of the newborns and 8 of 25 (32%) required intensive care. The mean length of hospital stays of 15.8 ± 10.8 days.[73] In another review of 26 articles published from December 1, 2019, to May 12, 2020, that included 38 SARS-CoV-2–positive confirmed neonates, 26 (68%) were symptomatic at a median age of 10 days (IQR, 2–19 days).[74] Clinical findings included fever in 50%, gastrointestinal symptoms in 26%, hypoxia in 20%, and cough in 20%. All newborns were discharged home after a median length of stay of 10 days (IQR, 6–14 days).[74] In a study by the national surveillance registry of

UK that included 66 newborns who tested positive, 16 (24%) were born preterm. The incidence of SARS-CoV-2 was estimated to be 5.6 per 10,000 live births. The most common symptoms were hyperthermia (35%), poor feeding/vomiting (33%), and coryza (26%). In terms of respiratory support, 33% required supplemental oxygen, 15% required noninvasive ventilation, and 5% required intubation.[75] In a large single-center study in New York including 101 newborns born to SARS-CoV-2–positive mothers, maternal severe or critical COVID-19 disease was associated with birth approximately 1 week before the due date (median gestational age, 37.9 weeks [IQR, 37.1–38.4 weeks] vs median, 39.1 weeks [IQR, 38.3–40.2 weeks]; $P = .02$) and an increased risk of requiring phototherapy (3 of 10 [30.0%] vs 6 of 91 [7.0%]; $P = .04$) compared with newborns of mothers with asymptomatic or mild COVID-19.[76] Interestingly, a preterm newborn delivered at 34 weeks of gestation developed late-onset fever, thrombocytopenia, and elevated inflammatory markers concerning for fetal inflammatory response syndrome, which was attributed to maternal SARS-CoV-2 infection. The neonate tested negative for SARS-CoV-2 by RT-PCR twice 24 hours apart. He subsequently developed pulmonary hypertension requiring inhaled nitric oxide with significant improvement and discharge home at 22 days of age.[77]

DEFINITION OF COVID-19 IN NEONATES

In February 2020, the Chinese Perinatal-neonatal 2019-nCoV Committee proposed the definition of suspected and confirmed neonatal cases after a systematic review of current and previous literature in their consensus statement.

Suspected COVID-19

All newborns born to SARS-CoV-2–positive confirmed mothers within 14 days before birth and 28 days after birth or newborns exposed directly to SARS-CoV-2–infected individuals (including family members, caregivers, medical staff, and visitors) are considered to be suspected cases.[8]

Confirmed COVID-19

Newborn in whom respiratory tract or blood specimens tested by RT-PCR are positive for SARS-CoV-2;
OR
Virus gene sequencing of the respiratory tract or blood specimens is highly homologous to that of the known SARS-CoV-2 specimens.[8]

Management

The majority of newborns with suspected and confirmed SARS-CoV-2 who require medical attention do so because of associated comorbidities of the perinatal period. All newborns with suspected or confirmed SARS-CoV-2 should be quarantined with droplet and contact precautions for at least 14 days. The management of these newborns is mainly supportive. Owing to a lack of evidence of the efficacy and safety profile of pharmaceutical agents such as hydroxychloroquine, azithromycin, and remdesivir in newborns, their use is not recommended.[5,8] Similarly, there is no evidence for the effectiveness of gamma globulin, hormonal therapy or interferon therapy.[8] However, owing to the widespread use of the COVID-19 vaccine, we expect to see an increase in the titers of anti-COVID-19 antibodies in intravenous immunoglobulin pooled from plasma donors that could be used for treating SARS-CoV-2 in the near future. Modifications in clinical practice made while caring for newborns with SARS-CoV-2 in terms of respiratory support, isolation, appropriate use of personal protective equipment, and KN95 masks by health care providers, laboratory and radiology staff and for discharge planning is summarized elsewhere in this article.

Respiratory support, personal protective equipment, and isolation

There are few neonates reported with suspected or confirmed SARS-CoV-2 requiring respiratory support so far.[9,78] Aerosolization of SARS-CoV-2 can be decreased by limiting and/or cautiously performing procedures such as ventilation (bag and mask, invasive and noninvasive), endotracheal intubation, and insertion of orogastric or nasogastric tubes.[5,15,40,79] For bag and mask ventilation, high-efficiency particulate air filters should be used between the mask and CO_2 detector to minimize aerosolization.[80,81] Dual limb conventional ventilators are a closed circuit containing in-built high-efficiency particulate air filters near the endotracheal tube and, therefore, are safer than bag and mask ventilation.[80,81] Suctioning should be performed using an in-line suction catheter.[80] The use of personal protective equipment, including a face mask, face shield, and gloves, while performing these aerosolization procedures and even otherwise is essential for health care workers to protect themselves and minimize spread while taking care of these newborns as recommended by the CDC.[82] Depending on the availability of infrastructure and resources, isolation or cohorting of confirmed newborns in a designated enclosed space in NICU is recommended.[8,40] Reusable monitoring tools such as stethoscope and thermometers should not be shared among patients.

Laboratory evaluation

Both the AAP and the CDC recommend testing for SARS-CoV-2 for all newborns delivered by suspected or confirmed SARS-CoV-2–positive mothers because it guides ongoing infection prevention and control, clinical observation of newborn, the need for isolation, discharge planning, and newborn outpatient follow-up visits.[45,82] The timing of first testing is usually between 24 and 48 hours after delivery, depending on the discharge plan for the newborn. If the results of the first test at 24 hours are negative, the AAP recommends repeat testing at 24 hours or later after the first test result because some tests in newborns become positive at a later time. If the first test performed at 24 hours is positive, then repeat testing at least 24 hours apart should be performed until 2 test results are negative.[45,82] This process will suggest clearance of the virus from the mucosal sites. RT-PCR from nasopharyngeal and throat swabs are recommended. Presently, the diagnostic role of antibody testing has not been well-established owing to inconclusive data.

Radiologic studies

A chest radiograph should be performed if clinically indicated. Radiologic findings in newborns are not specific and may include ground glass opacities, unilateral and bilateral subsegmental opacities and pneumothorax.[8,9,26] In a national surveillance registry from the UK, of the 26 newborns who were SARS-CoV-2 positive and had chest radiographs, 14 (56%) had abnormal findings, with ground-glass changes reported in 7 (28%); in addition. 4 of these 7 babies were born preterm.[75]

ROUTINE NEWBORN SURVEILLANCE AND NEWBORN/NEONATAL INTENSIVE CARE UNIT VISITATION BY FAMILY MEMBERS

In April 2020, the Vermont Oxford Network, in partnership with the AAP SONPM, conducted an audit to assess the impact of SARS-CoV-2 on neonates and their families.[83] Of the 332 hospitals, 54% reported shortages of equipment, testing, or personnel, 73% reported minor disruptions to care for infants and families, and 3% reported an inability to provide care to some, most, or all infants.[84] Owing to the ever-evolving evidence of SARS-CoV-2 transmission between asymptomatic carriers, varying policy changes have been made by many NICUs and newborn nurseries across the world to limit the entry of healthy family members. Owing to vulnerability of the infant's health in the NICU, the AAP recommends restricting parents and family members with COVID-19 for 14 to 20 days from the onset of disease symptoms or the first positive test.[45] Some NICUs made strict visitation policies with exceptions on a case-by-case basis. This difference led to disparities in the NICU visitation by family members and lack of parental participation in family-centered rounds.[83] The AAP strongly advocated that "any policy restricting visitors for pediatric patients should be applied equally regardless of children's race, ethnicity, socioeconomic status, culture, and religion" to minimize health disparities.[85] Nonetheless, various social, emotional, and psychological challenges were faced by family members during the separation of neonates staying for an extended duration in the NICU.[83] Parental stress arising from NICU admission has been associated with poor neurodevelopmental outcomes in preterm babies.[86] Especially in the pandemic, parental stress can worsen owing to restricted visitation. Owing to growing evidence of low transmission risk in the NICU, these restrictions have been alleviated to some extent in most NICUs and newborn nurseries across the country.[87] In a center where universal screening of neonates, parents, and staff was practiced, no SARS-CoV-2 infection among the neonates admitted to the NICU was noted in an area with a high incidence of SARS-CoV-2.[88] If parental visitation is restricted, the NICU should provide numerous ways to best support infants and their families to cope within this stressful environment.[89] As the literature on SARS-CoV-2 in neonates accumulates, evidence-based policies should be formulated to prevent horizontal spread of SARS-CoV-2 in the NICU that can be applicable universally.[90]

DISCHARGE PLANNING AND FOLLOW-UP

Routine newborn care including physical examination, vitamin K injection, administration of erythromycin eye ointment, performing hearing and critical congenital heart disease screens, and administering hepatitis B vaccine per the institutional policies should be completed before discharge, regardless of SARS-CoV-2 testing. If the newborn tests positive, remains positive on repeat testing, and is asymptomatic, then the newborn can be discharged with home quarantine for 10 days from the first positive test.[45] Care should be taken to prevent spread from the newborn to other members at home. Newborn visits can be arranged by telemedicine or phone. In-office visits should be avoided as far as possible to prevent spread. Some hospital centers, through charitable organizations, have been arranging and distributing electronic scales at discharge for assessing weight gain at home.[40] This practice may decrease the need for newborn in-office visits. If an in-office visit is necessary, parents should inform the clinic about the COVID-19 status of the newborn and the accompanying parent before arrival so that necessary precautions can be in place at the pediatrician's office. If the newborn is tested negative at discharge, then thorough parental counseling and additional infection prevention education should be provided to all the possible caregivers and household members after discharge. Other household members who may have been exposed to COVID-19 should maintain 6 or more feet of distance with the use of facemasks and adequate hand hygiene.[45] In a cohort analysis of 101 neonates born to mothers with perinatal SARS-CoV-2 infections at a single institution in New York, 55 who were seen at the newborn COVID-19 follow-up clinic remained healthy at 2 weeks of life. The appropriate duration of infection control practiced by the breastfeeding mother is unknown because a varying duration of viral shedding has been shown from different sites.[30] However, the AAP recommends that infection control be practiced for at least 10 days from the onset of symptoms and at least 24 hours from being afebrile without antipyretics.[7] Other precautionary measures as mentioned elsewhere in this article should be followed by mothers while breast-feeding. Parents should be educated regarding normal newborn care and common red flags concerning illness in newborns.[45]

CLINICS CARE POINTS

- While extensive research suggest horizontal transmission of COVID-19 from caregivers to neonates, there are few case reports demonstrating the rare possibility of vertical transmission.
- Although most of the neonates with SARS-CoV2 are asymptomatic or have a mild clinical course, there are rare case reports of severe disease manifestation in this age group.
- Most governing agencies have recommended mothers with COVID-19 to continue breast feeding, considering its long-term benefits.

DISCLOSURE

The authors have nothing to disclose.

REFERENCES

1. Lu R, Zhao X, Li J, et al. Genomic characterisation and epidemiology of 2019 novel coronavirus: implications for virus origins and receptor binding. Lancet 2020;395(10224):565–74.
2. Hui DS, E IA, Madani TA, et al. The continuing 2019-nCoV epidemic threat of novel coronaviruses to global health - The latest 2019 novel coronavirus outbreak in Wuhan, China. Int J Infect Dis 2020;91:264–6.
3. Li Q, Guan X, Wu P, et al. Early Transmission Dynamics in Wuhan, China, of Novel Coronavirus–Infected Pneumonia. N Engl J Med 2020;382(13):1199–207.
4. Shen K, Yang Y, Wang T, et al. Diagnosis, treatment, and prevention of 2019 novel coronavirus infection in children: experts' consensus statement. World J Pediatr 2020;16(3):223–31.
5. World Health Organization. Clinical management of COVID-19 2020. https://www.who.int/publications-detail/clinical-management-of-severe-acute-respiratory-infection-when-novel-coronavirus-(ncov)-infection-is-suspected.
6. Uddin M, Mustafa F, Rizvi TA, et al. SARS-CoV-2/COVID-19: viral genomics, epidemiology, vaccines, and therapeutic interventions. Viruses 2020;12(5).
7. Puopolo KM, Hudak ML, Kimberlin DW, et al. American Academy of pediatrics committee on fetus and newborn, section of neonatal-perinatal medicine & committee on infectious disease 2020. Initial guidance: management of infants born to mothers with COVID-19. Available at: https://downloads.aap.org/AAP/PDF/COVID%2019%20Initial%20Newborn%20Guidance.pdf. Accessed October 2, 2020.
8. Wang L, Shi Y, Xiao T, et al. Chinese expert consensus on the perinatal and neonatal management for the prevention and control of the 2019 novel coronavirus infection (First edition). Ann Transl Med 2020;8(3):47.

9. Zeng L, Xia S, Yuan W, et al. Neonatal Early-Onset Infection With SARS-CoV-2 in 33 Neonates Born to Mothers With COVID-19 in Wuhan, China. JAMA Pediatr 2020;174(7):722–5.

10. Shalish W, Lakshminrusimha S, Manzoni P, et al. COVID-19 and neonatal respiratory care: current evidence and practical approach. Am J Perinatol 2020;37(8): 780–91.

11. Juan J, Gil MM, Rong Z, et al. Effect of coronavirus disease 2019 (COVID-19) on maternal, perinatal and neonatal outcome: systematic review. Ultrasound Obstet Gynecol 2020;56(1):15–27.

12. Lim WS, Macfarlane JT, Colthorpe CL. Pneumonia and pregnancy. Thorax 2001; 56(5):398–405.

13. Schwartz DA. An analysis of 38 pregnant women with COVID-19, their newborn infants, and maternal-fetal transmission of SARS-CoV-2: maternal coronavirus infections and pregnancy outcomes. Arch Pathol Lab 2020;144(7):799–805.

14. Ellington S, Strid P, Tong VT, et al. Characteristics of Women of Reproductive Age with Laboratory-Confirmed SARS-CoV-2 Infection by Pregnancy Status - United States, January 22-June 7, 2020. MMWR Morb Mortal Wkly Rep 2020;69(25): 769–75.

15. Perlman J, Oxford C, Chang C, et al. Delivery Room Preparedness and Early Neonatal Outcomes During COVID-19 Pandemic in New York City. Pediatrics 2020;146(2).

16. Breslin N, Baptiste C, Gyamfi-Bannerman C, et al. Coronavirus disease 2019 infection among asymptomatic and symptomatic pregnant women: two weeks of confirmed presentations to an affiliated pair of New York City hospitals. Am J Obstet Gynecol MFM 2020;2(2):100118.

17. Sentilhes L, De Marcillac F, Jouffrieau C, et al. Coronavirus disease 2019 in pregnancy was associated with maternal morbidity and preterm birth. Am J Obstet Gynecol 2020;223(6):914 e911–5.

18. Delahoy MJ, Whitaker M, O'Halloran A, et al. Characteristics and Maternal and Birth Outcomes of Hospitalized Pregnant Women with Laboratory-Confirmed COVID-19 - COVID-NET, 13 States, March 1-August 22, 2020. MMWR Morb Mortal Wkly Rep 2020;69(38):1347–54.

19. Zambrano LD, Ellington S, Strid P, et al. Update: characteristics of symptomatic women of reproductive age with laboratory-confirmed SARS-CoV-2 infection by pregnancy status - United States, January 22-October 3, 2020. MMWR Morb Mortal Wkly Rep 2020;69(44):1641–7.

20. Hosier H, Farhadian SF, Morotti RA, et al. SARS-CoV-2 infection of the placenta. J Clin Invest 2020;130(9):4947–53.

21. Boelig RC, Saccone G, Bellussi F, et al. MFM guidance for COVID-19. Am J Obstet Gynecol MFM 2020;2(2):100106.

22. Suresh SC, MacGregor CA, Ouyang DW. Urgent Cesarean Delivery Following Nonstress Test in a Patient with COVID-19 and Pregestational Diabetes. Neoreviews 2020;21(9):e625–30.

23. Zeng LK, Tao XW, Yuan WH, et al. [First case of neonate with COVID-19 in China]. Zhonghua er ke Za Zhi Chin J Pediatr 2020;58(4):279–80.

24. Simões E, Silva AC, Leal CRV. Is SARS-CoV-2 vertically transmitted? Front Pediatr 2020;8:276.

25. Chen H, Guo J, Wang C, et al. Clinical characteristics and intrauterine vertical transmission potential of COVID-19 infection in nine pregnant women: a retrospective review of medical records. Lancet 2020;395(10226):809–15.

26. Zhu H, Wang L, Fang C, et al. Clinical analysis of 10 neonates born to mothers with 2019-nCoV pneumonia. Transl Pediatr 2020;9(1):51–60.

27. Fan C, Lei D, Fang C, et al. Perinatal transmission of 2019 coronavirus disease–associated severe acute respiratory syndrome coronavirus 2: should we worry? Clin Infect Dis 2021;72(5):862–4.

28. Chen R, Zhang Y, Huang L, et al. Safety and efficacy of different anesthetic regimens for parturients with COVID-19 undergoing Cesarean delivery: a case series of 17 patients. Can J Anaesth 2020;67(6):655–63.

29. Mullins E, Evans D, Viner RM, et al. Coronavirus in pregnancy and delivery: rapid review. Ultrasound Obstet Gynecol 2020;55(5):586–92.

30. Zheng S, Fan J, Yu F, et al. Viral load dynamics and disease severity in patients infected with SARS-CoV-2 in Zhejiang province, China, January-March 2020: retrospective cohort study. BMJ 2020;369:m1443.

31. Dong L, Tian J, He S, et al. Possible Vertical Transmission of SARS-CoV-2 From an Infected Mother to Her Newborn. JAMA 2020;323(18):1846–8.

32. Wang S, Guo L, Chen L, et al. A Case Report of Neonatal 2019 Coronavirus Disease in China. Clin Infect Dis 2020;71(15):853–7.

33. NPC-19 Registry update: AAP SONPM National Registry of Perinatal COVID 19 infection. 2020. Available at: https://my.visme.co/view/ojq9qq8e-npc-19-registry. Accessed February 20, 2021.

34. Woodworth KR, Olsen EO, Neelam V, et al. Birth and Infant Outcomes Following Laboratory-Confirmed SARS-CoV-2 Infection in Pregnancy - SET-NET, 16 Jurisdictions, March 29-October 14, 2020. MMWR Morb Mortal Wkly Rep 2020; 69(44):1635–40.

35. Centers for Disease Control and Prevention. COVID-19 ACIP vaccine recommendations. 2020. Available at: https://www.cdc.gov/vaccines/hcp/acip-recs/vacc-specific/covid-19.html. Accessed February 20, 2021.

36. American College of Obstetricians and Gynecologists' Immunization, Infectious Disease, and Public Health Preparedness Expert Work Group. Practice Advisory. Vaccinating pregnant and lactating patients against COVID-19 2021. Available at: https://www.acog.org/clinical/clinical-guidance/practice-advisory/articles/2020/12/vaccinating-pregnant-and-lactating-patients-against-covid-19. Accessed February 21, 2021.

37. Adhikari EH, Spong CY. COVID-19 Vaccination in Pregnant and Lactating Women. JAMA 2021;325(11):1039–40.

38. Flannery DD, Gouma S, Dhudasia MB, et al. Assessment of Maternal and Neonatal Cord Blood SARS-CoV-2 Antibodies and Placental Transfer Ratios. JAMA Pediatr 2021;175(6):594–600.

39. World Health Organization. The Moderna COVID-19 (mRNA-1273) vaccine: what you need to know 2021. Available at: https://www.who.int/news-room/feature-stories/detail/the-moderna-covid-19-mrna-1273-vaccine-what-you-need-to-know. Accessed February 2, 2021.

40. Amatya S, Corr TE, Gandhi CK, et al. Management of newborns exposed to mothers with confirmed or suspected COVID-19. J Perinatol 2020;40(7):987–96.

41. Altendahl M, Afshar Y, De St, et al. Perinatal maternal-fetal/neonatal transmission of COVID-19: a guide to safe maternal and neonatal care in the era of COVID-19 and physical distancing. NeoReviews 2020;21(12):e783–94.

42. van Doremalen N, Bushmaker T, Morris DH, et al. Aerosol and surface stability of HCoV-19 (SARS-CoV-2) compared to SARS-CoV-1 2020. 2020.2003.2009.20033217.

43. American College of Obstetricians and Gynecologists. COVID-19 FAQs for Obstetrician-Gynecologists, Obstetrics 2020. Available at: https://www.acog.org/clinical-information/physician-faqs/covid-19-faqs-for-ob-gyns-obstetrics. Accessed July 3, 2020.

44. Ovalı F. SARS-CoV-2 infection and the newborn. Front Pediatr 2020;8(294).

45. American Academy of Pediatrics Section on Neonatal-Perinatal Medicine. COVID-19 clinical guidance FAQs 2020. Available at: https://services.aap.org/en/pages/2019-novel-coronavirus-covid-19-infections/clinical-guidance/faqs-management-of-infants-born-to-covid-19-mothers/.

46. Zhang L, Jiang Y, Wei M, et al. Analysis of the pregnancy outcomes in pregnant women with COVID-19 in Hubei Province. Zhonghua fu chan ke za zhi 2020; 55(3):166–71.

47. Qi H, Luo X, Zheng Y, et al. Safe delivery for pregnancies affected by COVID-19. BJOG 2020;127(8):927–9.

48. Iqbal SN, Overcash R, Mokhtari N, et al. An Uncomplicated Delivery in a Patient with Covid-19 in the United States. N Engl J Med 2020;382(16):e34.

49. Ali Khan MM, Khan MN, Mustagir MG, et al. COVID-19 infection during pregnancy: a systematic review to summarize possible symptoms, treatments, and pregnancy outcomes 2020. 2020.2003.2031.20049304.

50. Academy of breastfeeding medicine statement on coronavirus 2019 (COVID-19). Available at: https://www.bfmed.org/abm-statement-coronavirus. Accessed February 20, 2021.

51. Pregnancy, Breastfeeding, and Caring for Newborns. 2020. Available at: https://www.cdc.gov/coronavirus/2019-ncov/need-extra-precautions/pregnancy-breastfeeding.html. Accessed January 2, 2021.

52. World Health Organization. Breastfeeding advice during the COVID-19 outbreak 2020. Available at: http://www.emro.who.int/nutrition/nutrition-infocus/breastfeeding-advice-during-covid-19-outbreak.html.

53. Davanzo R, Moro G, Sandri F, et al. Breastfeeding and coronavirus disease-2019: ad interim indications of the Italian Society of Neonatology endorsed by the Union of European Neonatal & Perinatal Societies. Matern Child Nutr 2020;16(3): e13010.

54. Sullivan SE, Thompson LA. Best Practices for COVID-19–Positive or Exposed Mothers—Breastfeeding and Pumping Milk. JAMA Pediatr 2020;174(12):1228.

55. Liu W, Wang J, Li W, et al. Clinical characteristics of 19 neonates born to mothers with COVID-19. Front Med 2020;14(2):193–8.

56. Li Y, Zhao R, Zheng S, et al. Lack of Vertical Transmission of Severe Acute Respiratory Syndrome Coronavirus 2, China. Emerg Infect Dis 2020;26(6):1335–6.

57. Wu Y, Liu C, Dong L, et al. Coronavirus disease 2019 among pregnant Chinese women: case series data on the safety of vaginal birth and breastfeeding. BJOG 2020;127(9):1109–15.

58. Groß R, Conzelmann C, Müller JA, et al. Detection of SARS-CoV-2 in human breastmilk. Lancet 2020;395(10239):1757–8.

59. Lugli L, Bedetti L, Lucaccioni L, et al. An Uninfected Preterm Newborn Inadvertently Fed SARS-CoV-2–Positive Breast Milk. Pediatrics 2020. e2020004960.

60. Bertino E, Moro GE, De Renzi G, et al. Detection of SARS-CoV-2 in Milk From COVID-19 Positive Mothers and Follow-Up of Their Infants. Front Pediatr 2020;8.

61. Darnell MER, Taylor DR. Evaluation of inactivation methods for severe acute respiratory syndrome coronavirus in noncellular blood products. Transfusion 2006; 46(10):1770–7.

62. Centers for Disease Control. Interim considerations for infection prevention and control of coronavirus disease 2019 (COVID-19) in inpatient obstetric healthcare settings 2020. Available at: https://www.cdc.gov/coronavirus/2019-ncov/hcp/inpatient-obstetric-healthcare-guidance.html.

63. Union of European Neonatal and Perinatal Societies. Breastfeeding and SARS-CoV infection 2020. Available at: https://www.uenps.eu/2020/03/16/sars-cov-2-infection-sin-recommendations-endorsed-by-uenps/. Accessed January 25, 2021.

64. Gonya J, Ray WC, Rumpf RW, et al. Investigating skin-to-skin care patterns with extremely preterm infants in the NICU and their effect on early cognitive and communication performance: a retrospective cohort study. BMJ Open 2017; 7(3):e012985.

65. Weber A, Harrison TM, Sinnott L, et al. Associations Between Nurse-Guided Variables and Plasma Oxytocin Trajectories in Premature Infants During Initial Hospitalization. Adv Neonatal Care 2018;18(1):E12–23.

66. Patil UP, Maru S, Krishnan P, et al. Newborns of COVID-19 mothers: short-term outcomes of colocating and breastfeeding from the pandemic's epicenter. J Perinatol 2020;40(10):1455–8.

67. Hoffmann M, Kleine-Weber H, Schroeder S, et al. SARS-CoV-2 Cell Entry Depends on ACE2 and TMPRSS2 and Is Blocked by a Clinically Proven Protease Inhibitor. Cell 2020;181(2):271–80.e278.

68. Diaz JH. Hypothesis: angiotensin-converting enzyme inhibitors and angiotensin receptor blockers may increase the risk of severe COVID-19. J Travel Med 2020;27(3).

69. Zhang ZJ, Yu XJ, Fu T, et al. Novel coronavirus infection in newborn babies aged <28 days in China. Eur Respir J 2020;55(6).

70. Rappaport L. Neonatal SARS-CoV-2 May Present With Hypoxemia Without Respiratory Distress. Medscape 2020.

71. Kamali Aghdam M, Jafari N, Eftekhari K. Novel coronavirus in a 15-day-old neonate with clinical signs of sepsis, a case report. Infect Dis (Lond) 2020; 52(6):427–9.

72. Dong Y, Mo X, Hu Y, et al. COVID-19 among child China. Epidemiol 2020;145(6): e20200702.

73. De Bernardo G, Giordano M, Zollo G, et al. The clinical course of SARS-CoV-2 positive neonates. J Perinatol 2020;40(10):1462–9.

74. Trevisanuto D, Cavallin F, Cavicchiolo ME, et al. Coronavirus infection in neonates: a systematic review. Arch Dis Child Fetal Neonatal Ed 2021;106(3):330–5.

75. Gale C, Quigley MA, Placzek A, et al. Characteristics and outcomes of neonatal SARS-CoV-2 infection in the UK: a prospective national cohort study using active surveillance. Lancet Child Adolesc Health 2021;5(2):113–21.

76. Dumitriu D, Emeruwa UN, Hanft E, et al. Outcomes of Neonates Born to Mothers With Severe Acute Respiratory Syndrome Coronavirus 2 Infection at a Large Medical Center in New York City. JAMA Pediatr 2021;175(2):157–67.

77. McCarty KL, Tucker M, Lee G, et al. Fetal Inflammatory Response Syndrome Associated with Maternal SARS-CoV-2 Infection. Pediatrics 2020. e2020010132.

78. Yu N, Li W, Kang Q, et al. Clinical features and obstetric and neonatal outcomes of pregnant patients with COVID-19 in Wuhan, China: a retrospective, single-centre, descriptive study. Lancet Infect Dis 2020;20(5):559–64.

79. Gupta M, Zupancic JAF, Pursley DM. Caring for newborns born to mothers with COVID-19: more questions than answers. Pediatrics 2020;146(2). e2020001842.

80. Cook TM, El-Boghdadly K, McGuire B, et al. Consensus guidelines for managing the airway in patients with COVID-19: guidelines from the Difficult Airway Society, the Association of Anaesthetists the Intensive Care Society, the Faculty of Intensive Care Medicine and the Royal College of Anaesthetists. Anaesthesia 2020; 75(6):785–99.

81. Edelson DP, Sasson C, Chan PS, et al. Interim guidance for basic and advanced life support in adults, children, and neonates with suspected or confirmed COVID-19: from the Emergency Cardiovascular Care Committee and Get With The Guidelines-Resuscitation Adult and Pediatric Task Forces of the American Heart Association. Circulation 2020;141(25):e933–43.

82. Centers for Disease Control. Evaluation and management considerations for neonates at risk for COVID-19 2020. Available at: https://www.cdc.gov/coronavirus/2019-ncov/hcp/caring-for-newborns.html. Accessed February 20, 2021.

83. Pang EM, Sey R, De Beritto T, et al. Advancing Health Equity by Translating Lessons Learned from NICU Family Visitations During the COVID-19 Pandemic. Neoreviews 2021;22(1):e1–6.

84. Horbar JD, Edwards EM, Soll RF, et al. COVID-19 and newborn care: April 2020. Pediatrics 2020. e2020002824.

85. Virani AK, Puls HT, Mitsos R, et al. Benefits and risks of visitor restrictions for hospitalized children during the COVID pandemic. Pediatrics 2020;146(2).

86. Turpin H, Urben S, Ansermet F, et al. The interplay between prematurity, maternal stress and children's intelligence quotient at age 11: a longitudinal study. Sci Rep 2019;9(1):450.

87. Salvatore CM, Han JY, Acker KP, et al. Neonatal management and outcomes during the COVID-19 pandemic: an observation cohort study. Lancet Child Adolesc Health 2020;4(10):721–7.

88. Cavicchiolo ME, Trevisanuto D, Lolli E, et al. Universal screening of high-risk neonates, parents, and staff at a neonatal intensive care unit during the SARS-CoV-2 pandemic. Eur J Pediatr 2020;179(12):1949–55.

89. Murray PD, Swanson JR. Visitation restrictions: is it right and how do we support families in the NICU during COVID-19? J Perinatol 2020;40:1576–81.

90. de Winter JP, De Luca D, Tingay DG. COVID-19 surveillance for all newborns at the NICU; conditio sine qua non? Eur J Pediatr 2020;179(12):1945–7.

The Effect of COVID-19 on Education

Jacob Hoofman, MS2[a], Elizabeth Secord, MD[b],*

KEYWORDS

- COVID-19 • Education • Virtual learning • Special education
- Medical school education

KEY POINTS

- Virtual learning has become a norm during COVID-19.
- Children requiring special learning services, those living in poverty, and those speaking English as a second language have lost more from the pandemic educational changes.
- For children with attention deficit disorder and no comorbidities, virtual learning has sometimes been advantageous.
- Math learning scores are more likely to be affected than language arts scores by pandemic changes.
- School meals, access to friends, and organized activities have also been lost with the closing of in-person school.

BACKGROUND

The transition to an online education during the coronavirus disease 2019 (COVID-19) pandemic may bring about adverse educational changes and adverse health consequences for children and young adult learners in grade school, middle school, high school, college, and professional schools. The effects may differ by age, maturity, and socioeconomic class. At this time, we have few data on outcomes, but many oversight organizations have tried to establish guidelines, expressed concerns, and extrapolated from previous experiences.

GENERAL EDUCATIONAL LOSSES AND DISPARITIES

Many researchers are examining how the new environment affects learners' mental, physical, and social health to help compensate for any losses incurred by this pandemic and to better prepare for future pandemics. There is a paucity of data at

[a] Wayne State University School of Medicine, 540 East Canfield, Detroit, MI 48201, USA;
[b] Department of Pediatrics, Wayne Pediatrics, School of Medicine, Pediatrics Wayne State University, 400 Mack Avenue, Detroit, MI 48201, USA
* Corresponding author.
E-mail address: esecord@med.wayne.edu

Pediatr Clin N Am 68 (2021) 1071–1079
https://doi.org/10.1016/j.pcl.2021.05.009
0031-3955/21/© 2021 Elsevier Inc. All rights reserved.
pediatric.theclinics.com

this juncture, but some investigators have extrapolated from earlier school shutdowns owing to hurricanes and other natural disasters.[1]

Inclement weather closures are estimated in some studies to lower middle school math grades by 0.013 to 0.039 standard deviations and natural disaster closures by up to 0.10 standard deviation decreases in overall achievement scores.[2] The data from inclement weather closures did show a more significant decrease for children dependent on school meals, but generally the data were not stratified by socioeconomic differences.[3,4] Math scores are impacted overall more negatively by school absences than English language scores for all school closures.[4,5]

The Northwest Evaluation Association is a global nonprofit organization that provides research-based assessments and professional development for educators. A team of researchers at Stanford University evaluated Northwest Evaluation Association test scores for students in 17 states and the District of Columbia in the Fall of 2020 and estimated that the average student had lost one-third of a year to a full year's worth of learning in reading, and about three-quarters of a year to more than 1 year in math since schools closed in March 2020.[5]

With school shifted from traditional attendance at a school building to attendance via the Internet, families have come under new stressors. It is increasingly clear that families depended on schools for much more than math and reading. Shelter, food, health care, and social well-being are all part of what children and adolescents, as well as their parents or guardians, depend on schools to provide.[5,6]

Many families have been impacted negatively by the loss of wages, leading to food insecurity and housing insecurity; some of loss this is a consequence of the need for parents to be at home with young children who cannot attend in-person school.[6] There is evidence that this economic instability is leading to an increase in depression and anxiety.[7] In 1 survey, 34.71% of parents reported behavioral problems in their children that they attributed to the pandemic and virtual schooling.[8]

Children have been infected with and affected by coronavirus. In the United States, 93,605 students tested positive for COVID-19, and it was reported that 42% were Hispanic/Latino, 32% were non-Hispanic White, and 17% were non-Hispanic Black, emphasizing a disproportionate effect for children of color.[9] COVID infection itself is not the only issue that affects children's health during the pandemic. School-based health care and school-based meals are lost when school goes virtual and children of lower socioeconomic class are more severely affected by these losses. Although some districts were able to deliver school meals, school-based health care is a primary source of health care for many children and has left some chronic conditions unchecked during the pandemic.[10]

Many families report that the stress of the pandemic has led to a poorer diet in children with an increase in the consumption of sweet and fried foods.[11,12] Shelter at home orders and online education have led to fewer exercise opportunities. Research carried out by Ammar and colleagues[12] found that daily sitting had increased from 5 to 8 hours a day and binge eating, snacking, and the number of meals were all significantly increased owing to lockdown conditions and stay-at-home initiatives. There is growing evidence in both animal and human models that diets high in sugar and fat can play a detrimental role in cognition and should be of increased concern in light of the pandemic.[13]

The family stress elicited by the COVID-19 shutdown is a particular concern because of compiled evidence that adverse life experiences at an early age are associated with an increased likelihood of mental health issues as an adult.[14] There is early evidence that children ages 6 to 18 years of age experienced a significant increase in their expression of "clinginess, irritability, and fear" during the early pandemic school shutdowns.[15] These emotions associated with anxiety may have a negative impact on the family unit, which was already stressed owing to the pandemic.

Another major concern is the length of isolation many children have had to endure since the pandemic began and what effects it might have on their ability to socialize. The school, for many children, is the agent for forming their social connections as well as where early social development occurs.[16] Noting that academic performance is also declining the pandemic may be creating a snowball effect, setting back children without access to resources from which they may never recover, even into adulthood.

Predictions from data analysis of school absenteeism, summer breaks, and natural disaster occurrences are imperfect for the current situation, but all indications are that we should not expect all children and adolescents to be affected equally.[4,5] Although some children and adolescents will likely suffer no long-term consequences, COVID-19 is expected to widen the already existing educational gap from socioeconomic differences, and children with learning differences are expected to suffer more losses than neurotypical children.[4,5]

SPECIAL EDUCATION AND THE COVID-19 PANDEMIC

Although COVID-19 has affected all levels of education reception and delivery, children with special needs have been more profoundly impacted. Children in the United States who have special needs have legal protection for appropriate education by the Individuals with Disabilities Education Act and Section 504 of the Rehabilitation Act of 1973.[17,18] Collectively, this legislation is meant to allow for appropriate accommodations, services, modifications, and specialized academic instruction to ensure that "every child receives a free appropriate public education . . . in the least restrictive environment."[17]

Children with autism usually have applied behavioral analysis (ABA) as part of their individualized educational plan. ABA therapists for autism use a technique of discrete trial training that shapes and rewards incremental changes toward new behaviors.[19] Discrete trial training involves breaking behaviors into small steps and repetition of rewards for small advances in the steps toward those behaviors. It is an intensive one-on-one therapy that puts a child and therapist in close contact for many hours at a time, often 20 to 40 hours a week. This therapy works best when initiated at a young age in children with autism and is often initiated in the home.[19]

Because ABA workers were considered essential workers from the early days of the pandemic, organizations providing this service had the responsibility and the freedom to develop safety protocols for delivery of this necessary service and did so in conjunction with certifying boards.[20]

Early in the pandemic, there were interruptions in ABA followed by virtual visits, and finally by in-home therapy with COVID-19 isolation precautions.[21] Although the efficacy of virtual visits for ABA therapy would empirically seem to be inferior, there are few outcomes data available. The balance of safety versus efficacy quite early turned to in-home services with interruptions owing to illness and decreased therapist availability owing to the pandemic.[21] An overarching concern for children with autism is the possible loss of a window of opportunity to intervene early. Families of children and adolescents with autism spectrum disorder report increased stress compared with families of children with other disabilities before the pandemic, and during the pandemic this burden has increased with the added responsibility of monitoring in-home schooling.[20]

Early data on virtual schooling children with attention deficit disorder (ADD) and attention deficit with hyperactivity (ADHD) shows that adolescents with ADD/ADHD found the switch to virtual learning more anxiety producing and more challenging than their peers.[22] However, according to a study in Ireland, younger children with ADD/ADHD and no other neurologic or psychiatric diagnoses who were stable on medication tended to report less anxiety with at-home schooling and their parents and caregivers reported improved behavior during the pandemic.[23] An unexpected benefit of shelter in home versus shelter in place may be to identify these stressors in face-to-face school for children with ADD/ADHD. If children with ADD/ADHD had an additional diagnosis of autism or depression, they reported increased anxiety with the school shutdown.[23,24]

Much of the available literature is anticipatory guidance for in-home schooling of children with disabilities rather than data about schooling during the pandemic. The American Academy of Pediatrics published guidance advising that, because 70% of students with ADHD have other conditions, such as learning differences, oppositional defiant disorder, or depression, they may have very different responses to in home schooling which are a result of the non-ADHD diagnosis, for example, refusal to attempt work for children with oppositional defiant disorder, severe anxiety for those with depression and or anxiety disorders, and anxiety and perseveration for children with autism.[25] Children and families already stressed with learning differences have had substantial challenges during the COVID-19 school closures.

HIGH SCHOOL, DEPRESSION, AND COVID-19

High schoolers have lost a great deal during this pandemic. What should have been a time of establishing more independence has been hampered by shelter-in-place recommendations. Graduations, proms, athletic events, college visits, and many other social and educational events have been altered or lost and cannot be recaptured.

Adolescents reported higher rates of depression and anxiety associated with the pandemic, and in 1 study 14.4% of teenagers report post-traumatic stress disorder, whereas 40.4% report having depression and anxiety.[26] In another survey adolescent boys reported a significant decrease in life satisfaction from 92% before COVID to 72% during lockdown conditions. For adolescent girls, the decrease in life satisfaction was from 81% before COVID to 62% during the pandemic, with the oldest teenage girls reporting the lowest life satisfaction values during COVID-19 restrictions.[27] During the school shutdown for COVID-19, 21% of boys and 27% of girls reported an increase in family arguments.[26] Combine all of these reports with decreasing access to mental health services owing to pandemic restrictions and it becomes a complicated matter for parents to address their children's mental health needs as well as their educational needs.[28]

A study conducted in Norway measured aspects of socialization and mood changes in adolescents during the pandemic. The opportunity for prosocial action was rated on a scale of 1 (not at all) to 6 (very much) based on how well certain phrases applied to them, for example, "I comforted a friend yesterday," "Yesterday I did my best to care for a friend," and "Yesterday I sent a message to a friend." They also ranked mood by rating items on a scale of 1 (not at all) to 5 (very well) as items reflected their mood.[29] They found that adolescents showed an overall decrease in empathic concern and opportunity for prosocial actions, as well as a decrease in mood ratings during the pandemic.[29]

A survey of 24,155 residents of Michigan projected an escalation of suicide risk for lesbian, gay, bisexual, transgender youth as well as those youth questioning their sexual orientation (LGBTQ) associated with increased social isolation. There was also a 66% increase in domestic violence for LGBTQ youth during shelter in place.[30] LGBTQ youth are yet another example of those already at increased risk having dispropor-tionate effects of the pandemic.

Increased social media use during COVID-19, along with traditional forms of educa-tion moving to digital platforms, has led to the majority of adolescents spending signif-icantly more time in front of screens. Excessive screen time is well-known to be associated with poor sleep, sedentary habits, mental health problems, and physical health issues.[31] With decreased access to physical activity, especially in crowded inner-city areas, and increased dependence on screen time for schooling, it is more difficult to craft easy solutions to the screen time issue.

During these times, it is more important than ever for pediatricians to check in on the mental health of patients with queries about how school is going, how patients are keeping contact with peers, and how are they processing social issues related to violence. Queries to families about the need for assistance with food insecurity, hous-ing insecurity, and access to mental health services are necessary during this time of public emergency.

MEDICAL SCHOOL AND COVID-19

Although medical school is an adult schooling experience, it affects not only the med-ical profession and our junior colleagues, but, by extrapolation, all education that re-quires hands-on experience or interning, and has been included for those reasons.

In the new COVID-19 era, medical schools have been forced to make drastic and quick changes to multiple levels of their curriculum to ensure both student and patient safety during the pandemic. Students entering their clinical rotations have had the most drastic alteration to their experience.

COVID-19 has led to some of the same changes high schools and colleges have adopted, specifically, replacement of large in-person lectures with small group activ-ities small group discussion and virtual lectures.[32] The transition to an online format for medical education has been rapid and impacted both students and faculty.[33,34] In a survey by Singh and colleagues,[33] of the 192 students reporting 43.9% found online lectures to be poorer than physical classrooms during the pandemic. In another report by Shahrvini and colleagues,[35] of 104 students surveyed, 74.5% students felt discon-nected from their medical school and their peers and 43.3% felt that they were unpre-pared for their clerkships. Although there are no pre-COVID-19 data for comparison, it is expected that the COVID-19 changes will lead to increased insecurity and feelings of poor preparation for clinical work.

Gross anatomy is a well-established tradition within the medical school curricu-lum and one that is conducted almost entirely in person and in close quarters around a cadaver. Harmon and colleagues[36] surveyed 67 gross anatomy educators and found that 8% were still holding in-person sessions and 34 ± 43% transitioned to using cadaver images and dissecting videos that could be accessed through the Internet.

Many third- and fourth-year medical students have seen periods of cancellation for clinical rotations and supplementation with online learning, telemedicine, or virtual rounds owing to the COVID-19 pandemic.[37] A study from Shahrvini and colleagues[38] found that an unofficial document from Reddit (a widely used social network platform with a subgroup for medical students and residents) reported that 75% of medical schools had canceled clinical activities for third- and fourth-year students for some part of 2020. In another survey by Harries and colleagues,[39] of the 741 students who responded, 93.7% were not involved in clinical rotations with in-person patient contact. The reactions of students varied, with 75.8% admitting to agreeing with the decision, 34.7% feeling guilty, and 27.0% feeling relieved.[39] In the same survey, 74.7% of students felt that their medical education had been disrupted, 84.1% said they felt increased anxiety, and 83.4% would accept the risk of COVID-19 infection if they were able to return to the clinical setting.[39]

Since the start of the pandemic, medical schools have had to find new and innovative ways to continue teaching and exposing students to clinical settings. The use of electronic conferencing services has been critical to continuing education. One approach has been to turn to online applications like Google Hangouts, which come at no cost and offer a wide variety of tools to form an integrative learning environment.[32,37,40] Schools have also adopted a hybrid model of teaching where lectures can be prerecorded then viewed by the student asynchronously on their own time followed by live virtual lectures where faculty can offer question-and-answer sessions related to the material. By offering this new format, students have been given more flexibility in terms of creating a schedule that suits their needs and may decrease stress.[37]

Although these changes can be a hurdle to students and faculty, it might prove to be beneficial for the future of medical training in some ways. Telemedicine is a growing field, and the American Medical Association and other programs have endorsed its value.[41] Telemedicine visits can still be used to take a history, conduct a basic visual physical examination, and build rapport, as well as performing other aspects of the clinical examination during a pandemic, and will continue to be useful for patients unable to attend regular visits at remote locations. Learning effectively now how to communicate professionally and carry out telemedicine visits may better prepare students for a future where telemedicine is an expectation and allow students to learn the limitations as well as the advantages of this modality.[41]

Pandemic changes have strongly impacted the process of college applications, medical school applications, and residency applications.[32] For US medical residencies, 72% of applicants will, if the pattern from 2016 to 2019 continues, move between states or countries.[42] This level of movement is increasingly dangerous given the spread of COVID-19 and the lack of currently accepted procedures to carry out such a mass migration safely. The same follows for medical schools and universities.

We need to accept and prepare for the fact that medial students as well as other learners who require in-person training may lack some skills when they enter their profession. These skills will have to be acquired during a later phase of training. We may have less skilled entry-level resident physicians and nurses in our hospitals and in other clinical professions as well.

SUMMARY

The COVID-19 pandemic has affected and will continue to affect the delivery of knowledge and skills at all levels of education. Although many children and adult learners will likely compensate for this interruption of traditional educational services and adapt to new modalities, some will struggle. The widening of the gap for those whose families cannot absorb the teaching and supervision of education required for in-home education because they lack the time and skills necessary are not addressed currently. The gap for those already at a disadvantage because of socioeconomic class, language, and special needs are most severely affected by the COVID-19 pandemic school closures and will have the hardest time compensating. As pediatricians, it is critical that we continue to check in with our young patients about how they are coping and what assistance we can guide them toward in our communities.

CLINICS CARE POINTS

- Learners and educators at all levels of education have been affected by COVID-19 restrictions with rapid adaptations to virtual learning platforms.
- The impact of COVID-19 on learners is not evenly distributed and children of racial minorities, those who live in poverty, those requiring special education, and children who speak English as a second language are more negatively affected by the need for remote learning.
- Math scores are more impacted than language arts scores by previous school closures and thus far by these shutdowns for COVID-19.
- Anxiety and depression have increased in children and particularly in adolescents as a result of COVID-19 itself and as a consequence of school changes.
- Pediatricians should regularly screen for unmet needs in their patients during the pandemic, such as food insecurity with the loss of school meals, an inability to adapt to remote learning and increased computer time, and heightened anxiety and depression as results of school changes.

DISCLOSURE

The authors have nothing to disclose.

REFERENCES

1. Harris D, Larsen M. The Effects of the New Orleans Post-Katrina Market-based School Reforms on Medium Term Student Outcomes. Education Research Alliance for New Orleans. New Orleans (LA): Tulane University; 2019. p. 160215. Available at: http://educationresearchalliancenola.org/files/publications/Harris-Larsen-Reform-Effects-2019-08-01.
2. Hansen D, Larden M. School year length and student performance: quasi experimental evidence. Social Sci Res Netw Paper 2011. https://doi.org/10.2139/ssrn.2269846.
3. Marcotte DE, Helmelt SW. Unscheduled school closings and student performance. Educ Finance Policy 2008;3(3):316–38.
4. Kuhfeld M, Soland J, Tarasawa B, et al. Projecting the potential impact of COVID-19 school closures on academic achievement. Educ Res 2020;49(8):549–65.
5. Kuhfeld M, Tarasawa B. The COVID-19 slide: what summer learning loss can tell us about the potential impact of school closures on student academic achievement. NWEA; 2020. ED609141.NWEA. Available at: eric.ed.gov/?id.
6. Wolfson JA, Leung CW. Food insecurity and COVID-19: disparities in early effects for US Adults. Nutrients 2020;12(6):1648.
7. Fegert JM, Vitiello B, Plener PL, et al. Challenges and burden of the coronavirus 2019 (COVID-19) pandemic for child and adolescent mental health: a narrative review to highlight clinical and research needs in the acute phase and the long return to normality. Child Adolesc Psychiatry Ment Health 2020;14:20.
8. Bobo E, Lin L, Acquaviva E, et al. How do children and adolescents with attention deficit hyperactivity disorder (ADHD) experience during the COVID-19 outbreak? Encephale 2020;46(3S).
9. Leeb RT, Price S, Sliwa S, et al. COVID-19 trends among school-aged children - United States, March 1-September 19, 2020. MMWR Morb Mortal Wkly Rep 2020; 69(39):1410–5.

10. Anderson S, Haeder S, Caseman K, et al. When adolescents are in school during COVID-19, coordination between school-based health centers and education is key. J Adolesc Health 2020;67(6):745–6.

11. Ruiz-Roso MB, de Carvalho Padilha P, Mantilla-Escalante DC, et al. Covid-19 confinement and changes of adolescent's dietary trends in Italy, Spain, Chile, Colombia and Brazil. Nutrients 2020;12(6):1807.

12. Ammar A, Brach M, Trabelsi K, et al. Effects of COVID-19 home confinement on eating behaviour and physical activity: results of the ECLB-COVID19 international online survey. Nutrients 2020;12(6):1583.

13. Yeomans M. Adverse effects of consuming high fat–sugar diets on cognition: Implications for understanding obesity. Proc Nutr Soc 2017;76(4):455–65.

14. Merrick MT, Ports KA, Ford DC, et al. Unpacking the impact of adverse childhood experiences on adult mental health. Child Abuse Negl 2017;69:10–9.

15. Singh S, Roy D, Sinha K, et al. Impact of COVID-19 and lockdown on mental health of children and adolescents: a narrative review with recommendations. Psychiatry Res 2020;293:113429.

16. Elkin F, Handel G. The child and society: the process of socialization. New York: Random House; 1972. The Child and Society: The Process of Socialization - Frederick Elkin, Gerald Handel - Google Books.

17. Keogh B. Celebrating PL 94-142: the education of All Handicapped Children Act of 1975. Issues Teach Educ Fall 2007;16(2):65–9.

18. United States Department of Education, Office of Special Education and Rehabilitative Services. History: twenty-five years of progress in educating children with disabilities through IDEA. Available at: http://www.ed.gov/policy/speced/leg/idea/history.pdf.

19. Spreat S. Chapter 10: behavioral treatments for children with ASDs. In: Reber M, editor. The autism Spectrum: Scientific Foundations and Treatment. Cambridge University Press; 2012. p. 239–57.

20. Cox DJ, Plavnick JB, Brodhead MT. A proposed process for risk mitigation during OID-19 pandemic. Behav Anal Pract 2020;13(2):299–305 (Behavior Analyst Certification Board.(2020) Ethics guidelines for ABA providers during COVID-19 pandemic. Available at: http://www.back.com/ethics-guidelines-for-aba-providers-during-covid-19-pandemic-2/.

21. Nicolson AC, Lazo-Pearson JF, Shandy J. ABA finding its heart during a pandemic: an exploration in social validity. Behav Anal Pract 2020;13:757–66.

22. Becker SP, Breaux R, Cusick C, et al. Remote learning during COVID-19: examining school practices, service continuation, and difficulties for adolescents with and without attention deficit hyperactivity disorder. J Adolesc Health 2020;67(6):769–77.

23. McGrath J. ADHD and COVID-19: current roadblocks and future opportunities. Ir J Psychol Med 2020;21:1–8.

24. Cortese S, Asherson P, Sonuga-Barke E, et al. ADHD management during the COVID-19 pandemic: guidance from the European ADHD Guidelines Group. Lancet Child Adolesc Health 2020;4(6):412–4.

25. Spinks-Franklin A. Available at: https://www.healthychildren.org/English/health-issues/conditions/COVID-19/Pages/ADHD-and-Learning-During-COVID-19.aspx. Accessed: January 27, 2021.

26. Liang L, Ren H, Cao R, et al. The effect of COVID-19 on youth mental health. Psychiatr Q 2020;91:841–52.

27. Soest TV, Bakken A, Pedersen W, et al. Life satisfaction among adolescents before and during the COVID-19 pandemic. Tidsskr Nor Laegeforen 2020;(10):140.
28. Lee J. Mental health effects of school closures during COVID-19 [published correction appears in Lancet Child Adolesc Health. 2020 Apr 17]. Lancet Child Adolesc Health 2020;4(6):421.
29. Van de Groep S, Zanolie K, Green KH, et al. A daily diary study on adolescents' mood, empathy, and prosocial behavior during the COVID-19 pandemic. PLoS One 2020;(10):15.
30. Edwards E, Janney CA, Mancuso A, et al. Preparing for the behavioral health impact of COVID-19 in Michigan. Curr Psychiatry Rep 2020;22(12):88.
31. Nagata JM, Abdel Magid HS, Gabriel KP. Screen time for children and adolescents during the COVID-19 pandemic. Obesity (Silver Spring) 2020;28:1582–3.
32. Rose S. Medical student education in the time of COVID-19. JAMA 2020;323(21): 2131–2.
33. Singh K, Srivastav S, Bhardwaj A, et al. Medical education during the COVID-19 pandemic: a single institution experience. Indian Pediatr 2020;57(7):678–9.
34. Wilcha RJ. Effectiveness of virtual medical teaching during the COVID-19 crisis: systematic review. JMIR Med Educ 2020;6(2):e20963.
35. Shahrvini B, Baxter SL, Coffey CS, et al. Pre-clinical remote undergraduate medical education during the COVID-19 pandemic: a survey study. Preprint Res Sq 2020;rs.3:rs-33870.
36. Harmon DJ, Attardi SM, Barremkala M, et al. An analysis of anatomy education before and during Covid-19: May-August 2020. Anat Sci Educ 2021;2:132–47.
37. Sandhu P, de Wolf M. The impact of COVID-19 on the undergraduate medical curriculum. Med Educ Online 2020;25(1):1764740.
38. Shahrvini B, Baxter SL, Coffey CS, et al. Pre-clinical remote undergraduate medical education during the COVID-19 pandemic: a survey study. BMC Med Educ 2021;21:13.
39. Harries AJ, Lee C, Jones L, et al. Effects of the COVID-19 pandemic on medical students: a multicenter quantitative study. BMC Med Educ 2021;21(1):14.
40. Moszkowicz D, Duboc H, Dubertret C, et al. Daily medical education for confined students during coronavirus disease 2019 pandemic: a simple videoconference solution. Clin Anat 2020;33(6):927–8.
41. Iancu AM, Kemp MT, Alam HB. Unmuting medical students' education: utilizing telemedicine during the COVID-19 pandemic and beyond. J Med Internet Res 2020;22(7):e19667.
42. Byrne LM, Holmboe ES, Combes JR, et al. From medical school to residency: transitions during the COVID-19 pandemic. J Grad Med Educ 2020;12(4): 507–11.

Neurological Effects of COVID-19 in Children

Tuhina Govil-Dalela, MD[a,b,c], Lalitha Sivaswamy, MD[c,d,e],*

KEYWORDS

- COVID-19 • SARS CoV-2 • Neurologic manifestations • Children

KEY POINTS

- COVID-19 is predominantly a respiratory disease that affects children less commonly and less seriously than adults.
- Neurologic manifestations, although more common in adults, are also being seen in children infected with the virus, especially those with multisystem inflammatory syndrome in children.
- Neurologic features of the virus are highly variable, involving the central as well as the peripheral nervous system.
- Multiple mechanisms of neurologic involvement by the virus have been postulated, including attachment to the neuronal ACE-2 receptors, via the olfactory nerve or immune-mediated pathogenesis. These mechanisms lead individually or collectively to an "endotheliopathy" with resultant neurologic symptoms.
- No specific treatments for the central or peripheral nervous system involvement are available to date; however, caution must be advised in administering immunotherapy where required, as this may decrease the body's innate immunity to fight the virus.

INTRODUCTION

In December 2019, a novel coronavirus, now designated as severe acute respiratory syndrome coronavirus 2 (SARS-CoV-2), was reported to cause a severe form of pneumonia in adults living in the Wuhan province of China in December 2019. The resultant clinical syndrome, termed COVID-19, has since been declared a pandemic, and cases have been reported from every country in the world.[1] In this article, the authors

The authors have no financial relationships to disclose.
a Department of Pediatrics, Children's Hospital of Michigan, Wayne State University, Detroit, MI, USA; b Department of Neurology, Children's Hospital of Michigan, Wayne State University, Detroit, MI, USA; c Department of Pediatric Neurology, Children's Hospital of Michigan Specialty Center, 2nd Floor, 3950 Beaubien Street, Detroit, MI 48202, USA; d Department of Pediatrics, Central Michigan University, Pleasant, MI, USA; e Department of Neurology, Central Michigan University, Pleasant, MI, USA
* Corresponding author. Department of Pediatric Neurology, Children's Hospital of Michigan Specialty Center, 2nd Floor, 3950 Beaubien Street, Detroit, MI 48202.
E-mail address: lsivaswamy@med.wayne.edu

describe the current state of knowledge regarding the neurologic complications of COVID-19 in children.

EPIDEMIOLOGY

Although children were initially thought to be immune from COVID-19, it is now known that children can indeed develop the disease and shed the virus, although a smaller proportion of the pediatric population suffers from disease-related morbidity and mortality compared with adults.[2] Children form only about 1% to 5% of all COVID-19 infections worldwide, and 80% of them are either asymptomatic or have mild infection.[3] In the largest published cohort thus far, 1% of affected children were less than 10 years of age and 1% were between 10 and 18 years of age.[4] The youngest reported patient was a 1-day-old.[5] In a study of more than 700 children from China who tested positive for the SARS-CoV-2 virus, less than 6% had severe symptoms requiring supplemental oxygen or admission to the hospital.[6]

In an adult cohort in Wuhan, 36.4% of patients with COVID-19 had neurologic manifestations, including headache, dizziness, stroke, or seizures.[7] Neurologic manifestations were mostly noted in those with severe underlying infection, suggested by more deranged laboratory markers like lymphopenia, D-dimer, and therefore, neurologic features may suggest a higher disease burden and possibly a higher viral load. In a Chinese study of 171 children, no neurologic manifestations were reported, whereas an Italian study reported only nonspecific headaches in 4% to 28% of affected children.[3,8] Incidence of neurologic manifestations in children with COVID-19 was reported as 9.2% in a meta-analysis of 28 pediatric studies, with a total of 199 children included.[9] However, with the recently described multisystem inflammatory syndrome in children (MIS-C), which may be a postinfectious immune response to prior infection, the incidence of neurologic manifestations has reportedly increased to 34%.[10]

PATHOPHYSIOLOGY

SARS-CoV-2 may enter the central nervous system (CNS) through hematogenous spread or retrograde transmission (**Fig. 1**).

SARS-CoV-2 appears to have neurotropic potential similar to SARS-CoV and MERS (Middle East respiratory syndrome) viruses as well as other respiratory viruses, such as

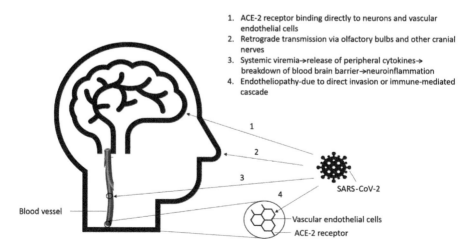

1. ACE-2 receptor binding directly to neurons and vascular endothelial cells
2. Retrograde transmission via olfactory bulbs and other cranial nerves
3. Systemic viremia→release of peripheral cytokines→ breakdown of blood brain barrier→neuroinflammation
4. Endotheliopathy-due to direct invasion or immune-mediated cascade

Fig. 1. Proposed mechanisms of neuroinvasion by SARS-CoV-2.

influenza, respiratory syncytial virus, Human Herpes Virus (HHV)-6 and -7, echovirus, and coxsackie virus. Autopsy reports of edema in the medulla oblongata with microscopic evidence of neuronal degeneration in this part of the brain stem may explain the depressed respiratory drive in infected patients.[11] Indirect evidence of neurotropism with resultant astrocytic and neuronal injury is provided by studies demonstrating elevated serum levels of biomarkers such as glial fibrillary acidic protein (GFAP) and neurofilament (nFL). GFAP is a marker of glial activation, whereas nFL is indicative of neuronal injury.[12] More importantly, in vitro replicability of SARS-CoV-2 has been demonstrated in pulmonary, intestinal, hepatic, renal, and neuronal cells.[13]

Evidence for hematogenous spread is obtained from electron microscopic studies noting the presence of viral particles in the endothelial cells of the brain capillaries.[14] Angiotensin converting enzyme 2 (ACE2) has gathered interest as the binding target receptor of CoV-2 on the vascular endothelium. SARS-CoV-2 differs from SARS-CoV because of 380 amino-acid substitutions that lead to differences in the viral spike protein (S), which forms a key part of the receptor binding domain. These changes cause the novel SARS virus to have greater binding affinity with the ACE2 receptor, which is expressed on a variety of cells, including neurons.[15] The entry of the virus into cells is facilitated by the interaction between the trimeric viral S protein with the extracellular domain of the transmembrane ACE2 protein. ACE2, in turn, constitutes an important mechanism for negative regulation of the renin angiotensin pathway (RAS). The disinhibition of the RAS pathway that is caused by binding of the virus to ACE2 leads to direct loss of ACE2 receptors and via proteolytic processing and shedding, may drive the systemic manifestations of COVID-19, making it a far more serious disease than SARS-CoV that primarily led to an acute respiratory distress syndrome phenotype.[16]

Retrograde axonal transmission predominantly via the olfactory bulb has been proposed as another potential mechanism to explain the spread of SARS-CoV-2 to the CNS. Experiments in mice have demonstrated that intranasal infection with SARS-CoV can lead to disruption of the nasal epithelium and subsequent neuroinvasion.[17] The presence of anosmia in infected individuals may also lend credence to this theory of neuroinvasion via the olfactory cells, the only part of the CNS not protected by dura mater. Retrograde transmission through other cranial nerves has also been postulated via the tongue through cranial nerve VII, IX, and X to the nucleus of tractus solitarius, the thalamus, and then the cortex, or through the corneal and buccal epithelium via cranial nerve V.[18]

In addition to the above proposed mechanisms, the neurologic effects of SARS-CoV-2 may also be related to release of inflammatory agents that can occur with systemic viremia. These inflammatory chemicals may lead to partial break down of the blood-brain barrier (BBB), thereby allowing peripheral cytokines to gain access to the CNS, which in turn can exacerbate or trigger neuroinflammation.[19,20] In the pediatric population, this mechanism may assume special importance as a systemic inflammatory/autoinflammatory response with multiorgan dysfunction and has been widely reported.[21,22] Therefore, in a sense, the CNS manifestations of SARS-CoV-2 may be due to an "endotheliopathy,"-either because of direct invasion of the endothelial cells in the vasculature of the BBB or because of an immune-mediated cascade that causes swelling or inflammation of these cells.[23]

CLINICAL FEATURES
Central Nervous System

Manifestations described in children and adults

1. *Meningitis/encephalitis/encephalopathy*: In a meta-analysis of 187 children with MIS-C, 64 (34%) were reported to have symptoms suggestive of meningitis or

encephalitis, including headache, positive meningeal signs, and altered mental status. Of these children, only 8 had evaluation of the cerebrospinal fluid (CSF). Five of them showed CSF pleocytosis, but none had SARS-CoV-2 isolated via CSF reverse transcription-polymerase chain reaction (RT-PCR).[10] In another study of 27 children with COVID-19 based in the United Kingdom, 4 (15%) had altered mentation, encephalopathy, headaches, and brainstem and cerebellar ataxia.[24] One of the youngest reported children with COVID-19–related neurologic involvement was a 6-week-old infant who has episodes of bilateral leg stiffening and sustained upward gaze.[25] Several reported cases of adults with altered mental status, meningismus, seizures, and occasionally focal neurologic deficits, including facial weakness, diplopia, and oscillopsia, have also been described.[26] Some of these patients demonstrated a positive CSF RT-PCR for SARS-CoV-2.[27] Apart from the neurotropism of the virus itself, another possible mechanism of the encephalopathy may be the severe hypoxia seen in these patients, which may cause cerebral vasodilation and eventually diffuse cerebral edema.[28]

2. *Seizures*: In a multicenter Italian study on children with SARS-CoV-2, 3% of children were noted to have seizures, with 60% of these children having an underlying diagnosis of epilepsy.[29] The seizures were not associated with fever in all cases. A detailed description of seizure semiology or duration was not provided in these cases either. In a case series of 8 critically ill pediatric patients, a 10-month-old was described who had intussusception, multiorgan dysfunction disseminated intravascular coagulation, toxic encephalopathy, and status epilepticus.[30] Seizures were also reported along with fever, cough, and vomiting, in a 2-year-old girl with RT-PCR–confirmed COVID-19 by nasopharyngeal swab.[31]

3. *Stroke*: Acute cerebrovascular disease in COVID-19 may manifest as intraparenchymal hemorrhage, large vessel occlusion, or venous sinus thrombosis. A 16-year-old boy with aseptic meningitis, cavernous sinus thrombosis, followed by left middle cerebral artery stroke and eventual death was described in the French literature.[32] However, it is not clear if arterial strokes are predominantly due to large or small vessel disease. It is postulated that SARS-CoV-2 leads to vessel thrombosis secondary to endothelial dysfunction, stasis, platelet activation, or inflammation.[33]

4. *Possible developmental delay*: Vertical transmission of the virus from mother to fetus has not been demonstrated; however, the effects of fetal exposure to chronic maternal viremia in utero on long-term neurodevelopmental outcomes are unknown at this time.[18]

5. *Loss of sense of smell and taste (anosmia and ageusia)*: Anosmia is commonly seen in the adults who have milder disease. A reported incidence of 34% to 89% has been noted in studies involving adults. Anosmia and ageusia have also been occasionally reported in the pediatric population.[34,35] The incidence in children was estimated to be about 0.5% in a meta-analysis of 199 children.[9] Another case series reported children presenting solely with anosmia and ageusia in the absence of any other manifestations of the disease.[36]

Manifestations described only in adults so far

6. *Acute disseminated encephalomyelitis (ADEM) and myelitis*: Two case reports have described adults with encephalopathy and focal neurologic deficits (one with dysphagia and dysarthria; the other with seizures), normal CSF, and hyperintensities on MRI.[37,38] Both patients improved with immunotherapy (steroids and intravenous immunoglobulin [IVIg], respectively). A case report from Wuhan, China described the only case of COVID and myelitis with acute flaccid paraparesis,

incontinence, hyporeflexia, and a sensory level in the thoracic spine.[39] MRI was not performed in this case because of high infectivity during the pandemic.

7. *Acute necrotizing hemorrhagic encephalopathy*: A single case of symmetric, multifocal involvement of the brain parenchyma, including the thalamus, in an adult patient has been described.[40] This is a known, rare entity seen postviral infections, usually in the pediatric age group and is thought to occur secondary to a cytokine storm with breakdown of BBB.

8. *Neuropsychiatric disorders (including neurocognitive) and dementia-like syndrome*: Presenting as altered mental status, this manifestation was described in a surveillance study of 153 patients with neurologic features from the United Kingdom.[41]

Peripheral Nervous System

Manifestations described in children and adults

1. *Guillain-Barré syndrome (GBS)*: Several case reports have been published describing classic GBS a few days to weeks after a severe infection with SARS-CoV-2. Common presenting symptoms included lower limb/all limb weakness, paresthesia, and ataxia.[42] Electrophysiological studies were consistent with demyelinating disease or axonal disease. Two such cases have also been described in children.[43,44] These children were 11 and 15 years old, respectively, and developed weakness about 3 weeks after upper respiratory infection symptoms, and both cases had nerve conduction velocity studies consistent with GBS.

2. *Nonspecific peripheral nervous system*: Global proximal muscle weakness and hyporeflexia were described in 15% and 7% of the children, respectively, in a small UK-based study.[24]

3. *Muscle injury and rhabdomyolysis*: There have been 2 case reports of adolescents presenting with rhabdomyolysis as one of the initial symptoms, one presented with isolated rhabdomyolysis and later developed other symptoms, while the other had associated fever and shortness of breath from the onset of the disease. There has been at least 1 pediatric case of rhabdomyolysis albeit a 16 year old.[45] Cases with rhabdomyolysis with elevated creatine kinase resulting from muscle injury have also been described in adults as a late manifestation of COVID-19.[46,47]

Aside from the clinical manifestations of the disease itself, it should also be recognized that the features and impact of the disease may be different in patients with underlying comorbidities. Patients with neuromuscular disease should be considered at a higher risk of complications, because of possible involvement of breathing and swallowing muscles.[48] Infection with SARS-CoV-2 may also cause exacerbation or progression of underlying myasthenia gravis and spinal muscular atrophy.[49] A French study described a 17-year-old girl with underlying severe neonatal encephalopathy and epilepsy, who presented with severe respiratory distress secondary to COVID-19. The decision to withdraw care and not intubate was made because of underlying severe comorbidities and poor quality of life.[32]

INVESTIGATIONS
MRI of the Brain

MRI of the brain in children with neurologic manifestations of COVID-19 has been reported to demonstrate acute lesions in the splenium of the corpus callosum.[24] Such lesions may be representative of intra-myelin edema and as such may occur in a variety of disorders, including other forms of viral encephalitis, demyelination, or CNS malignancies, such as lymphoma.[50] Larger case series in adults who have involvement of the CNS in COVID-19 point to the presence of acute/subacute infarcts, leukoencephalopathy involving the subcortical and deep white matter, cortical abnormalities on fluid-attenuated inversion recovery sequences, microhemorrhages, and leptomeningeal enhancement as the more common features. Posterior reversible encephalopathy syndrome–like features, acute hemorrhagic necrotizing encephalopathy, and dural venous sinus thrombosis were less frequently reported, and only 15% patients had normal imaging.[51] However, because large case series of this nature are lacking in children, it cannot be stated with certainty if similar findings are likely to be present in the pediatric age group. It is possible that certain radiological findings may only be present in adults with COVID-19. For instance, although a temporary increase in the size of the olfactory bulbs, signal changes, and contrast uptake has been reported in certain adults with COVID-19–related anosmia, no such changes could be documented in children with anosmia.[52] A few reports commenting on the use of other imaging modalities, such as PET, are emerging in adults but not yet in the pediatric age group.[53]

Electroencephalography

EEG features of COVID-19 appear to be nonspecific and consist of generalized slowing.[24]

Cerebrospinal Fluid Studies

CSF has been reported to be acellular in most reported cases, with negative SARS-CoV-2 cultures and no other evidence of inflammatory disease process, such as presence of oligoclonal bands. RT-PCR presence of SARS-CoV-2 in CSF has been reported to be positive in rare cases of adults with encephalitis, but no such cases have been reported yet in children.[42]

Histopathology

Histopathological correlates are now emerging, and cases with ADEM-like pathologic condition are being reported with axonal injury, perivascular lymphocytic infiltration, neuronal loss, and interstitial inflammatory changes.[54]

TREATMENT OPTIONS
Treatment of Neurologic Complications of COVID-19

No specific treatment exists for the neurologic manifestations, and the treating physician must depend on symptom-based management. IVIg and plasmapheresis have been used in the treatment of ADEM and GBS, as they are in non-COVID–based situations. Antiepileptics must be used for the management of seizures. Critically ill children may require management of airway and circulation issues in a critical care unit.

Treatment of Other Neurologic Conditions During the COVID-19 Pandemic

Medications used for migraines in pediatric patients are considered safe for use during the pandemic, with the initial reservations regarding the use of nonsteroidal anti-inflammatory drugs, including ibuprofen, having been dismissed by the World Health Organization and European Medicines Agency.[55,56]

Treatment of Patients with Underlying Neuroimmunologic Disorders

An important consideration is the treatment of patients with underlying neuroimmunologic diseases, including multiple sclerosis and neuromyelitis optica spectrum disorder. It is not entirely clear if these patients are at a higher risk of severe COVID-19 infection and complications compared with the general population and depending on the specific medications they are on. Alemtuzumab, cladribine, fingolimod, and B-cell–depleting agents (used in individuals with multiple sclerosis) may increase risk of infection, whereas glatiramer, dimethyl fumarate, and teriflunomide should not.[45] In general, it has been proposed that steroids, IVIg, and plasmapheresis are safe to administer during the pandemic in the case of an exacerbation of the underlying condition. Patients who are already on immunosuppressive therapy should continue the same therapy during the pandemic and even if they develop mild symptoms. Those with a severe COVID-19 infection may need to stop immunosuppressants, but this is best determined based on the specific situation and underlying factors.

Drug Interactions Between COVID-19 Therapy and Drugs Used in Neurologic Conditions

Treatments for the COVID-19 disease are constantly evolving, and several medications have been suggested and studied. In general, they include anti-inflammatory agents (usually corticosteroids), antivirals (remdesivir, favipiravir), and in most cases, anticoagulation drugs (usually aspirin or clopidogrel).[57] Other medications, like hydroxychloroquine and ivermectin, were also suggested at the beginning of the pandemic, but their efficacy in this infection is not well proven. Some patients on chloroquine have been shown to have seizures.[58] Chloroquine and hydroxychloroquine have also been shown to prolong QTc and should be used with caution in patients on tricyclic antidepressants (used in children with migraine or depression), which have the same side effect.

Hydroxychloroquine, chloroquine, and remdesivir carry the risk of drug interactions and enzymatic induction/inhibition when combined with carbamazepine, phenytoin, phenobarbital, and primidone, which are commonly used antiepileptic agents.[28] Ritonavir, also used in some cases, can lead to induction of CYP450.[59] Azithromycin should be used with caution in patients with myasthenia gravis, as it may exacerbate symptoms or cause new-onset myasthenia gravis.[60] Tocilizumab and anakinra have not been associated with any CNS side effects or interactions with any drugs. Patients with preexisting neurologic conditions requiring infliximab can generally be continued without significant adverse effects or increased risk for COVID-19. However, enough data are not available, and registries are required to collect more information.[1]

DIFFERENTIAL DIAGNOSIS

There is an extensive list of differential diagnoses for the neurologic complications of the virus. It includes several other respiratory viruses, as well as noninfectious causes that may be associated with each symptom. It is important, however, to consider COVID-19 or a COVID-19 postinflammatory syndrome, such as MIS-C, when evaluating a patient with any of the manifestations described above. It is important to note that the sensitivity and specificity of the testing process are not 100%, leading to possible missed diagnoses. In addition, case reports of different and novel findings are being published on a daily basis.

SUMMARY

The COVID-19 pandemic has affected upwards of 93 million people worldwide, causing more than 2 million deaths so far (as of January 15, 2021). It has affected adults more than children; however, the disease affects people of different age groups in a dissimilar manner, resulting in protean manifestations. The proportion of children with CNS and peripheral nervous system involvement in those infected with COVID-19 may be low; however, the sheer number of patients infected with the virus could make the absolute number of patients with these complications exceptionally large. Therefore, continued collection of accurate data, detailed descriptions of various neurologic manifestations, along with efforts to isolate the virus from CSF and autopsy samples will provide more answers in the future. Up until that point, management decisions will have to be made according to available evidence on a case-by-case basis.

CLINICS CARE POINTS

- Management of neurologic complications of COVID-19 is similar to that of non-COVID-19–affected patients, including intravenous immunoglobulin and plasmapheresis for inflammatory demyelination and antiepileptic drugs for seizures.

- Medications for migraines are generally considered to be safe. There are no limitations to using nonsteroidal anti-inflammatory drugs in severe acute respiratory syndrome coronavirus 2–infected patients.

- In those with underlying neuroimmunologic conditions, steroids, intravenous immunoglobulins, and plasmapheresis are safe to administer during the pandemic in the case of an exacerbation of the underlying condition. Patients who are already on immunosuppressive therapy should continue the same therapy during the pandemic and even if they develop mild symptoms of COVID-related disease. Those with severe COVID-19 infection may need to temporarily suspend immunosuppressants, but this is best determined based on the specific situation and underlying factors.

REFERENCES

1. Cucinotta D, Vanelli M. WHO declares COVID-19 a pandemic. Acta Biomed 2020;91(1):157–60.
2. Christy A. COVID-19: a review for the pediatric neurologist. J Child Neurol 2020; 35(13):934–9.
3. Parri N, Lenge M, Buonsenso D. Children with Covid-19 in pediatric emergency departments in Italy. N Engl J Med 2020;383(2):187–90.
4. Wu Z, McGoogan JM. Characteristics of and important lessons from the coronavirus disease 2019 (COVID-19) outbreak in China: summary of a report of 72 314 cases from the Chinese Center for Disease Control and Prevention. JAMA 2020; 323(13):1239–42.
5. Lorenz N, Treptow A, Schmidt S, et al. Neonatal early-onset infection with SARS-CoV-2 in a newborn presenting with encephalitic symptoms. Pediatr Infect Dis J 2020;39(8):e212.
6. Dong Y, Mo X, Hu Y, et al. Epidemiology of COVID-19 among children in China. Pediatrics 2020;145(6):e20200702.
7. Mao L, Jin H, Wang M, et al. Neurologic manifestations of hospitalized patients with coronavirus disease 2019 in Wuhan, China. JAMA Neurol 2020;77(6): 683–90.
8. Lu X, Zhang L, Du H, et al. SARS-CoV-2 infection in children. N Engl J Med 2020; 382(17):1663–5.
9. Pousa PA, Mendonça TSC, Oliveira EA, et al. Extrapulmonary manifestations of COVID-19 in children: a comprehensive review and pathophysiological considerations. J Pediatr (Rio J). 2020;97(2):116–39.
10. Chen TH. Neurological involvement associated with COVID-19 infection in children. J Neurol Sci 2020;418:117096.

11. Li YC, Bai WZ, Hashikawa T. The neuroinvasive potential of SARS-CoV2 may play a role in the respiratory failure of COVID-19 patients. J Med Virol 2020;92(6): 552–5.

12. Kanberg N, Ashton NJ, Andersson LM, et al. Neurochemical evidence of astrocytic and neuronal injury commonly found in COVID-19. Neurology 2020; 95(12):e1754–9.

13. Chu H, Chan JF, Yuen TT, et al. Comparative tropism, replication kinetics, and cell damage profiling of SARS-CoV-2 and SARS-CoV with implications for clinical manifestations, transmissibility, and laboratory studies of COVID-19: an observational study. Lancet Microbe 2020;1(1):e14–23.

14. Paniz-Mondolfi A, Bryce C, Grimes Z, et al. Central nervous system involvement by severe acute respiratory syndrome coronavirus-2 (SARS-CoV-2). J Med Virol 2020;92(7):699–702.

15. Hamming I, Timens W, Bulthuis ML, et al. Tissue distribution of ACE2 protein, the functional receptor for SARS coronavirus. A first step in understanding SARS pathogenesis. J Pathol 2004;203(2):631–7.

16. Gheblawi M, Wang K, Viveiros A, et al. Angiotensin-converting enzyme 2: SARS-CoV-2 receptor and regulator of the renin-angiotensin system: celebrating the 20th anniversary of the discovery of ACE2. Circ Res 2020;126(10):1456–74.

17. Desforges M, Le Coupanec A, Dubeau P, et al. Human coronaviruses and other respiratory viruses: underestimated opportunistic pathogens of the central nervous system? Viruses 2019;12(1):14.

18. Stafstrom CE, Jantzie LL. COVID-19: neurological considerations in neonates and children. Children (Basel) 2020;7(9):133.

19. Platt MP, Bolding KA, Wayne CR, et al. Th17 lymphocytes drive vascular and neuronal deficits in a mouse model of postinfectious autoimmune encephalitis. Proc Natl Acad Sci U S A 2020;117(12):6708–16.

20. Cain MD, Salimi H, Diamond MS, et al. Mechanisms of pathogen invasion into the central nervous system. Neuron 2019;103(5):771–83.

21. Nakra NA, Blumberg DA, Herrera-Guerra A, et al. Multi-system inflammatory syndrome in children (MIS-C) following SARS-CoV-2 infection: review of clinical presentation, hypothetical pathogenesis, and proposed management. Children (Basel) 2020;7(7):69.

22. Kaushik S, Aydin SI, Derespina KR, et al. Multisystem inflammatory syndrome in children associated with severe acute respiratory syndrome coronavirus 2 infection (MIS-C): a multi-institutional study from New York City. J Pediatr 2020; 224:24–9.

23. Varga Z, Flammer AJ, Steiger P, et al. Endothelial cell infection and endotheliitis in COVID-19. Lancet 2020;395(10234):1417–8.

24. Abdel-Mannan O, Eyre M, Löbel U, et al. Neurologic and radiographic findings associated with COVID-19 infection in children. JAMA Neurol 2020;77(11): 1440–5.

25. Dugue R, Cay-Martínez KC, Thakur KT, et al. Neurologic manifestations in an infant with COVID-19. Neurology 2020;94(24):1100–2.

26. Wong PF, Craik S, Newman P, et al. Lessons of the month 1: a case of rhombencephalitis as a rare complication of acute COVID-19 infection. Clin Med (Lond) 2020;20(3):293–4.

27. Moriguchi T, Harii N, Goto J, et al. A first case of meningitis/encephalitis associated with SARS-coronavirus-2. Int J Infect Dis 2020;94:55–8.

28. Orsini A, Corsi M, Santangelo A, et al. Challenges and management of neurological and psychiatric manifestations in SARS-CoV-2 (COVID-19) patients. Neurol Sci 2020;41(9):2353–66.
29. Garazzino S, Montagnani C, Donà D, et al. Multicentre Italian study of SARS-CoV-2 infection in children and adolescents, preliminary data as at 10 April 2020. Euro Surveill 2020;25(18):2000600.
30. Sun D, Li H, Lu XX, et al. Clinical features of severe pediatric patients with coronavirus disease 2019 in Wuhan: a single center's observational study. World J Pediatr 2020;16(3):251–9.
31. Tan X, Huang J, Zhao F, et al. [Clinical features of children with SARS-CoV-2 infection: an analysis of 13 cases from Changsha, China]. Zhongguo Dang Dai Er Ke Za Zhi 2020;22(4):294–8.
32. Oualha M, Bendavid M, Berteloot L, et al. Severe and fatal forms of COVID-19 in children. Arch Pediatr 2020;27(5):235–8.
33. Connors JM, Levy JH. COVID-19 and its implications for thrombosis and anticoagulation. Blood 2020;135(23):2033–40.
34. Giacomelli A, Pezzati L, Conti F, et al. Self-reported olfactory and taste disorders in patients with severe acute respiratory coronavirus 2 infection: a cross-sectional study. Clin Infect Dis 2020;71(15):889–90.
35. Lechien JR, Chiesa-Estomba CM, De Siati DR, et al. Olfactory and gustatory dysfunctions as a clinical presentation of mild-to-moderate forms of the coronavirus disease (COVID-19): a multicenter European study. Eur Arch Otorhinolaryngol 2020;277(8):2251–61.
36. Mak PQ, Chung K-S, Wong JS-C, et al. Anosmia and ageusia: not an uncommon presentation of COVID-19 infection in children and adolescents. Pediatr Infect Dis J 2020;39(8):e199–200.
37. Zanin L, Saraceno G, Panciani PP, et al. SARS-CoV-2 can induce brain and spine demyelinating lesions. Acta Neurochir (Wien) 2020;162(7):1491–4.
38. Zhang T, Hirsh E, Zandieh S, et al. COVID-19-Associated acute multi-infarct encephalopathy in an asymptomatic CADASIL patient. Neurocritical care 2020;1–4.
39. Zhao K, Huang J, Dai D, et al. Acute myelitis after SARS-CoV-2 infection: a case report. MedRxiv 2020. [Epub ahead of print].
40. Poyiadji N, Shahin G, Noujaim D, et al. COVID-19-associated acute hemorrhagic necrotizing encephalopathy: imaging features. Radiology 2020;296(2):E119–20.
41. Varatharaj A, Thomas N, Ellul MA, et al. Neurological and neuropsychiatric complications of COVID-19 in 153 patients: a UK-wide surveillance study. Lancet Psychiatry 2020;7(10):875–82.
42. Ellul MA, Benjamin L, Singh B, et al. Neurological associations of COVID-19. Lancet Neurol 2020;19(9):767–83.
43. Khalifa M, Zakaria F, Ragab Y, et al. Guillain-Barré syndrome associated with severe acute respiratory syndrome coronavirus 2 detection and coronavirus disease 2019 in a child. J Pediatr Infect Dis Soc 2020;9(4):510–3.
44. Frank CHM, Almeida TVR, Marques EA, et al. Guillain-Barré syndrome associated with SARS-CoV-2 infection in a pediatric patient. J Trop Pediatr 2020. https://doi.org/10.1093/tropej/fmaa044.
45. Korsukewitz C, Reddel SW, Bar-Or A, et al. Neurological immunotherapy in the era of COVID-19 - looking for consensus in the literature. Nat Rev Neurol 2020;16(9):493–505.
46. Jin M, Tong Q. Rhabdomyolysis as potential late complication associated with COVID-19. Emerg Infect Dis 2020;26(7):1618–20.

47. Suwanwongse K, Shabarek N. Rhabdomyolysis as a presentation of 2019 novel coronavirus disease. Cureus 2020;12(4):e7561.
48. Guidon AC, Amato AA. COVID-19 and neuromuscular disorders. Neurology 2020;94(22):959–69.
49. Gummi RR, Kukulka NA, Deroche CB, et al. Factors associated with acute exacerbations of myasthenia gravis. Muscle Nerve 2019;60(6):693–9.
50. Doherty MJ, Jayadev S, Watson NF, et al. Clinical implications of splenium magnetic resonance imaging signal changes. Arch Neurol 2005;62(3):433–7.
51. Gulko E, Oleksk ML, Gomes W, et al. MRI brain findings in 126 patients with COVID-19: initial observations from a descriptive literature review. AJNR Am J Neuroradiol 2020;41(12):2199–203.
52. Hatipoglu N, Mine Yazici Z, Palabiyik F, et al. Olfactory bulb magnetic resonance imaging in SARS-CoV-2-induced anosmia in pediatric cases. Int J Pediatr Otorhinolaryngol 2020;139:110469.
53. Delorme C, Paccoud O, Kas A, et al. Covid-19-related encephalopathy: a case series with brain FDG-PET/CT findings. Eur J Neurol 2020;27(12):2651–7.
54. Paterson RW, Brown RL, Benjamin L, et al. The emerging spectrum of COVID-19 neurology: clinical, radiological and laboratory findings. Brain 2020;143(10):3104–20.
55. Szperka CL, Ailani J, Barmherzig R, et al. Migraine care in the era of COVID-19: clinical pearls and plea to insurers. Headache 2020;60(5):833–42.
56. Agency EM. EMA gives advice on the use of non-steroidal anti-inflammatories for COVID-19. The Netherlands: European Medicines Agency; 2020.
57. Jean SS, Lee PI, Hsueh PR. Treatment options for COVID-19: the reality and challenges. J Microbiol Immunol Infect 2020;53(3):436–43.
58. Mülhauser P, Allemann Y, Regamey C. Chloroquine and nonconvulsive status epilepticus. Ann Intern Med 1995;123(1):76–7.
59. Brooks J, Daily J, Schwamm L. Protease inhibitors and anticonvulsants. AIDS Clin Care 1997;9(11):87–90.
60. May EF, Calvert PC. Aggravation of myasthenia gravis by erythromycin. Ann Neurol 1990;28(4):577–9.

Care of Pediatric Patients with Diabetes During the Coronavirus Disease 2019 (COVID-19) Pandemic

Colleen Buggs-Saxton, MD, PhD*

KEYWORDS

- Pediatric type 1 diabetes • COVID-19 pandemic • Diabetic ketoacidosis
- Telemedicine

KEY POINTS

- During the COVID-19 pandemic pediatric patients with new-onset diabetes often presented with more severe diabetic ketoacidosis (DKA).
- Most pediatric patients with type 1 diabetes (T1D) who developed COVID-19 had mild disease or were asymptomatic similar to children without diabetes.
- Stay-at-home initiatives and school closures often resulted in improved glycemic control for children with diabetes secondary to closer parental monitoring.
- Improved telemedicine adaptations for pediatric diabetic teams will likely continue to support care for these children after the pandemic.

CORONAVIRUS DISEASE 2019 AND DIABETES

The coronavirus disease 2019 (COVID-19), which is caused by the severe acute respiratory syndrome coronavirus-2 (SARS-CoV-2), created a pandemic in March 2020 with now more than 120 million cases and more than 2.5 million deaths worldwide. Early observations from studies in China, Italy, England, and the United States reported that adults with diabetes were more vulnerable to developing severe complications of COVID-19 including severe acute respiratory syndrome (SARS) with multiorgan failure and death.[1–3] As type 2 diabetes (T2D) is the more common form of diabetes in adults, it was unclear during the early phase of the pandemic if there was a similar increased risk of morbidity among individuals with type 1 diabetes (T1D) and COVID-19. One study of hospitalized adult patients with COVID-19 in the United Kingdom reported that of the 23,698 patients who died, one-third had diabetes with 31.4% T2D compared with 1.5% T1D.[4] Observations in adults with T2D and

Department of Pediatrics, Wayne Pediatrics, Wayne State University School of Medicine, 400 Mack Avenue, Suite 1East, Detroit, MI 48201, USA
* Corresponding author.
E-mail address: cbuggs@med.wayne.edu

Pediatr Clin N Am 68 (2021) 1093–1101
https://doi.org/10.1016/j.pcl.2021.05.014
0031-3955/21/© 2021 Elsevier Inc. All rights reserved.

pediatric.theclinics.com

COVID-19 reported higher morbidity in individuals with a history of microvascular and macrovascular complications associated with diabetes.[5] Therefore, early during the COVID-19 pandemic diabetes was one of the major pre-existing conditions associated with increased morbidity and mortality.

It was important to further understand factors that contributed to lower rates of hospitalization among individuals with T1D during the COVID-19 pandemic. First, T1D is more common in younger individuals, whereas higher rates of hospitalization and mortality were seen in elderly patients with COVID-19. Second, individuals with T1D typically receive ongoing education about management of diabetes when ill to help avoid hospitalization. Third, the immune system in patients with T1D may provide an advantage to decrease disease severity from SARS-CoV-2. T1D and COVID-19 are both associated with inflammatory changes. The destruction of the pancreatic β-cells in T1D is mediated by Th1 immunity, which may protect against pathogens like SARS-CoV-2.[6,7] On the other hand, diabetic ketoacidosis (DKA), a well-known complication frequently seen in T1D that can result in significant morbidity and mortality, may be associated with Th1-type cytokines. DKA is characterized by hyperglycemia with metabolic acidosis and ketosis. DKA causes inflammatory changes that increase cytokines, including interleukin (IL)-6, tumor necrosis factor-α, and IL-β, that together exacerbate the cytokine storm associated with COVID-19 that is mediated by high levels of IL-6. IL-6 is one of the cytokines that is involved in Th1 autoimmunity of T1D.[8]

SARS infection is associated with glucose dysregulation. Review of historical data from individuals without diabetes who were infected with SARS showed a transient fasting hyperglycemia.[9] One proposed mechanism through which SARS coronavirus may impair insulin secretion is by damaging the pancreas by binding to angiotensin-converting enzyme-2 (ACE2) receptors in the pancreatic β-cells. However, this proposed mechanism is based on limited data showing detection of ACE2 protein in the pancreas from single donor and ACE2 mRNA expression in a pooled pancreas sample from 3 donors.[9,10] An additional study showed that SARS-CoV-2 binds to ACE2 and infects pancreatic β-cells derived from human pluripotent stem cells.[11] Therefore, these observations together support a direct effect of SARS-CoV-2 in the pancreatic β-cell that may contribute to impairment of insulin secretion, which can lead to hyperglycemia and increase morbidity among patients with diabetes.

INITIAL CONCERNS ABOUT CORONAVIRUS DISEASE IN PEDIATRIC PATIENTS WITH TYPE 1 DIABETES

Owing to increased morbidity among adult patients with diabetes and COVID-19, concerns were raised about whether children with T1D could become very ill from COVID-19 as well. One study collected data on children living in 4 areas affected early by the COVID-19 pandemic: (1) Wuhan, China; (2) Catalonia, Spain; (3) Italy; and (4) San Francisco-Bay Area in the United States.[12] Although these 4 locations included large populations, there was only one patient who required hospitalization, a 20-year-old female from Spain with uncontrolled T1D (hemoglobin A_{1C} [HbA_{1C}] 11%) developed bilateral pneumonia and was intubated but was subsequently discharged from the hospital within 2 weeks. Wuhan reported no cases of children with T1D and COVID-19, whereas San Francisco reported 2 pediatric patients with T1D and COVID-19, but they did not require hospitalization. The Italian Society of Pediatric Endocrinology and Diabetes registry collected data on 15,500 pediatric patients with T1D from March 1, 2020, to August 31, 2020. Only 11 patients with T1D tested positive for COVID-19, and 5 of these patients had mild symptoms including fever, cough, conjunctivitis, anosmia, and transient hyperglycemia. Three patients with COVID-19 were admitted to the hospital: 2 required extensive education for new-onset T1D and one of these patients also had DKA without any COVID-related complications. The third patient who was admitted to the hospital had moderate DKA but recent glycemic control as close to target goal (HbA$_{1C}$ 7.8% with target less than 7.5%). Therefore, this early observation on the effects of COVID-19 in pediatric patients with T1D showed that most children have mild disease compared with adults with diabetes.

A survey conducted by the T1D Quality Improvement Collaborative (T1DX-QI) along with 49 other endocrinology clinics in the United States identified 33 patients with COVID-19 early in the pandemic.[13] In this group of patients, the mean age was 24.8 years with the youngest patient aged 7 years and most patients had hyperglycemia and mild symptoms including fever, cough, fatigue, and shortness of breath. The most common comorbidities among these patients were obesity and hypertension/cardiovascular, and one death was reported in a patient with DKA. Overall, the study concluded that children and adolescents with T1D and COVID-19 had a similar disease course as other children with COVID-19 who did not have diabetes. Taken together, these studies show that most pediatric patients with T1D do not become severely ill with COVID-19, unlike adults with diabetes and COVID-19.

THE IMPACT OF CORONAVIRUS DISEASE 2019 IN PEDIATRIC PATIENTS WITH NEWLY DIAGNOSED TYPE 1 DIABETES

Although the clinical course among pediatric patients already diagnosed with diabetes and COVID-19 was not as severe as expected, some reports examined whether COVID-19 had any impact on the initial diagnosis of T1 in pediatric patients. It is well known that there is a seasonal variation associated with new-onset T1D with increased cases during the fall and winter when exposure to viruses increase.[14–17] One study examined the effect of the COVID-19 pandemic on the new diagnosis of T1D in pediatric patients in Italy.[18] A cross-sectional analysis of pediatric diabetes centers in Italy examined data from children diagnosed with new-onset T1D or established patients with T1D presenting with DKA during 2 time periods: February 20, 2019, to April 14, 2019, and February 20, 2020, to April 14, 2020. In 2020 there were 160 newly diagnosed patients compared with 208 patients in 2019. The 23% decrease in new cases of T1D during the pandemic was attributed to effects of social distancing requirements and school closures, which together reduced exposure to seasonal viruses. The study also, however, reported a significantly higher proportion of patients presenting with severe DKA (pH < 7.1 and bicarbonate < 5 mmol/L) during the COVID-19 pandemic compared with the previous year (44.3% compared with 36%, P value < .03). Eight patients were diagnosed with COVID-19, 4 had mild symptoms, and the others were asymptomatic. The investigators concluded that several factors may have contributed to fewer cases of new-onset T1D but increased number of patients with severe DKA during the COVID-19 pandemic. First, lockdown restrictions implemented during the pandemic decreased exposure to seasonal viruses, which are associated with new-onset T1D. Second, families were more hesitant in seeking medical care early when children became ill due to fear of exposure to COVID-19. Finally, other reports highlighted the impact of unintended consequences of the pandemic on routine care at clinics and acute care in emergency room, which together contributed to a delay in diagnosis of diabetes causing more severe DKA in children in several countries.[19–21]

Two other studies also examined changes in pediatric T1D during the COVID-19 pandemic. First, a study that included 30 pediatric patients in the United Kingdom reported an increase in the number of new cases of T1D by 80% compared with previous years.[22] This observation was limited to only patients admitted to 2 of 5 inpatient units included in the study. Furthermore, there was no evidence that the increase in new cases of T1D was statistically significant or directly linked to exposure to SARS-CoV-2. Similar to observations in Italy during the COVID-19 pandemic, most patients with new-onset T1D presented with DKA (70%), of which 52% had severe DKA. Only 21 patients were screened for SARS-CoV-2 and 3 of 5 patients who tested positive presented with severe DKA complicated by refractory hypokalemia. One of these patients with severe hypokalemia had a cardiac arrest but survived. Although hypokalemia is the common electrolyte abnormality seen during DKA, the investigators proposed that SARS-CoV-2 might exacerbate hypokalemia by modulating the renin-angiotensin system (RAS).[23] SARS-CoV-2 enters the cell by binding to ACE2, which also plays an important role in decreasing RAS activity to limit the effects of angiotensin II and aldosterone. In patients with COVID-19 decreased regulation of RAS activity by ACE2 contributes to prolonged effects of angiotensin II and aldosterone, which increases potassium excretion, which is the major cause of hypokalemia.[24] An increase in the prevalence of hypokalemia was also reported in adults who were critically ill with COVID-19.[24]

A study conducted in Germany also examined the impact of COVID-19 on the incidence of pediatric T1D. This study included patients from 216 centers diagnosed with T1D between March 13 and May 13 yearly from 2011 to 2020 and estimated the incidence per 100,000 patient-years.[25] Although the incidence of pediatric T1D increased significantly from 2011 to 2019 (16.4–22.2, respectively, P value = .04), there was no significant change in the incidence of T1D among 532 patients in 2020 compared with predicted incidence (23.4 vs 22.1). This study concludes that during the COVID-19 pandemic there was no significant increase in the incidence of pediatric T1D among children in Germany, which is similar to observations in Italy but not those in the United Kingdom.

CORONAVIRUS DISEASE 2019 IN PEDIATRIC PATIENTS WITH A HISTORY OF TYPE 1 DIABETES

Studies in Italy and the United Kingdom reported no significant increase in hospitalization among pediatric patients with a history of T1D, although there were some reported cases of DKA.[18,22] Others had also reported overall fewer cases of severe illness among pediatric patients with diabetes.[12] Patients with a history of T1D receive extensive education regarding management of diabetes during illnesses. These specific instructions called *sick day guidelines* provide important tools to help patients avoid hospitalization, which may have contributed to decreased disease severity among these patients during the pandemic. In addition, stay-at-home orders and school closures likely promoted more engagement among patients and their caregivers with diabetes management at home. Therefore, parents had more time to supervise their children with testing blood glucose, monitoring food intake, and administering insulin, which together may have helped to decrease emergency room visits and hospitalizations in patients with a history of T1D.

Although most pediatric patients with T1D and COVID-19 had mild disease, some patients required hospitalization and had significant morbidity. Two studies provided early characteristics of pediatric patients with COVID-19 admitted to pediatric intensive care units (PICUs). The first study reported 48 children admitted to 14 PICUs in the United States of which 83% had pre-existing health conditions and 8% had T1D with 75% of T1D patients presenting with DKA.[26] The second study reported that among pediatric patients admitted to PICU with COVID-19, those with T1D had increased need for respiratory support including use of high-flow nasal cannula as well as mechanical and high-flow frequency ventilation.[27]

As COVID-19 hospitalizations increased in the United States, reports showed that socioeconomic factors contributed to worse health outcomes, and some ethnic minorities had more severe outcomes.[28,29] A cross-sectional multisite study of patients with T1D and COVID-19 in the United States examined differences in DKA presentation among different ethnic groups.[30] Of the 180 patients, 44% were non-Hispanic (NH) white, 31% were NH black, and 26% were Hispanic with 42% patients being in the pediatric group (age $\leq$ 19 years). NH blacks and Hispanics had significantly elevated HbA1c compared with NH whites (11.7% and 9.7%, compared with 8.3%, P value = .001 and .01, respectively) and were more likely to present with DKA compared with NH whites (55% and 33% compared with 13%, respectively). After adjusting for age, sex, glycemic control, and insurance status, NH blacks were 3.7 times more likely than NH whites to present with DKA during the COVID-19 pandemic, but there was no statistical difference between Hispanics and NH whites. The study suggests that multiple factors may contribute to ethnic disparities in DKA: social determinants of health, inadequate access to health care services, inability to self-manage diabetes especially when ill, and delay in seeking medical assistance if condition worsens. This study also highlights that health disparity that existed among patients with T1D and DKA before the COVID-19 pandemic persisted and became more evident among patients with COVID-19. Although the study highlights the need to provide more targeted approach to vulnerable patients with T1D, no new insights were identified that could be immediately implemented especially during the pandemic.

CHALLENGES WITH OUTPATIENT MANAGEMENT OF PEDIATRIC TYPE 1 DIABETES DURING THE CORONAVIRUS DISEASE 2019 PANDEMIC

During the COVID-19 pandemic, the implementation of social distancing and stay-at-home orders or lockdown in many countries directly impacted how health care providers interacted with their patients to provide routine care, which was particularly challenging for pediatric patients with T1D. Most clinics had to implement changes quickly to accommodate the needs of patients and their caregivers while simultaneously redefining roles and responsibilities of health care team members to navigate the complexity of shifting from in-person clinic visits to a telemedicine platform as the primary mode of care. Many pediatric patients with T1D use advanced diabetes devices including continuous subcutaneous insulin infusion (insulin pumps) and continuous glucose monitors (CGMs). Both insulin pumps and CGMs use Web-based management software to collect and store data that can be shared between patients and their health care team members. This remote monitoring aspect of diabetes is used routinely throughout pediatric clinics even before the COVID-19 pandemic allowing for frequent insulin dose adjustments in the growing child. In addition, remote access to data is particularly helpful to assist with management of emergencies including hypoglycemia and hyperglycemia. Although this remote technology was used in many pediatric diabetes clinics before COVID-19, several adaptations were needed to provide ongoing care for patients during the pandemic. Before the pandemic families were not always expected to upload data from diabetes devices before coming to clinic and therefore needed assistance from the health care team as well as technical support from the diabetes device company. Families also needed access to the Internet and a computer at home to upload data that could be reviewed by their health care team. Finally, owing to limitations with in-person clinic visits during the COVID-19 pandemic, many patients and their families had to participate in virtual visits (telemedicine) to receive ongoing care for diabetes management. Several studies have examined the impact of telemedicine visits on glycemic control in pediatric patients with T1D, and the results are promising and indicate that telemedicine may become an important component of routine care for outpatient management of diabetes (see following paragraphs).

Some studies examined the use of telemedicine in pediatric diabetes clinics during the COVID-19 pandemic. One study conducted a survey analyzing the impact of changes in pediatric diabetes clinics on the patients and their providers from different countries.[31] There were several major concerns about telemedicine visits. Accessing patient data was challenging for providers who often had to help guide family with specific instructions to share data from insulin pumps and glucose monitoring devices. The ability to retrieve data often depended on good Internet connection as well as access to electronic devices. Providers were initially concerned about the increased risk of DKA in children with T1D during the COVID-19 pandemic, but many clinics did not report any significant morbidity among their patients. Providers observed more health care disparities among vulnerable patients who had limited access to the Internet to connect with the health care team virtually as well as lack of close follow-up by social worker and assistance with diabetes care by school nurses. This study also identified some benefits of telemedicine that included the following: educating families about data sharing, improving efficiency during patient interactions, and improving adherence to diabetes management plan. Overall, the COVID-19 pandemic forced health care team to quickly implement changes to use telemedicine as a tool to provide ongoing care for pediatric patient with diabetes.

Several other studies examined the impact of telemedicine on metrics used to assess improvement in glycemic control in pediatric patients during the COVID-19 pandemic. A study in Italy examined changes in glycemic control 3 weeks before and after the lockdown was implemented during the pandemic.[32] A total of 62 pediatric patients with T1D using the Dexcom G6 CGM device (Dexcom, Inc) were followed via telemedicine during 2 time periods: November 26, 2019 to February 23, 2020, and February 24, 2020, to May 18, 2020. Although patients were more sedentary, there was a significant increase in the median time that glucose levels were in the target range (60.5% to 63.5%) and a decrease in the time that glucose levels were above the target range (37.3% to 34.1%) and below the target range (1.85 to 1.45%). A multicenter study conducted in Israel among 195 children with T1D (mean age 14.6 ± 5.3 years) examined changes in time in range 2 weeks before and after telemedicine visits during the Israeli lockdown from March 15, 2020, to April 12, 2020.[33] Among the 121 patients who completed the telemedicine visit, time in range improved (62.9% compared with 59%) during the 2-week period after the telemedicine visit. Therefore, the use of telemedicine together with remote monitoring of diabetes during the COVID-19 pandemic showed positive changes in metrics that directly impact glycemic control.

Finally, pediatric endocrinologists at the University of Pittsburgh Medical Center in the United States provided some recommendations and insights for using telemedicine services to provide ongoing patient care during the COVID-19 pandemic.[34] First, a representative from each member of the health care team should always be part of the development and assessment of telemedicine services that will be offered to patients. Second, different telemedicine platforms may be required to communicate with patients/families effectively and when possible choose one that can integrate with the electronic medical record. Third, one should remember to address any concerns about billing requirements when conducting telemedicine visits. Fourth, administrative staff will need to provide clear instructions for patients to use during the telemedicine visit. Fifth, it is important to continue to integrate different members of the health care team during the telemedicine visit including pediatric endocrinologist, trainees on team, diabetes nurse, certified diabetes educator, registered dietitian, and social worker. Sixth, problems encountered with telemedicine services related to institutional policies as well as limitations inherent to conducting virtual visits should be identified and steps should be taken to quickly resolve them (eg, inability to perform a comprehensive examination or laboratory testing). Finally, it is important that both health care team members and families attempt to maintain a positive attitude when implementing telemedicine to provide ongoing care for pediatric patients with diabetes especially during the COVID-19 pandemic.

In summary, during the COVID-19 pandemic pediatric patients with new-onset diabetes presented with more severe DKA. Most pediatric patients with a history of T1D who developed COVID-19 had mild disease or were asymptomatic similar to their peers without diabetes. Children with T1D and COVID-19 clearly had less severe disease than adults with diabetes and COVID-19. Telemedicine was successfully used to provide ongoing care for pediatric patients with T1D and provide some insights about positive changes in glycemic control during the pandemic. Lessons learned about management of diabetes during the COVID-19 pandemic should help to provide better care for pediatric patients with T1D and improve their health outcomes.

CLINICS CARE POINTS

- Most pediatric patients with T1D do not become severely ill with COVID-19, unlike adults with diabetes and COVID-19.
- Delay in access to medical care during the COVID-19 pandemic contributed to an increase in cases of severe DKA among pediatric patients with newly diagnosed T1D.
- The use of remote technology and telemedicine in pediatric diabetes clinics during the COVID-19 pandemic had a positive impact on glycemic control.

DISCLOSURE STATEMENT

Dr Buggs-Saxton has the following disclosures:

- Coinvestigator for NIH/NIDDK RO1 DK110075: Effectiveness of an E-Health Intervention to Support Diabetes in Minority Youth
- Data Safety Monitoring Board Member: Defining the role of management factors in outcome disparity in pediatric T1D

REFERENCES

1. Bode B, Garrett V, Messler J, et al. Glycemic Characteristics and Clinical Outcomes of COVID-19 Patients Hospitalized in the United States. J Diabetes Sci Technol 2020;14(4):813–21.
2. Huang I, Lim MA, Pranata R, et al. Diabetes mellitus is associated with increased mortality and severity of disease in COVID-19 pneumonia - A systematic review, meta-analysis, and meta-regression. Diabetes Metab Syndr 2020;14(4):395–403.
3. Williamson EJ, Walker AJ, Bhaskaran K, et al. Factors associated with COVID-19-related death using OpenSAFELY. Nature 2020;584(7821):430–6.
4. Barron E, Bakhai C, Kar P, et al. Associations of type 1 and type 2 diabetes with COVID-19-related mortality in England: a whole-population study. Lancet Diabetes Endocrinol 2020;8(10):813–22.

5. Apicella M, Campopiano MC, Mantuano M, et al. COVID-19 in people with diabetes: understanding the reasons for worse outcomes. Lancet Diabetes Endocrinol 2020;8(9):782–92.
6. Iughetti L, Trevisani V, Cattini U, et al. COVID-19 and Type 1 Diabetes: Concerns and Challenges. Acta Biomed 2020;91(3):e2020033.
7. Tatti P, Tonolo G, Zanfardino A, et al. Is it fair to hope that patients with Type 1 Diabetes (autoimmune) may be spared by the infection of Covid-19? Med Hypotheses 2020;142:109795.
8. Hundhausen C, Roth A, Whalen E, et al. Enhanced T cell responses to IL-6 in type 1 diabetes are associated with early clinical disease and increased IL-6 receptor expression. Sci Transl Med 2016;8(356).
9. Yang JK, Lin SS, Ji XJ, et al. Binding of SARS coronavirus to its receptor damages islets and causes acute diabetes. Acta Diabetol 2010;47(3):193–9.
10. Harmer D, Gilbert M, Borman R, et al. Quantitative mRNA expression profiling of ACE 2, a novel homologue of angiotensin converting enzyme. FEBS Lett 2002;532(1-2):107–10.
11. Yang L, Lin SS, Ji XJ, et al. A Human Pluripotent Stem Cell-based Platform to Study SARS-CoV-2 Tropism and Model Virus Infection in Human Cells and Organoids. Cell Stem Cell 2020;27(1):125–36.e127.
12. Cardona-Hernandez R, Cherubini V, Iafusco D, et al. Children and youth with diabetes are not at increased risk for hospitalization due to COVID-19. Pediatr Diabetes 2021;22(2):202–6.
13. Ebekozien OA, Noor N, Gallagher MP, et al. Type 1 Diabetes and COVID-19: Preliminary Findings From a Multicenter Surveillance Study in the U.S. Diabetes Care 2020;43(8):e83–5.
14. Knip M, Veijola R, Virtanen SM, et al. Environmental triggers and determinants of type 1 diabetes. Diabetes 2005;54(Suppl 2):S125–36.
15. Craig ME, Nair S, Stein H, et al. Viruses and type 1 diabetes: a new look at an old story. Pediatr Diabetes 2013;14(3):149–58.
16. Elding Larsson H, Vehik K, Gesualdo P, et al. Children followed in the TEDDY study are diagnosed with type 1 diabetes at an early stage of disease. Pediatr Diabetes 2014;15(2):118–26.
17. Laitinen OH, Honkanen H, Pakkanen O, et al. Coxsackievirus B1 is associated with induction of beta-cell autoimmunity that portends type 1 diabetes. Diabetes 2014;63(2):446–55.
18. Rabbone I, Schiaffini R, Cherubini V, et al. Has COVID-19 Delayed the Diagnosis and Worsened the Presentation of Type 1 Diabetes in Children? Diabetes Care 2020;43(11):2870–2.
19. Cella AM,F, Iughetti L, Di Biase AR, et al. Italian COVID-19 epidemic: effects on paediatric emergency attendance—a survey in the Emilia Romagna region. BMJ Paediatrics 2020;4(1).
20. Cherubini V, Gohil A, Addala A, et al. Unintended Consequences of Coronavirus Disease-2019: Remember General Pediatrics. J Pediatr 2020;223:197–8.
21. Scaramuzza A, Tagliaferri F, Bonetti L, et al. Changing admission patterns in paediatric emergency departments during the COVID-19 pandemic. Arch Dis Child 2020;105(7):704–6.
22. Unsworth R, Wallace S, Oliver NS, et al. New-Onset Type 1 Diabetes in Children During COVID-19: Multicenter Regional Findings in the U.K. Diabetes Care 2020;43(11):e170–1.
23. Pal R, Bhansali A. COVID-19, diabetes mellitus and ACE2: The conundrum. Diabetes Res Clin Pract 2020;162:108132.

24. Chen D, Li X, Song Q, et al. Assessment of Hypokalemia and Clinical Characteristics in Patients With Coronavirus Disease 2019 in Wenzhou, China. JAMA Netw Open 2020;3(6):e2011122.
25. Tittel SR, Rosenbauer J, Kamrath C, et al. Did the COVID-19 Lockdown Affect the Incidence of Pediatric Type 1 Diabetes in Germany? Diabetes Care 2020;43(11): e172–3.
26. Shekerdemian LS, Mahmood NR, Wolfe KK, et al. Characteristics and Outcomes of Children With Coronavirus Disease 2019 (COVID-19) Infection Admitted to US and Canadian Pediatric Intensive Care Units. JAMA Pediatr 2020;174(9):868–73.
27. Loomba RS, Villarreal EG, Farias JS, et al. Pediatric Intensive Care Unit Admissions for COVID-19: Insights Using State-Level Data. Int J Pediatr 2020;2020: 9680905.
28. Laurencin CT, McClinton A. The COVID-19 Pandemic: a Call to Action to Identify and Address Racial and Ethnic Disparities. J Racial Ethn Health Disparities 2020; 7(3):398–402.
29. Wiemers EE, Abrahams S, AlFakhri M, et al. Disparities in Vulnerability to Severe Complications from COVID-19 in the United States. Res Soc Stratif Mobil 2020; 69:100553.
30. Ebekozien O, Agarwal S, Noor N, et al. Full Inequities in Diabetic Ketoacidosis among Patients with Type 1 diabetes and COVID-19: Data from 52 US Clinical Centers. J Clin Endocrinol Metab 2021;106(4).
31. Sarteau AC, Souris KJ, Wang J, et al. Changes to care delivery at nine international pediatric diabetes clinics in response to the COVID-19 global pandemic. Pediatr Diabetes 2021;2021:1–6.
32. Predieri B, Leo F, Candia F, et al. Glycemic Control Improvement in Italian Children and Adolescents With Type 1 Diabetes Followed Through Telemedicine During Lockdown Due to the COVID-19 Pandemic. Front Endocrinol (Lausanne) 2020;11:595735.
33. Rachmiel M, Lebenthal Y, Mazor-Aronovitch K, et al. Glycaemic control in the paediatric and young adult population with type 1 diabetes following a single telehealth visit - what have we learned from the COVID-19 lockdown? Acta Diabetol 2021;58(6):697–705.
34. March CA, Flint A, DeArment D, et al. Paediatric diabetes care during the COVID-19 pandemic: Lessons learned in scaling up telemedicine services. Endocrinol Diabetes Metab 2020;e00202.

Avoidance of COVID-19 for Children and Adolescents and Isolation Precautions

Shipra Gupta, MD[a],*, Layne Smith, PharmD[b], Adriana Diakiw, MD[a]

KEYWORDS

- COVID-19 transmission • Prevention • Children • Household transmission

KEY POINTS

- Infections caused by severe acute respiratory syndrome coronavirus-2 (SARS-CoV-2) are spread mainly by person-to-person transmission via respiratory droplets.
- Household transmission has been well documented, and spread from presymptomatic and symptomatic individuals is a key driver for transmission.
- SARS-CoV-2–related illness has usually been mild in children, with rare complications leading to mortality.
- Various investigations and published experiences have shown that schools and day care centers have been safely opened with implementation of guidance of mask wearing, maintaining distance, and hand hygiene.
- Vaccination against SARS-CoV-2 offers a way to reduce rates of severe illness and mortality from the disease.

INTRODUCTION

Prevention is better than cure has been the dictum driving the public health response to the novel coronavirus, which was first reported in China toward the end of 2019.[1] Full-length genomic sequencing from virus identified from infected patients was 96% identical to a bat coronavirus. The novel coronavirus shared 79.6% sequence identity with the severe acute respiratory syndrome (SARS) coronavirus and, therefore, was named SARS coronavirus-2 (SARS-CoV-2).[2] The virus has since spread worldwide and was declared a pandemic by the World Health Organization (WHO) on March 11, 2020.[3,4]

Initial emphasis had been on containment measures to curb community spread, with widespread lockdowns, school closures, and nonpharmaceutical interventions

[a] West Virginia University School of Medicine, One Medical Center Drive, HSC 9214, Morgantown, WV 26506, USA; [b] West Virginia University School of Pharmacy, One Medical Center Drive, Morgantown, WV 26506, USA
* Corresponding author.
E-mail address: Shipra.gupta@hsc.wvu.edu

Pediatr Clin N Am 68 (2021) 1103–1118
https://doi.org/10.1016/j.pcl.2021.05.011
0031-3955/21/© 2021 Elsevier Inc. All rights reserved.

pediatric.theclinics.com

such as masking and social distancing. There have been multiple reports of familial clusters and studies on household transmission.[5-14] However, there is limited guidance on prevention measures once a household member is diagnosed with or exposed to the virus. This article highlights available data on transmission of SARS-CoV-2 and reviews preventive measures to reduce transmission of the virus both in the community and the household setting.

Epidemiology

Transmission and incubation period

The acquisition of SARS-CoV-2 occurs when a susceptible host comes in contact with respiratory secretions from an infected individual. Most transmission occurs through large droplets and occasionally small droplets via airborne spread.[15-18] Airborne transmission can occur in enclosed spaces, poorly ventilated areas with improper air handling and prolonged or higher exposure dose of respiratory particles, as with expiratory exertion during exercise or singing.[19-22] Theoretically, transmission can occur through contaminated surfaces; however, this is infrequent. Virus has been detected in stool specimens; however, viable virus has not been isolated from stool samples.[23] The incubation period for SARS-CoV-2 is up to 14 days from the time of exposure, and about 50% of people exposed have symptoms by day 4 or 5 and 98% by day 12 from exposure.[24-29]

The window of contagiousness for a symptomatic individual starts about 2 to 3 days before onset of symptoms, peaks at symptoms onset, and declines over the following 7 days in most cases.[30-33] Therefore, presymptomatic transmission seems to be a significant driver of spread of infection in the community and households. Early on during the pandemic, asymptomatic carriers were thought to be significant spreaders, especially in the household setting.[34,35] However, recent data from Wuhan, China, showed that there was no SARS-CoV-2 detected by polymerase chain reaction (PCR) in 1174 close household contacts of the 300 asymptomatic persons.[36] The role of asymptomatic spreaders remains controversial, with recent modeling data suggesting that 50% of new infections were estimated to have been acquired from asymptomatic spreaders.[37] The period of contagiousness for asymptomatic individuals is not clearly understood and, for purposes of contact tracing, the cutoff is 48 hours before the positive test date is applied for identification of individuals who had potential exposure.

Secondary Attack Rates and Household Transmission

Secondary attack rate (SAR) is defined as the proportion of infections that occur among susceptible individuals following contact with an infected person within the incubation period.[38] The SAR for SARS-CoV-2 varies in different contact and exposure settings. Recent meta-analysis showed a pooled SAR for SARS-CoV-2 in diverse contact settings of 7% (95% confidence interval [CI], 3%–12%).[39] This study also highlighted low SAR in health care facilities, public transport, and work settings compared with the high SAR in households and exposures in social gatherings.

Crowded indoor environments and close contact among household members are high-risk settings for transmission of SARS-CoV-2. Initial reports out of China described SAR of 12.4% among household contacts when defined by close relatives and 17.1% when they shared the same residential address.[8] Recent systemic review and meta-analysis estimated household SAR of 16.6% (95% CI, 14.0%–19.3%).[40] Most published literature reports increased SAR from symptomatic index cases compared with asymptomatic index cases as well as in spouses compared with other family contacts.[40,41]

Lewis and colleagues[9] reported that 31 out of the 58 households from Utah and Wisconsin had secondary transmission and 52 of 188 household contacts tested positive by either polymerase chain reaction (PCR) assay or serologic testing, giving a secondary infection rate of 28%. This study was done during March to April 2020 when there was low community prevalence at the study sites to reduce risk of additional community exposure. A higher secondary infection rate of 53% (95% CI, 46%–60%) was detected in households in a study done in Tennessee and Wisconsin in April to September 2020.[6]

Various retrospective studies have identified black ethnicity, male gender, smoking, and obesity as risk factors associated with higher risk of infection.[42–44] Higher rates of infection have been reported in older household contacts (age $\geq$ 60 years) compared with younger contacts.[5,8] Multiple reports described lower SAR for children compared with adults.[5,8–10,40,41] Hu and colleagues[45] performed a retrospective review of secondary cases and reported that secondary cases had less severe symptoms such as fever, cough, sore throat, and myalgia compared with the index cases.

Transmission from Children

Prolonged shedding of respiratory viruses after viral illness has been described in children younger than 5 years compared with older participants.[46] With most children having no symptoms or mild symptoms, it was thought that children could serve as a silent reservoir for SARS-CoV-2. However, multiple studies of outbreaks in familial clusters have shown that children are rarely the index case and are often identified after an adult has tested positive. Similar findings were confirmed from outbreaks at childcare facilities that were linked to index cases in adults.[47] In a large, multicenter, cross-sectional investigation in Germany, the estimated SARS-CoV-2 seroprevalence was low in parents and 3-fold lower in children.[48] Follow-up interviews with families of children who were hospitalized for coronavirus disease 2019 (COVID-19) illness were performed 6 weeks after the child became ill and showed there were no reported illnesses in the households and 1 case of child-to-child transmission.[49]

School and Day Care Attendance

Schools across the United States were preemptively closed to in-person classes and transitioned to virtual learning early during the pandemic to mitigate spread of SARS-CoV-2. However, as months passed, certain states allowed in-person learning options along with the remote option. With the help of the local health department and guidance from Centers for Disease Control and Prevention (CDC), there have been multiple reports published for safe reopening of schools. A recent study showed that attending school or childcare 2 weeks before the testing date was not associated with an increased probability of a positive SARS-CoV-2 test.[47] Parents of cases and controls reported 64% and 76% consistent mask use respectively for both children and staff at schools or childcare facilities. Most of the children (<18 years old) who tested positive for SARS-CoV-2 were more likely to have attended gatherings with people outside their households 14 days before testing positive. Similar results were reported from North Carolina schools over a period of 9 weeks with extensive contact tracing where there was limited secondary transmission and zero child-to-adult transmission noted within the school.[50] These studies highlight that in-person teaching at schools can be achieved with consistent mask wearing, hand hygiene, and maintaining a distance of 2 m (6 feet) as well as screening and early detection of infection.

Nonpharmaceutical Interventions for Prevention of Severe Acute Respiratory Syndrome Coronavirus-2

Nonpharmaceutical interventions recommended to reduce transmission of SARS-CoV-2 include mask wearing, social distancing, hand hygiene, disinfection of frequently touched surfaces, improved ventilation, self-isolation, and quarantine.

Mask Wearing

Face masks are thought to reduce viral transmission from both the source and target of infection; they reduce the exhalation of respiratory particles by an infected person[51,52] and reduce the inhalation of these particles by a susceptible host.[52,53] Evidence supporting face mask use comes from epidemiologic data, observational studies, mathematical models, and laboratory studies.

Like SARS and Middle Eastern Respiratory Syndrome (MERS) Coronavirus, SARS-CoV-2 is a member of the Betacoronavirus genus, but it resembles the 2009 H1N1 influenza virus in its high degree of upper respiratory tract shedding, its propensity for asymptomatic and presymptomatic transmission, and the scope of its global spread.[54] The WHO sponsored a systematic review and meta-analysis that concluded that face mask use could significantly decrease the risk of SARS-CoV-2 infection.[55] In their systematic review and meta-analysis, Li and colleagues found that mask wearing significantly reduced the risk of COVID-19 infection, with a pooled odds ratio of 0.38 and 95% CI of 0.21 to 0.69.[56] A retrospective cohort study of households in Beijing, China, showed a 79% reduction in transmission if both the index case and family contacts wore masks before onset of symptoms in the index case.[57]

Epidemiologic studies support the widespread use of face masks to prevent community transmission of SARS-CoV-2. Early in the course of the pandemic, Cheng and colleagues[58] compared the epidemiology of SARS-CoV-2 in the Hong Kong Special Administrative Region (HKSAR), where community-wide compliance with face mask use was 96.6%, with selected countries in North America, Europe, and Asia having similar population density but without universal masking. The incidence of SARS-CoV-2 was significantly lower in HSKAR.[58] A cross-sectional population-level study in the United States showed that self-reported face mask use was correlated with increased odds of transmission control, and that the effect of mask use was higher with increased levels of physical distancing.[59]

Laboratory studies of airborne transmission provide additional evidence for the role of mask wearing in preventing the spread of COVID-19. Ueki and colleagues[52] examined the efficacy of cotton, surgical, and N95 masks in blocking the transmission of infectious droplets and aerosols of SARS-CoV-2 using an airborne transmission simulator. All types of masks were protective against transmission of infectious particles, with a stronger effect noted when the mask was worn by the source of the virus.[52] A study of the aerosol filtration efficiency of cloth masks showed that snugly fitted masks could provide good protection from a range of aerosol particle sizes. Filtration efficiency was significantly higher in masks made from multiple layers of tightly woven fabric, particularly when different types of fabric were combined in the same mask. Of note, filtration efficiency in poorly fitted masks was found to decrease by more than 60%, highlighting the importance of proper mask fitting to reduce transmission of respiratory particles.[53]

Current evidence-based guidelines from the CDC emphasize the importance of consistent and correct face mask use to decrease transmission of SARS-CoV-2 in the community. The CDC recommends using fabric masks made with 2 or 3 layers of tightly woven, breathable fabric (such as cotton), or disposable, single-use nonmedical masks. Regardless of the type of mask used, it should be snugly fitted around the nose and chin, without large gaps at the sides or top. Masks with exhalation valves or vents should not be used, because they may allow passage of respiratory particles. In order to prevent critical supply shortages, surgical masks and respirators should be avoided in the community setting. Outside the home, face masks should be worn while indoors in public places, and in crowded outdoor areas where interpersonal distance is less than 2 m.[60]

Physical Distancing

Studies of COVID-19 outbreaks occurring in community settings outside the home have shown that increased infection risk is associated with close contact with other members of the community, particularly in enclosed spaces.[60] A contact tracing study of train passengers in China found that risk of SARS-CoV-2 transmission increased with spatial proximity to the index case, as well as increased duration of shared travel time.[61]

Epidemiologic studies lend support to public health guidance on physical distancing to slow the spread of the pandemic. The WHO's systematic review and meta-analysis of nonpharmaceutical measures to prevent SARS-CoV-2 transmission found that the risk of viral infection decreased as interpersonal distancing increased, and concluded that physical separation of at least 1 m was beneficial, but separation of 2 m might be more effective in decreasing the risk of infection.[55]

The COVID-19 Pandemic Pulse Study evaluated self-reported movement patterns and nonpharmaceutical intervention use with SARS-CoV-2 positivity in Maryland in June of 2020. Although this study failed to show a statistically significant effect for indoor mask use, it did show a significant association between strict social distancing and decreased risk of SARS-CoV-2 infection. Of note, after adjusting for social distancing and demographic variables, the types of movement that significantly correlated with increased infection risk were use of public transportation and visiting a place of worship within the previous 2 weeks.[62]

Physical distancing to reduce the spread of SARS-CoV-2 has reduced the incidence of other respiratory viruses. A Mayo Clinic study that reviewed community transmission of respiratory viruses in Arizona found that enactment of distancing policies coincided with a marked reduction in both the overall number of respiratory panel tests and the percentage of positive test results for common respiratory viruses during April through July of 2020, compared with the equivalent time frame in 2017 through 2019.[63]

Based on the available evidence regarding transmission patterns, unnecessary interactions with persons outside the household should be limited while SARS-CoV-2 is circulating in the community.[60] When outside the home, physical distance of at least 2 m should be maintained from nonhousehold members. Unnecessary exposure to indoor environments should be avoided, particularly those associated with increased transmission risk, such as indoor restaurant dining, worship services, and exercise classes. Nonessential use of public transportation should be avoided whenever possible. Because there is emerging evidence of SARS-CoV-2 transmission occurring in large outdoor gatherings, exposure to crowded outdoor venues should also be avoided.[60,64] Limiting contact with other members of the community is especially important for persons at high risk for severe COVID-19 illness, and those who share a household with someone at high risk. With the advent of widespread immunization for COVID-19, the CDC has issued revised guidelines for indoor visits or small gatherings in private residences. Fully vaccinated people do not need to wear masks or maintain physical distancing during indoor visits with other fully vaccinated people, or with unvaccinated people from a single household who are at low risk for severe COVID-19. If any of the unvaccinated people or their household members are at increased risk of severe COVID-19, or if the unvaccinated people come from multiple households, fully vaccinated people should continue to wear masks, maintain physical distance of at least 2 m, and visit outdoors or in a well-ventilated indoor space.[65] Unvaccinated individuals should continue to limit the number of unvaccinated visitors allowed inside the home, ensure that masks are worn by unvaccinated visitors and members of the household alike, maintain at least 2 m of separation from unvaccinated visitors at all times, and limit the amount of time spent visiting indoors.[66] All people, regardless of their immunization status, should continue to avoid medium-sized or large gatherings, regardless of their immunization status.[65]

The CDC recommends that people postpone travel while SARS-CoV-2 is prevalent in the community. Those who do travel should be tested for SARS-CoV-2 from 1 to 3 days before departure and retested 3 to 5 days after arrival. On return, travelers should self-isolate and monitor for symptoms at home for 7 days if tested, even if test results are negative, and for 10 days if not tested. If other members of the household did not accompany the traveler, both the traveler and other members of the household should wear masks in shared household spaces for 14 days.[67]

Hand Hygiene

Although there are several case reports of suspected transmission of SARS-CoV-2 via contact with contaminated surfaces, there is currently no definitive evidence of transmission via direct contact or fomites.[68] Studies of nonpharmaceutical interventions to prevent the spread of respiratory viruses have shown mixed results on the efficacy of hand washing alone. A systematic review and meta-analysis of influenza virus transmission in the community found that frequent hand hygiene plus mask wearing significantly decreased transmission of influenza, but hand hygiene alone did not.[69] However, these reviews considered the impact of hand hygiene on transmission of respiratory viruses but not SARS-CoV-2. These results may not correspond with the real-world transmission dynamics of SARS-CoV-2, which is significantly more stable than influenza virus.[70] A modeling study by Przekwas and Chen[71] described how SARS-CoV-2 might be inoculated onto respiratory epithelium via deposition of viral particles on the face by contaminated hands, and concluded that washing of the face and hands might prevent infection.

Because SARS-CoV-2 is a lipid-enveloped RNA virus, it is susceptible to inactivation by agents that disrupt the integrity of its lipid envelope, such as alcohol and hand soap.[72] A review of commonly used hand sanitizers found that most alcohol-based hand sanitizers were successful at inactivating enveloped viruses, including coronavirus, but that washing with soap and water was superior to sanitizers in removing pathogens and debris from hands.[73] A laboratory study by Hirose and colleagues[70] determined that hand sanitizer containing 80% ethanol completely inactivated SARS-CoV-2 on skin within 15 seconds of exposure.

Disinfection of Frequently Touched Surfaces

Although less likely, transmission by fomites remains a possibility, and disinfection of frequently touched surfaces may help to decrease the risk of infection. A retrospective cohort study of households in Beijing, China, found that daily use of a disinfectant containing chlorine or ethanol was 77% effective in decreasing household transmission of SARS-CoV-2.[57]

A literature review that examined the effectiveness of various cleaning products in disinfecting surfaces contaminated by human coronaviruses concluded that the virus was successfully inactivated by solutions of 62% to 71% ethanol, 0.5% hydrogen peroxide, or 0.1% sodium hypochlorite within 1 minute. For household disinfection, the investigators recommend a 1:50 dilution of standard household bleach; alternatively, a solution of 62% to 70% ethanol may be used for disinfection of small surfaces.[74] Current guidance for prevention of COVID-19 from WHO recommends the use of 0.1% sodium hypochlorite solution or 70% to 90% ethanol for household disinfection.[75]

Ventilation

Respiratory particles emitted by humans span a continuum of sizes, from large droplets to tiny aerosols. Conventional wisdom holds that droplets more than 5 μm in diameter fall to the ground within 1 to 2 m of the source, whereas smaller aerosols remain suspended in the air; however, this is now understood to be a false dichotomy. The duration of time that a particle remains suspended in the air depends not only on its diameter but also on the velocity at which it is emitted, and a host of environmental factors, including the temperature, humidity, speed, and direction of ambient airflow.[76] Therefore, both proximity and ventilation have emerged as key determinants of transmission risk for SARS-CoV-2.[68] A mathematical model of indoor transmission found that increasing ventilation rate was correlated with decreasing infection probability. Of note, the model also predicted that mask wearing indoors significantly decreased infection probability, even at lower rates of air exchange.[77] Using the principles of fluid mechanics, Bhagat and colleagues[78] assessed the impact of ventilation on the movement of infectious particles in an enclosed space, and concluded that displacement ventilation was most effective in removing contaminated air and decreasing the exposure risk. Displacement ventilation consists of exhaust fans or vents installed on or near the ceiling of the room, as can be found in the kitchens and bathrooms of most modern homes.

Preventive Measures When Household Member Has Been Diagnosed with COVID-19 and Is at Home

Given the high secondary attack rate of SARS-CoV-2 in households, special care must be taken to reduce the risk of transmission to household contacts when an infected person is quarantined at home. The CDC provides detailed recommendations for preventive measures when a member of the household is symptomatic with COVID-19 and is cared for at home. The same recommendations apply when a household member has tested positive for the virus but remains asymptomatic or presymptomatic. Affected persons should be isolated from other members of the household and, if possible, should use a separate bedroom and bathroom, and eat meals in their rooms. Caregivers should limit exposure to the individual and try to maintain at least 2 m of interpersonal distance. The affected persons and their household contacts should wear masks whenever they are near each other; however, masks should not be worn by children less than 2 years of age, people who are unable to remove them without assistance, or anyone with respiratory distress.[79] Prevention of airborne transmission is particularly important in household settings. Current CDC guidance emphasizes the importance of good ventilation to decrease the concentration of potentially infectious airborne particles in shared indoor spaces. Recommendations for improving household ventilation include the following[80]:

- Open doors and windows as much as possible to introduce fresh air from outside.
- Increase air circulation in the home using portable fans, ceiling fans, or central heating, ventilation, and air conditioning fan setting.

- Install high-efficiency pleated filters in central heating, ventilation, and air conditioning systems. Filter indoor air using a portable air cleaner or high-efficiency particulate air filter.
- Turn on exhaust fans in kitchen and bathroom, or place portable fans blowing outward near open doors and windows, to move stale air outdoors.

To decrease transmission through direct contact and fomites, the CDC advises that household members wash their hands frequently with soap and water for at least 20 seconds, or use hand sanitizer containing at least 60% alcohol, and avoid touching the eyes, nose, or mouth with unwashed hands. Frequently touched surfaces, such as light switches, doorknobs, desks, tables, electronics, sinks, faucets, and toilets, should be cleaned and disinfected daily. If the affected person uses a shared bathroom, the person should clean and disinfect it after use if are able to do so; if not, the caregiver should wait as long as possible before entering the bathroom to clean and disinfect it. Caregivers should wear gloves to prevent contact with the affected person's secretions, bodily fluids, or stool. Gloves should also be worn when handling contaminated items, washing dishes, or doing laundry. Dishes should be washed with soap and hot water, or in a dishwasher. Dirty laundry may be combined with laundry from other household members but should be washed and dried on the hottest settings possible. Used gloves, masks, and other contaminated items should be discarded in a trash can with a disposable liner, preferably one set aside for use by the affected person, and gloves should be worn when handling and disposing of contaminated trash. Caregivers should wash their hands after removing gloves.[79]

Because the estimated incubation period of SARS-CoV-2 can last up to 14 days, the CDC recommends that caregivers and close household contacts of the affected person quarantine at home for 14 days after their last exposure to the affected person, or 14 days after the affected person meets criteria to end isolation. Close contact is defined as being within 2 m of the infected person for a total of 15 minutes or more, direct physical contact such as hugging or kissing, sharing the same utensils for eating or drinking, or direct exposure to respiratory droplets from coughing or sneezing. Caregivers and close household contacts with a history of laboratory-confirmed COVID-19 infection and recovery within the past 3 months or fully vaccinated contacts are exempted from the quarantine requirement, and do not require repeat testing unless they become symptomatic.[81] Public health departments establish quarantine guidelines within their jurisdictions based on local circumstances and resources, and may recommend alternative guidelines to shorten the duration of quarantine.[81]

Pharmaceutical Interventions

Throughout the pandemic, there have been ongoing efforts to evaluate the antiviral properties of medications that could prevent SARS-CoV-2 infection following exposure. Examples include antiparasitic drugs such as ivermectin, antimalarials such as hydroxychloroquine, antiviral medications such as amantadine, and antiretroviral medications.[82] None of the therapeutics have shown a clear benefit and none have been approved/recommended for early prevention of COVID-19 infection.

In addition, there are various ongoing clinical studies to understand the role of early therapeutic interventions to prevent progression of disease in the early phase of illness. Anti–SARS-CoV-2 monoclonal antibodies such as bamlanivimab and the combination of casirivimab and imdevimab received an emergency use authorization (EUA) by the US Food and Drug Administration (FDA) as preventive management for nonhospitalized patients at high risk of disease progression who have mild to moderate illness. The interim results of a phase 2, randomized, placebo-controlled trial showed that a single infusion of bamlanivimab increased the viral RNA clearance and decreased rates of hospitalization compared with a placebo group.[83] The current EUAs for both bamlanivimab and the combination of casirivimab and imdevimab include pediatric patients at least 12 years of age who weigh at least 40 kg.

Vitamin D and vitamin C have been studied as potential immunomodulatory agents to prevent infection with SARS-CoV-2. However, data on prevention of COVID-19 with supplements containing vitamin D and vitamin C are limited to observational studies. Vitamin D increases innate immunity by secretion of antiviral peptides, which improve mucosal defenses. Various systematic reviews and meta-analyses of observational data have shown that low levels of serum vitamin D are associated with increase in respiratory tract infections, including influenza and pneumonia. A recent study evaluated the association between average levels of vitamin D and mortality caused by COVID-19 and number of cases of COVID-19. This study was limited to European countries and found a negative correlation between levels of vitamin D and number of cases of COVID-19 as well as mortality caused by COVID-19, showing that low vitamin D level may be associated with COVID-19 infection and complications.[84] Another study of patients in European countries found a significant negative correlation between average vitamin D levels and COVID-19 cases, but not with death.[85] Because of the limited ability to generalize from these trials and lack of studies in pediatric patients, supplementation with vitamin D to prevent SARS-CoV-2 infection is currently not recommended. However, vitamin D supplementation may be warranted in pediatric patients with known vitamin D deficiency.

Ascorbic acid, or Vitamin C, has been studied as potential immunomodulatory agent. Vitamin C has been evaluated in patients with serious infections and sepsis with inconsistent results.[86,87] Although there are many ongoing clinical trials evaluating its place in therapy, it is currently not routinely recommended for prevention of SARS-CoV-2 in pediatric patients.

Zinc supplementation has also been studied as a preventive as well as for management of COVID-19 in ongoing clinical trials. In vitro studies have shown that increased intracellular zinc concentrations decrease replication in RNA viruses such as rhinoviruses and coronaviruses.[88,89]

Topical Agents

The nose and mouth are significant entry portals for the virus, because infection is primarily transmitted by inhalation of, or contact with, infected droplets. In addition, the nasal cavity and nasopharynx contains the highest viral load. Therefore, topical nasal irrigations and oral rinses have been identified as potential options to prevent SARS-CoV-2 infection.

There is currently limited evidence regarding the use of topical therapies in the prevention of SARS-CoV-2 infection specifically. However, available data to support these agents in other viral illnesses may help guide preventive measures for SARS-CoV-2.[90] Regular use of saline nasal irrigation in children has been shown to prevent symptoms of rhinitis and associated complications.[91] In addition, use of hypertonic saline nasal irrigation and gargling was associated with decreased duration of illness, over-the-counter medication use, transmission within household contacts, and viral load of many viruses, including rhinovirus, enterovirus, influenza A virus, and coronavirus (not SARS-CoV-2).[92]

Povidone-iodine (PVP-1) is another topical agent identified for potential use in the prevention of SARS-CoV-2 infections. PVP-1 is a solution that disrupts microbial metabolic pathways, destabilizes structural components of cell membranes, and leads to irreversible damage to pathogens. PVP-1 has been shown to achieve almost

100% virucidal activity against SARS-CoV-2 within 30 seconds of contact in the laboratory.[93] Another in vitro study found that PVP-1 at diluted concentrations of 0.5%, 1.25%, and 2.5% completely inactivated SARS-CoV-2 within 15 seconds of contact.[94] Although neither of these studies was done in humans, a review of PVP-1 use in sinonasal and oral cavities found that PVP-1 is safe to use in the nose up to a strength of 1.25% for 5 months and in the mouth up to a strength of 5% for 6 months.[95] However, the over-the-counter product is commercially available at a strength of 10%, so this product should not be used in the nose or mouth. Until a commercially available diluted solution is available and clinical trials have been completed, PVP-1 should not be used to prevent SARS-CoV-2 infections in children.

There is currently insufficient evidence to support the use of topical therapies to prevent COVID-19 in children. Risks associated with these therapies include irritation, loss of smell, and destruction of microorganisms in the nose or mouth that are useful in preventing infection. In addition, if nasal spray solutions are used on multiple children without sterilizing the bottle or product, spread of disease may increase. There are currently multiple trials underway to determine the safety and efficacy of topical agents in prevention of COVID-19 infection and transmission.

Vaccines

Vaccines offer the best preventive strategy to contain the SARS-CoV-2 pandemic. Several vaccines using different methodologies are being developed across the world. Recently, 2 nucleoside-modified RNA vaccines encoding the SARS-CoV-2 spike protein were shown to be efficacious in preventing COVID-19 illness, including severe disease.[96,97] These 2 vaccines received an EUA by the FDA and are being used across the United States to vaccinate health care workers and people at high risk of severe disease. The Pfizer-BioNTech COVID-19 vaccine and MODERNA COVID-19 vaccine also received an interim recommendation for immunization of individuals greater than or equal to 16 years and greater than or equal to 18 years of age respectively.[98,99] However, there are clinical trials being done to evaluate safety and efficacy in younger children.

There are limited data on the effect of vaccine on asymptomatic transmission, and therefore the current recommendation is to continue practicing masking and social distancing until most the population is immunized.

SUMMARY

Prevention of exposure to SARS-CoV-2 and, most recently, vaccination against the virus have been the mainstay of efforts to control the spread of the virus. Children have been reported to have mild illness, with few developing complications and having poor outcomes. Children have also been noted to not spread or acquire the virus as much as adults. Childcare settings and schools have been safely reopened with minimal transmission noted among children with safety measures of masking, maintaining distance, and hand washing. Transmission in outdoor settings is low and indoor transmission can be reduced in the household setting by increasing ventilation along with other mitigation strategies. Pharmaceutical interventions other than vaccination have not been shown to prevent infection with SARs-CoV-2.

CLINICS CARE POINTS

- Nonpharmaceutical interventions such as social distancing, masking, and hand hygiene have been the primary preventive strategies to avoid infection with SARS-CoV-2.

- Early and rapid identification of infected individuals and tracing of contacts, as well as isolation and quarantine, are effective measures to curb the spread of infection.
- Systematic development of effective vaccines to prevent severe illness caused by COVID-19 offer a path forward to containing the pandemic and reducing the burden of severe disease Other pharmaceutical interventions are still under investigation and so far have not shown benefit in preventing COVID-19.

DISCLOSURE

The authors have no commercial or financial conflicts of interest or funding sources.

REFERENCES

1. Zhu N, Zhang D, Wang W, et al. A Novel Coronavirus from Patients with Pneumonia in China, 2019. N Engl J Med 2020;382(8):727–33.
2. Zhou P, Yang XL, Wang XG, et al. A pneumonia outbreak associated with a new coronavirus of probable bat origin. Nature 2020;579(7798):270–3.
3. Director-General's opening remarks at the media briefing on COVID19. World Health Organization WHO; 2020.
4. Coronavirus disease 2019 (COVID-19) Situation report - 3.11.2020. World Health Organization WHO. Available at: https://www.who.int/docs/default-source/coronaviruse/situation-reports/20200302-sitrep-42-covid-19.pdf?sfvrsn=224c1add_2. Accessed June 4, 2021.
5. Fung HF, Martinez L, Alarid-Escudero F, et al. The household secondary attack rate of SARS-CoV-2: A rapid review. Clin Infect Dis 2020. https://doi.org/10.1093/cid/ciaa1558.
6. Grijalva CG, Rolfes MA, Zhu Y, et al. Transmission of SARS-COV-2 Infections in Households - Tennessee and Wisconsin, April-September 2020. MMWR Morb Mortal Wkly Rep 2020;69(44):1631–4.
7. Jing QL, Liu MJ, Yuan J, et al. Household Secondary Attack Rate of COVID-19 and Associated Determinants. medRxiv 2020. https://doi.org/10.1101/2020.04.11.20056010.
8. Jing QL, Liu MJ, Zhang ZB, et al. Household secondary attack rate of COVID-19 and associated determinants in Guangzhou, China: a retrospective cohort study. Lancet Infect Dis 2020;20(10):1141–50.
9. Lewis NM, Chu VT, Ye D, et al. Household Transmission of SARS-CoV-2 in the United States. Clin Infect Dis 2020. https://doi.org/10.1093/cid/ciaa1166.
10. Li W, Zhang B, Lu J, et al. Characteristics of Household Transmission of COVID-19. Clin Infect Dis 2020;71(8):1943–6.
11. Wang Z, Ma W, Zheng X, et al. Household transmission of SARS-CoV-2. J Infect 2020;81(1):179–82.
12. Xu X, Liu X, Wang L, et al. Household transmissions of SARS-CoV-2 in the time of unprecedented travel lockdown in China. medRxiv 2020. https://doi.org/10.1101/2020.03.02.20029868.
13. Yang MC, Hung PP, Wu YK, et al. A three-generation family cluster with COVID-19 infection: should quarantine be prolonged? Public Health 2020;185:31–3.
14. Yung CF, Kam KQ, Chong CY, et al. Household Transmission of Severe Acute Respiratory Syndrome Coronavirus 2 from Adults to Children. J Pediatr 2020;225:249–51.
15. Kang M, Wei J, Yuan J, et al. Probable Evidence of Fecal Aerosol Transmission of SARS-CoV-2 in a High-Rise Building. Ann Intern Med 2020;173(12):974–80.

16. Miller SL, Nazaroff WW, Jimenez JL, et al. Transmission of SARS-CoV-2 by inhalation of respiratory aerosol in the Skagit Valley Chorale superspreading event. Indoor Air 2020. https://doi.org/10.1111/ina.12751.
17. Yu IT, Li Y, Wong TW, et al. Evidence of airborne transmission of the severe acute respiratory syndrome virus. N Engl J Med 2004;350(17):1731–9.
18. WHO. WHO. Transmission of SARS-CoV-2: implications for infection prevention precautions. Available at: https://www.who.int/news-room/commentaries/detail/transmission-of-sars-cov-2-implications-for-infection-prevention-precautions. Accessed June 6,2021.
19. Bae S, Kim H, Jung TY, et al. Epidemiological Characteristics of COVID-19 Outbreak at Fitness Centers in Cheonan, Korea. J Korean Med Sci 2020;35(31):e288.
20. Brlek A, Vidovič Š, Vuzem S, et al. Possible indirect transmission of COVID-19 at a squash court, Slovenia, March 2020: case report. Epidemiol Infect 2020;148:e120.
21. Lu J, Gu J, Li K, et al. COVID-19 Outbreak Associated with Air Conditioning in Restaurant, Guangzhou, China, 2020. Emerg Infect Dis 2020;26(7):1628–31.
22. Li Y, Leung GM, Tang JW, et al. Role of ventilation in airborne transmission of infectious agents in the built environment - a multidisciplinary systematic review. Indoor Air 2007;17(1):2–18.
23. Xu Y, Li X, Zhu B, et al. Characteristics of pediatric SARS-CoV-2 infection and potential evidence for persistent fecal viral shedding. Nat Med 2020;26(4):502–5.
24. Guan WJ, Ni ZY, Hu Y, et al. Clinical Characteristics of Coronavirus Disease 2019 in China. N Engl J Med 2020;382(18):1708–20.
25. Li Q, Guan X, Wu P, et al. Early Transmission Dynamics in Wuhan, China, of Novel Coronavirus-Infected Pneumonia. N Engl J Med 2020;382(13):1199–207.
26. Lauer SA, Grantz KH, Bi Q, et al. The Incubation Period of Coronavirus Disease 2019 (COVID-19) From Publicly Reported Confirmed Cases: Estimation and Application. Ann Intern Med 2020;172(9):577–82.
27. He X, Lau EHY, Wu P, et al. Author Correction: Temporal dynamics in viral shedding and transmissibility of COVID-19. Nat Med 2020;26(9):1491–3.
28. He X, Lau EHY, Wu P, et al. Temporal dynamics in viral shedding and transmissibility of COVID-19. Nat Med 2020;26(5):672–5.
29. Team C-I. Clinical and virologic characteristics of the first 12 patients with coronavirus disease 2019 (COVID-19) in the United States. Nat Med 2020;26(6):861–8.
30. Zou L, Ruan F, Huang M, et al. SARS-CoV-2 Viral Load in Upper Respiratory Specimens of Infected Patients. N Engl J Med 2020;382(12):1177–9.
31. To KK, Tsang OT, Leung WS, et al. Temporal profiles of viral load in posterior oropharyngeal saliva samples and serum antibody responses during infection by SARS-CoV-2: an observational cohort study. Lancet Infect Dis 2020;20(5):565–74.
32. Wölfel R, Corman VM, Guggemos W, et al. Author Correction: Virological assessment of hospitalized patients with COVID-2019. Nature 2020;588(7839):E35.
33. Wölfel R, Corman VM, Guggemos W, et al. Virological assessment of hospitalized patients with COVID-2019. Nature 2020;581(7809):465–9.
34. Jiang XL, Zhang XL, Zhao XN, et al. Transmission Potential of Asymptomatic and Paucisymptomatic Severe Acute Respiratory Syndrome Coronavirus 2 Infections: A 3-Family Cluster Study in China. J Infect Dis 2020;221(12):1948–52.
35. Ye F, Xu S, Rong Z, et al. Delivery of infection from asymptomatic carriers of COVID-19 in a familial cluster. Int J Infect Dis 2020;94:133–8.

36. Cao S, Gan Y, Wang C, et al. Post-lockdown SARS-CoV-2 nucleic acid screening in nearly ten million residents of Wuhan, China. Nat Commun 2020;11(1):5917.
37. Johansson MA, Quandelacy TM, Kada S, et al. SARS-CoV-2 Transmission From People Without COVID-19 Symptoms. JAMA Netw Open 2021;4(1):e2035057.
38. Palmer CR. Encyclopedia of biostatistics. BMJ 1999;318(7182):542.
39. Tian T, Huo X. Secondary attack rates of COVID-19 in diverse contact settings, a meta-analysis. J Infect Dev Ctries 2020;14(12):1361–7.
40. Madewell ZJ, Yang Y, Longini IM, et al. Household Transmission of SARS-CoV-2: A Systematic Review and Meta-analysis. JAMA Netw Open 2020;3(12): e2031756.
41. Koh WC, Naing L, Chaw L, et al. What do we know about SARS-CoV-2 transmission? A systematic review and meta-analysis of the secondary attack rate and associated risk factors. PLoS One 2020;15(10):e0240205.
42. Niedzwiedz CL, O'Donnell CA, Jani BD, et al. Ethnic and socioeconomic differences in SARS-CoV-2 infection: prospective cohort study using UK Biobank. BMC Med 2020;18(1):160.
43. Sattar N, Ho FK, Gill JM, et al. BMI and future risk for COVID-19 infection and death across sex, age and ethnicity: Preliminary findings from UK biobank. Diabetes Metab Syndr 2020;14(5):1149–51.
44. Engin AB, Engin ED, Engin A. Two important controversial risk factors in SARS-CoV-2 infection: Obesity and smoking. Environ Toxicol Pharmacol 2020;78: 103411.
45. Hu P, Ma M, Jing Q, et al. Retrospective study identifies infection related risk factors in close contacts during COVID-19 epidemic. Int J Infect Dis 2020. https:// doi.org/10.1016/j.ijid.2020.12.011.
46. Byington CL, Ampofo K, Stockmann C, et al. Community Surveillance of Respiratory Viruses Among Families in the Utah Better Identification of Germs-Longitudinal Viral Epidemiology (BIG-LoVE) Study. Clin Infect Dis 2015;61(8): 1217–24.
47. Lopez AS, Hill M, Antezano J, et al. Transmission Dynamics of COVID-19 Outbreaks Associated with Child Care Facilities — Salt Lake City, Utah, April–July 2020. MMWR Morb Mortal Wkly Rep 2020;1319–23.
48. Tönshoff B, Müller B, Elling R, et al. Prevalence of SARS-CoV-2 Infection in Children and Their Parents in Southwest Germany. JAMA Pediatr 2021. https://doi. org/10.1001/jamapediatrics.2021.0001.
49. Pitman-Hunt C, Leja J, Jiwani ZM, et al. SARS-CoV-2 Transmission in an Urban Community: The Role of Children and Household Contacts. J Pediatr Infect Dis Soc 2020. https://doi.org/10.1093/jpids/piaa158.
50. Zimmerman KO, Akinboyo IC, Brookhart MA, et al. Incidence and Secondary Transmission of SARS-CoV-2 Infections in Schools. Pediatrics 2021. https://doi. org/10.1542/peds.2020-048090.
51. Leung NHL, Chu DKW, Shiu EYC, et al. Respiratory virus shedding in exhaled breath and efficacy of face masks. Nat Med 2020;26(5):676–80.
52. Ueki H, Furusawa Y, Iwatsuki-Horimoto K, et al. Effectiveness of Face Masks in Preventing Airborne Transmission of SARS-CoV-2. mSphere 2020;5(5). https:// doi.org/10.1128/mSphere.00637-20.
53. Konda A, Prakash A, Moss GA, et al. Aerosol Filtration Efficiency of Common Fabrics Used in Respiratory Cloth Masks. ACS Nano 2020;14(5):6339–47.
54. Wu Z, Harrich D, Li Z, et al. The unique features of SARS-CoV-2 transmission: Comparison with SARS-CoV, MERS-CoV and 2009 H1N1 pandemic influenza virus. Rev Med Virol 2020;e2171.

55. Chu DK, Akl EA, Duda S, et al. Physical distancing, face masks, and eye protection to prevent person-to-person transmission of SARS-CoV-2 and COVID-19: a systematic review and meta-analysis. Lancet 2020;395(10242):1973–87.

56. Li Y, Liang M, Gao L, et al. Face masks to prevent transmission of COVID-19: A systematic review and meta-analysis. Am J Infect Control 2020. https://doi.org/10.1016/j.ajic.2020.12.007.

57. Wang Y, Tian H, Zhang L, et al. Reduction of secondary transmission of SARS-CoV-2 in households by face mask use, disinfection and social distancing: a cohort study in Beijing, China. BMJ Glob Health 2020;5(5). https://doi.org/10.1136/bmjgh-2020-002794.

58. Cheng VC, Wong SC, Chuang VW, et al. The role of community-wide wearing of face mask for control of coronavirus disease 2019 (COVID-19) epidemic due to SARS-CoV-2. J Infect 2020;81(1):107–14.

59. Rader B, White LF, Burns MR, et al. Mask-wearing and control of SARS-CoV-2 transmission in the USA: a cross-sectional study. Lancet Digit Health 2021. https://doi.org/10.1016/S2589-7500(20)30293-4.

60. Honein MA, Christie A, Rose DA, et al. Summary of Guidance for Public Health Strategies to Address High Levels of Community Transmission of SARS-CoV-2 and Related Deaths, December 2020. MMWR Morb Mortal Wkly Rep 2020; 69(49):1860–7.

61. Hu M, Lin H, Wang J, et al. The risk of COVID-19 transmission in train passengers: an epidemiological and modelling study. Clin Infect Dis 2020. https://doi.org/10.1093/cid/ciaa1057.

62. Clipman SJ, Wesolowski AP, Gibson DG, et al. Rapid real-time tracking of non-pharmaceutical interventions and their association with SARS-CoV-2 positivity: The COVID-19 Pandemic Pulse Study. Clin Infect Dis 2020. https://doi.org/10.1093/cid/ciaa1313.

63. Freeman CM, Rank MA, Bolster LaSalle CM, et al. Effectiveness of Physical Distancing: Staying 6 Feet Over to Put Respiratory Viruses 6 Feet Under. Mayo Clin Proc 2021;96(1):148–51.

64. Bulfone TC, Malekinejad M, Rutherford GW, et al. Outdoor Transmission of SARS-CoV-2 and Other Respiratory Viruses, a Systematic Review. J Infect Dis 2020;29. https://doi.org/10.1093/infdis/jiaa742.

65. Prevention CfDCa. Interim public health recommendations for fully vaccinated people 2021. Available at: https://www.cdc.gov/coronavirus/2019-ncov/vaccines/fully-vaccinated-guidance.html#anchor_1615143393075. Accessed March 23, 2021.

66. Prevention CfDCa. Personal and Social Activities. 2021. Available at: https://www.cdc.gov/coronavirus/2019-ncov/daily-life-coping/personal-social-activities.html. Accessed March 24, 2021.

67. Prevention CfDCa. Travel During COVID-19. 2021. Available at: https://www.cdc.gov/coronavirus/2019-ncov/travelers/travel-during-covid19.html. Accessed February 6, 2021.

68. Meyerowitz EA, Richterman A, Gandhi RT, et al. Transmission of SARS-CoV-2: A Review of Viral, Host, and Environmental Factors. Ann Intern Med 2021;174(1):69–79.

69. Wong VW, Cowling BJ, Aiello AE. Hand hygiene and risk of influenza virus infections in the community: a systematic review and meta-analysis. Epidemiol Infect 2014;142(5):922–32.

70. Hirose R, Ikegaya H, Naito Y, et al. Survival of SARS-CoV-2 and influenza virus on the human skin: Importance of hand hygiene in COVID-19. Clin Infect Dis 2020. https://doi.org/10.1093/cid/ciaa1517.

71. Przekwas A, Chen Z. Washing hands and the face may reduce COVID-19 infection. Med Hypotheses 2020;144:110261.

72. Rundle CW, Presley CL, Militello M, et al. Hand hygiene during COVID-19: Recommendations from the American Contact Dermatitis Society. J Am Acad Dermatol 2020;83(6):1730–7.

73. Golin AP, Choi D, Ghahary A. Hand sanitizers: A review of ingredients, mechanisms of action, modes of delivery, and efficacy against coronaviruses. Am J Infect Control 2020;48(9):1062–7.

74. Kampf G, Todt D, Pfaender S, et al. Persistence of coronaviruses on inanimate surfaces and their inactivation with biocidal agents. J Hosp Infect 2020;104(3): 246–51.

75. Organization WH. Cleaning and disinfection of environmental surfaces in the context of COVID-19: Interim guidance. 2020. Available at: https://www.who.int/publications/i/item/cleaning-and-disinfection-of-environmental-surfaces-inthe-context-of-covid-19. Accessed February 10, 2021.

76. Tang JW, Bahnfleth WP, Bluyssen PM, et al. Dismantling myths on the airborne transmission of severe acute respiratory syndrome coronavirus (SARS-CoV-2). J Hosp Infect 2021. https://doi.org/10.1016/j.jhin.2020.12.022.

77. Dai H, Zhao B. Association of the infection probability of COVID-19 with ventilation rates in confined spaces. Build Simul 2020;4:1–7.

78. Bhagat R, Davies Wykes M, Dalziel S, et al. Effects of ventilation on the indoor spread of COVID-19. J Fluid Mech 2020;903:F1.

79. Prevention CfDCa. Caring for someone Sick at home: Advice for caregivers in non-healthcare settings. 2021. Available at: https://www.cdc.gov/coronavirus/2019-ncov/if-you-are-sick/care-for-someone.html. Accessed March 24, 2021.

80. Prevention CfDCa. Improving ventilation in Your home. 2021. Available at: https://www.cdc.gov/coronavirus/2019-ncov/prevent-getting-sick/Improving-Ventilation-Home.html. Accessed January 26, 2021.

81. Prevention CfDCa. When to Quarantine: Stay home if you might have been exposed to COVID-19 2020. Available at: https://www.cdc.gov/coronavirus/2019-ncov/if-you-are-sick/quarantine.html. Accessed January 27, 2021.

82. Andrade BS, Rangel FS, Santos NO, et al. Repurposing Approved Drugs for Guiding COVID-19 Prophylaxis: A Systematic Review. Front Pharmacol 2020; 11:590598.

83. Chen P, Nirula A, Heller B, et al. SARS-CoV-2 Neutralizing Antibody LY-CoV555 in Outpatients with Covid-19. N Engl J Med 2021;384(3):229–37.

84. Ilie PC, Stefanescu S, Smith L. The role of vitamin D in the prevention of coronavirus disease 2019 infection and mortality. Aging Clin Exp Res 2020;32(7): 1195–8.

85. Ali N. Role of vitamin D in preventing of COVID-19 infection, progression and severity. J Infect Public Health 2020;13(10):1373–80.

86. Aranow C. Vitamin D and the immune system. J Investig Med 2011;59(6):881–6.

87. Wei XB, Wang ZH, Liao XL, et al. Efficacy of vitamin C in patients with sepsis: An updated meta-analysis. Eur J Pharmacol 2020;868:172889.

88. Korant BD, Kauer JC, Butterworth BE. Zinc ions inhibit replication of rhinoviruses. Nat 1974;248(449):588–90.

89. te Velthuis AJ, van den Worm SH, Sims AC, et al. Zn(2+) inhibits coronavirus and arterivirus RNA polymerase activity in vitro and zinc ionophores block the replication of these viruses in cell culture. PLoS Pathog 2010;6(11):e1001176.

90. Casale M, Rinaldi V, Sabatino L, et al. Could nasal irrigation and oral rinse reduce the risk for COVID-19 infection? Int J Immunopathol Pharmacol 2020;34. 2058738420941757.

91. Slapak I, Skoupá J, Strnad P, et al. Efficacy of isotonic nasal wash (seawater) in the treatment and prevention of rhinitis in children. Arch Otolaryngol Head Neck Surg 2008;134(1):67–74.

92. Ramalingam S, Graham C, Dove J, et al. A pilot, open labelled, randomised controlled trial of hypertonic saline nasal irrigation and gargling for the common cold. Sci Rep 2019;9(1):1015.

93. Anderson DE, Sivalingam V, Kang AEZ, et al. Povidone-Iodine Demonstrates Rapid In Vitro Virucidal Activity Against SARS-CoV-2, The Virus Causing COVID-19 Disease. Infect Dis Ther 2020;9(3):669–75.

94. Frank S, Brown SM, Capriotti JA, et al. In Vitro Efficacy of a Povidone-Iodine Nasal Antiseptic for Rapid Inactivation of SARS-CoV-2. JAMA Otolaryngol Head Neck Surg 2020. https://doi.org/10.1001/jamaoto.2020.3053.

95. Frank S, Capriotti J, Brown SM, et al. Povidone-Iodine Use in Sinonasal and Oral Cavities: A Review of Safety in the COVID-19 Era. Ear Nose Throat J 2020;99(9): 586–93.

96. Polack FP, Thomas SJ, Kitchin N, et al. Safety and Efficacy of the BNT162b2 mRNA Covid-19 Vaccine. N Engl J Med 2020;383(27):2603–15.

97. Baden LR, El Sahly HM, Essink B, et al. Efficacy and Safety of the mRNA-1273 SARS-CoV-2 Vaccine. N Engl J Med 2020. https://doi.org/10.1056/ NEJMoa2035389.

98. Oliver SE, Gargano JW, Marin M, et al. The Advisory Committee on Immunization Practices' Interim Recommendation for Use of Pfizer-BioNTech COVID-19 Vaccine - United States, December 2020. MMWR Morb Mortal Wkly Rep 2020; 69(50):1922–4.

99. Oliver SE, Gargano JW, Marin M, et al. The Advisory Committee on Immunization Practices' Interim Recommendation for Use of Moderna COVID-19 Vaccine - United States, December 2020. MMWR Morb Mortal Wkly Rep 2021;69(5152): 1653–6.

The Impact of Coronavirus Disease 2019 on Pediatric Asthma in the United States

Aishwarya Navalpakam, MD[a], Elizabeth Secord, MD[b],
Milind Pansare, MD[c],*

KEYWORDS

- COVID-19 • Pediatric asthma • United States

KEY POINTS

- The COVID-19 pandemic caused morbidities and mortalities of historic proportion and disrupted health-care delivery in the United States.
- The elderly and patients with chronic illnesses including asthma are at increased risks of poor outcomes.
- Limited data in the United States indicate children with asthma have done well despite multiple challenges to health-care delivery.
- It is important to adhere to asthma treatment guidelines to maintain asthma control in children during the pandemic.

INTRODUCTION

Coronaviruses are a common cause of upper respiratory infections in children.[1] A novel human coronavirus, severe acute respiratory syndrome coronavirus 2 (SARS-CoV-2), mutated in bats in Wuhan, China, and has been attributed to be the cause of a global pandemic leading to illness and death in 2020.[2] Initially, asthma was thought to be a risk factor for poor clinical outcomes in adult patients with coronavirus disease 2019 (COVID-19). However, limited data currently available have not shown significant COVID-19 illness or increase in asthma exacerbations in children during the pandemic. In this article, we aim to outline impact of COVID-19 on pediatric asthma in the United States and current recommendations for asthma care.

[a] Division of Allergy and Immunology, Department of Pediatrics, Pediatric Specialty Center, Children's Hospital of Michigan, 4th Floor, 3950 Beaubien Boulevard, Detroit, MI 48236, USA; [b] Department of Pediatrics, Wayne State University, Detroit, MI, USA; [c] Department of Pediatrics, Division of Allergy and Immunology, Pediatric Specialty Center, Children's Hospital of Michigan, Central Michigan University, Suite # 4018, 4th Floor, 3950 Beaubien Boulevard, Detroit, MI 48236, USA
* Corresponding author.
E-mail address: mpansare@dmc.org

Pediatr Clin N Am 68 (2021) 1119–1131
https://doi.org/10.1016/j.pcl.2021.05.012   pediatric.theclinics.com

IMPACT OF COVID-19 IN THE UNITED STATES

The United States has become an epicenter during the pandemic, reporting the highest number of cases and deaths due to COVID-19. In the United States alone by December 31, 2020, a total aggregate count of COVID-19 cases of 19,663,976 and total deaths of 341,199 were reported by states and territorial jurisdictions to the Centers for Disease Control and Prevention (CDC). These numbers continue to increase. In the age-group of 0 to 17 years, the total number of reported COVID-19 cases was 1,500,972 (10.5% estimated from the age reported in 14,226,540 cases) and the death count was 211 (<0.2% estimated from the age reported in 237,889 deaths) during the same period.[3] The CDC had listed asthma as a risk factor for COVID-19 outcomes, particularly morbidity and mortality.[4] Asthma is the most common chronic respiratory disease in children, affecting about 6 million children in the United States in ages 0 to 17 years. Every year, one in 6 children with asthma visits the ED and about 1 in 20 children with asthma is hospitalized for the same condition (https://cdc.gov.asthma). Practitioners and parents alike anticipated and rapidly prepared for the significant impact of SARS-CoV-2 infections in children with asthma. The reality was not what was anticipated.

RESPIRATORY VIRUSES AND ASTHMA

Asthma in children is often triggered by respiratory viruses. It is theorized that the type I interferon production, which is important for defense against viruses, is decreased in asthmatic individuals and is inhibited by Th2 inflammation seen in allergic asthma.[5] Studies also suggest that in atopic individuals, certain respiratory viruses such as respiratory syncytial virus (RSV) or human rhinovirus (RV), owing to the formation of specific IgE, may cause exacerbations.[5] RSV and RV have actually been implicated in the development of asthma. Other viruses such as influenza, coronavirus, adenovirus, parainfluenza virus, and metapneumovirus are considered risk factors for asthma exacerbations. At the advent of the COVID-19 pandemic, there was a concern that SARS-CoV-2 infection may also result in increased asthma exacerbations in children, which surprisingly did not occur.

PATHOPHYSIOLOGY OF SEVERE ACUTE RESPIRATORY SYNDROME CORONAVIRUS-2

COVID-19 is caused by the novel coronavirus SARS-CoV-2. It is a single-stranded RNA virus (ssRNA) that contains a spike protein (S protein) that binds to angiotensin-converting enzyme 2 (ACE2) receptors found on human cells. The ssRNA is inserted into the airway epithelial cells, where it replicates causing local inflammation, tissue damage, and cytokine release. The majority of these ACE2 receptors are located on type II alveolar epithelial cells. There are other associated receptors such as type II cellular transmembrane serine protease (TMPRSS2) that activate S protein and allow for the fusion of the viral membrane into the host cell.[6]

POTENTIAL ASTHMA-PROTECTIVE FACTORS AGAINST COVID-19

The pathophysiologic hallmark of asthma is chronic airway inflammation. Generally, two types of inflammatory asthma are described: type 2-high (T2) asthma and type 2-low (T1) asthma, based on the expression of T helper cell type 2 (TH2) cytokines. Type 2-high asthma is characterized by eosinophilic airway inflammation, elevated levels of cytokines such as interleukin (IL) 4, IL-5, and IL-13, and elevated levels of IgE. This is also known as allergic asthma that appears earlier in life, is responsive to corticosteroids, and is a common phenotype in children. The type 2 low asthma phenotype is more common in adults, has later disease onset, has less allergic comorbidities, and is less responsive to corticosteroids.

ACE2 receptor expression appears to vary with asthma phenotype. A study of two large adult asthma cohorts identified increased expression of the ACE2 gene in the bronchial epithelium of patients with type 2-low or T1-high asthma.[7] Interestingly, these patients also tended to have higher known risk factors for COVID-19 including hypertension, lymphopenia, and male gender.[7,8] This suggests that the T2-low phenotype is likely associated with higher risk of COVID-19. Another study of cohort of children with asthma, the Urban Environment and Childhood Asthma (URECA) cohort, revealed that allergic sensitization in children (positive IgE tests for allergens, either skin or serum testing) with asthma was associated with decreased ACE2 expression in children.[9] The type 2-high asthma phenotype characterized by the elevated serum IgE level, fractional exhaled nitric oxide (FeNO), and IL-13 expression was associated with decreased ACE2 receptor expression in this URECA cohort.[9] It suggests that T2 high-asthma and allergic sensitization is associated with decreased ACE2 receptor expression and may be a cause of decreased SARS-CoV-2 infection in these patients. This may be important to pediatric patients with asthma who tend to have the T2-high asthma phenotype. Children, when compared to adults, have lower ACE2 receptors in their nasal epithelium. This may account for the decreased incidence of COVID-19 in children.[10]

The use of inhaled corticosteroids (ICSs) may also provide a protective role for asthma from COVID-19. Cultures of human nasal and tracheal epithelial cells reveal that the combination of glycopyrronium, a long-acting muscarinic antagonist, formoterol, a long-acting beta-2 agonist, and budesonide, an ICS, inhibits replication of HCoV-229E, a virus that causes common cold by preventing receptor expression and decreases virus-induced airway inflammation.[11] When gene expression of ACE2 and TMPRSS2 was analyzed in sputum cells from patients with severe asthma, it was found that the use of ICSs was associated with lower expression of these receptors.[12] These studies suggests patients with asthma who are adherent to their ICSs thus may have decreased risk of COVID-19.

COVID-19 AND ASTHMA PREVALENCE

The number of adult patients with asthma hospitalized owing to COVID-19 across the world is low, with incidence reported from 1% to 2.7%.[13] An online questionnaire sent to 91 pediatric practitioners in 27 countries attempted to estimate the incidence of clinically relevant COVID-19 in pediatric patients with asthma. They noted that incidence is 12.8 times less frequent in children than in adults.[14] A retrospective study of a large cohort in Israel also showed that patients with asthma have a lower susceptibility for COVID-19 in pediatric and adult patients. The study did not find any difference in the rate of hospitalization in patients with COVID-19 with or without asthma.[15] A nationwide study in Japan examining asthma during the COVID-19 outbreak found decreased asthma admissions in 2020 compared with previous years for children and adults.[16] A study of 212 children with allergic asthma in Spain found no significant difference in asthma control or severity between patients with and without COVID-19.[17]

In the United States, adult data suggest that there is no significant increased risk of mortality associated with a history of asthma. A matched cohort study of adult patients with asthma admitted to Massachusetts General Hospital with COVID-19 found that patients with asthma were less likely to require intensive care and mechanical ventilation and did not have increased risk of mortality.[18] A large COVID-19 registry with 11,405 patients from the Mount Sinai Health System in NYC revealed that of the

54.8% of patients who were COVID-19 positive, only 4.4% had asthma, suggesting there was no significant association between asthma history and disease.[19]

The early data from Wuhan regarding hospitalized pediatric patients and those with severe COVID-19 do not list asthma as a risk factor.[20,21] As per the CDC, in the United States, as of January 2021, 10.8% of 16,212,877 COVID-19 cases are found in children. However, these data are changing and not necessarily accurate of the true incidence in children owing to lack of prioritization of testing in this population. Hospitalization is reported to be low among children when compared with adults (CDC). Owing to a paucity of data, there has been an urgent call for further studies in childhood asthma in the current pandemic.[22]

Asthma exacerbations have a seasonal pattern, generally have increased prevalence in the late fall and spring, and are seen across North America and known as the September peak or asthma epidemic.[23,24] This is attributed to viral upper respiratory infections (URI), air pollutants, weather changes, and increase in aeroallergens.[25] Viral infections particularly account for asthma exacerbations in children during the start of school in early fall. Although respiratory viruses are a risk factor for asthma exacerbations, this did not seem to pertain to the current SARS-CoV-2 infection outbreak. Previously, SARS-CoV infection, which caused the first SARS outbreak in 2002, did not appear to be associated with an increase in asthma exacerbations in children.[26] However, there are very few studies published evaluating incidence, trends, hospitalization, and mortality related to pediatric asthma with COVID-19 in the United States. Some of the published studies in the US population are summarized in **Table 1**.[27-31]

IMPACT ON PEDIATRIC ASTHMA: MORBIDITY AND MORTALITY

Various studies from around the world, including China, Brazil, Italy, Switzerland, and the United States, reveal that asthma is not associated with increased risk of mortality in adult patients with COVID-19.[13] The Morbidity and Mortality Weekly Report from October 2020 that evaluated COVID-19 trends among school-age children (N = 277, 285) noted that 1.2% were hospitalized, 0.1% had intensive care unit (ICU) admissions, and less than 0.1% died. Of those patients (hospitalized, ICU admissions, died owing to COVID-19), each had at least one underlying medical condition, and 55% of the underlying conditions were accounted for by chronic lung disease including asthma, emphysema, and chronic obstructive pulmonary disease (COPD).[32] The final determination of COVID-19 impact toward pediatric asthma morbidity and mortality remains to be seen owing to lack of sufficiently powered studies providing significant data.

IMPACT ON PEDIATRIC ASTHMA: CLINICAL CARE

As the pandemic surged worldwide, international and governmental agencies of countries across all the continents responded by implementing control measures to contain the spread of virus. In the United States, federal, state, and local governments passed many unprecedented regulations including stay-at-home orders; the closing of local businesses, universities, and schools; social distancing; and face mask mandates. In the initial surge of disease, health resources were targeted toward the care of seriously ill patients with COVID-19, and nonurgent care was deferred to the alternate delivery model. The federal government declared a public health emergency and also allocated resources to provide medical care. The Health Insurance Portability and Accountability Act was relaxed, which allowed physicians to use their personal electronic devices to communicate with their patients during the pandemic.[33] The Centers

Table 1
Summary of pediatric asthma and COVID-19 studies

Study	Timeline	Asthma Findings
Kenyon et al,[27] 2020 Initial ED impact of COVID-19 in pediatric asthma • Retrospective chart review • Compared daily ED visits for asthma for the January–April period in 2020 to years 2016–2019	January to April from years 2016 to 2020	• ED utilization for asthma decreased by 3 standard deviations below the mean in year 2020 as compared with years 2016–2019. • Decreased ED visits by 76% in March–April 2020 (COVID) as compared with January–March 2020 (pre-COVID-19)
Taquechel et al,[28] 2020 Asthma health-care utilization during COVID-19 • Retrospective chart review • Compared outpatient, inpatient, and ED visits for asthma for the January to May period from years 2015–2020	January to May from years 2015 to 2020	Until March 17, 2020, similar visits (when compared with 2015–2019) After March 17, 2020: • Outpatient in-person asthma encounters decreased by 87%. • Hospital encounters decreased by 84%. • Telephone encounters increased by 19%. • TM visits increased by 61%. Other findings: • Decreased asthma-related steroid prescriptions. • Decreased frequency of rhinovirus infections.

Bandi et al,[29] 2020
Risks of COVID-19 in asthma in children aged <18 y evaluated by the TM clinic
• Tested for SARS-CoV-2 (PCR)
• Documented asthma status
	March 12, 2020, to April 20, 2020	474 patients tested → 5.2% tested positive for SARS-CoV-2
		• Rate of asthma in SARS-CoV-2–positive cases: 12%
		• Rate of asthma in SARS-CoV-2–negative cases:10%
		  ○ No significant difference
		  ○ Asthma not a risk factor for infection

Bailey et al,[30] 2020 SARS-CoV-2 testing in US children • Retrospective cohort study	January 1, 2020, to September 8, 2020	135794 patients tested for SARS-CoV-2 → 4% positive • 7% had severe illness (ICU care, increased length of stay, ventilation). • 0.2% died. • Asthma had a negative association with SARS-CoV-2 positive test results (SR, 0.86 [95% CI, 0.80–0.91]).

(continued on next page)

Table 1
(continued)

Study	Timeline	Asthma Findings
Secord et al,[31] 2021 ED visits for pediatric asthma • Retrospective chart review	March 15 to May 31 in 2019 and in 2020	Asthma ED visits significantly decreased during school closure from March 15 to May 31, 2020, when compared with the same period in 2019. • Average daily ED visits for asthma of 17 in 2019 vs 3.5 in 2020 • Total ED visits for asthma of 1304 in 2019 vs 260 in 2020 ($P = .001$)

Abbreviations: ED, emergency department; PCR, polymerase chain reaction; SR, standardized ratio.

for Medicare & Medicaid Services also promoted telemedicine (TM) by waiving previous restrictions of patient qualification for TM visits, by permitting office-based and home-based video encounters on personal devices with patients, and by improving reimbursements.[34]

In the United States, practitioners actively responded by establishing virtual clinics and using telehealth tools in all medical specialties to curb the pandemic.[35] An ad hoc expert panel of allergy/immunology specialists from the United States and Canada developed a consensus document to guide specialists in lieu of reduced services due to the pandemic.[36] The guidelines on COVID-19 and allergy contingency planning noted "If the allergy/immunology office does not have personal protective equipment available, it would be recommended that no patients with co-potential for asthma exacerbation and COVID-19 be seen at the office; the patient should instead be seen at a facility capable of isolation and equipped for asthma care." These recommendations are expected to be adjusted based on disease prevalence. Most ambulatory allergy services in the country restricted new patient appointments and procedures. The established patients were evaluated in virtual platforms. Sick patients were referred to facilities equipped with personnel protection, laboratory testing for SARS-CoV-2, and high acuity care treatments. Diagnostic testing and therapeutic interventions for allergic disease and asthma were restricted owing to concerns of the spread of the virus. This included testing for allergic sensitization, lung functions, FeNO, and nebulized treatments and allergy injections.[36,37] Clinicians considered health-care delivery during the pandemic to be suboptimal and are eager to resume face-to-face encounters as soon as possible. Parents were also unwilling to bring their children to hospitals and clinics for fear of contracting the virus during the pandemic. Many raised concerns about inhaled or oral steroids and risks of COVID-19 infections. Despite the multiple challenges of wildly spreading disease and misinformation, the patient outcomes with asthma were not worse and have been better than expected, generally. This is likely due to initial fear of susceptibility to severe COVID-19 with asthma, which prompted families to adopt health safety measures and improve adherence to asthma medications. A study at a health system in Wisconsin using electronic medication monitors noted a 14.5% relative increase in asthma controller adherence across all age-groups from January to March 2020.[38] The increased adherence is due to parental concern about asthma control during the outbreak.[39] School closures in particular also reduced exposures to allergens and viruses among children, which are important triggers of asthma, thus enabling improved asthma control.

COVID-19 AND ASTHMA TREATMENT GUIDELINES

There were some initial concerns about continuing ICSs and oral corticosteroids for asthma owing to fear of contracting the virus because steroids can impair immune responses. A meta-analysis of 39 trials revealed that ICS use was not associated with higher risk of pneumonia or respiratory infection due to COVID-19.[40] A study of RNA expression in bronchial brushes of a cohort of adult patients with asthma in the United Kindgom found that there was no significant difference in expression of ACE2 receptor and TMPRSS between healthy controls and patients with moderate and severe asthma undergoing varying corticosteroid treatment.[41] There was no greater risk for asthmatics than the general population for risk of COVID-19, regardless of the severity of asthma and various corticosteroid treatment intensities. This supports the use of inhaled steroids in the management of asthma.

In response to the pandemic, the Global Initiative for Asthma (GINA) updated guidelines on asthma care during the pandemic.[42] The guideline emphasized the importance of optimal asthma management and medication adherence in reducing the risk of asthma exacerbations. The guidelines also recommend continuing prescribed medications including daily ICSs and biologic therapy.[42] The American Academy of Allergy, Asthma, and Immunology also reiterated that patients with asthma should continue to use their medications and aim for good control.[43] Both recommended the controller medication dose not be reduced or discontinued during the pandemic unless there is clear-cut benefit after careful consideration of risk/benefit for the child.[36,42,43] Systemic or oral steroids are recommended for use in moderate to severe asthma exacerbations that are unimproved with bronchodilators.[42,43] There is no evidence to suggest impairment of immune response to COVID-19 in patients treated with biologics for asthma. It is reasonable to continue administration of these agents during the pandemic.[42–44] Allergen immunotherapy used as an adjunct is also recommended to be continued with adjustment in doses and duration.[43]

COVID-19: USE OF NEBULIZERS AND SPIROMETRY

Many national and international societies including the GINA, National Asthma Council Australia, and American College of Allergy, Asthma and Immunology recommend against using nebulizers to reduce the risk of spreading the virus, with a preference for pressurized metered dose inhalers (MDIs).[42,43] SARS-CoV-2 is transmitted via droplets and aerosols. Owing to aerosol treatments, SARS-CoV-2 may persist in the air for up to 2 hours and may be recirculated and remain on dependent surfaces, promoting virus spread.[45] There is also concern that the particles that are generated with nebulization may stimulate cough in patients, which can spread the pathogen.[46] Use of the albuterol MDI (90 mcg/puff), 4 to 8 puffs every 20 minutes for 3 doses and then inhalation using the valved holding chamber every 1 to 4 hours, has shown to be as effective as nebulized therapy for mild to moderate asthma exacerbation in children.[47] MDIs with spacers have comparable efficacy with nebulizers, take shorter time for delivery, are more portable, and are less likely to spread the virus during the pandemic. Nebulizer treatments may still be necessary in very young or sick children and are

---

Box 1
Guidelines for minimizing risk of SARS-CoV-2 transmission[42]

Follow CDC guidelines[a]

Follow state and local directives on public health measures to control disease.

CDC guidelines for schools and childcare program.

Social and physical distancing measures
- Avoid close contact from other people—remain six feet away from others at all times.
- Practice self-isolation if you are in a high-risk group or if you are sick.
- Stay home and avoid large crowds and indoor spaces.

Face mask and personal protection measures:
- Wash hands using a sanitizing handwash containing at least 60% alcohol.
- Refrain from touching your face.
- Cover your mouth/nose when coughing with your elbow or a tissue.
  - Dispose of your tissue immediately afterward.
- Wear a face mask or face covering in public settings (now recommended by the CDC).
- Clean and disinfect surfaces regularly.

[a]https://www.cdc.gov/coronavirus/2019-ncov/prevent-getting-sick/prevention.html.

preferred in settings equipped with infection control measures. Most hospitals and clinics have rapidly adapted to the change of using MDIs to help control the pandemic without compromising asthma outcomes.

Spirometry is an important tool of asthma management but poses a considerable risk for the spread of infection to individuals and the surrounding surfaces within and around the test areas. The American Thoracic Society recommends prioritizing patients' clinical status by screening for urgent cases, ensuring protection of the health-care worker, and using in-line filters for spirometry.[48] The full operation of lung function services can resume when virus prevalence is low.[48] General guidelines for infection control and daily asthma management adapted from GINA guidelines are highlighted in **Box 1** and **Table 2**. The Food and Drug Administration under the Emergency Use Authorization approved two mRNA vaccines for ages more than 18 years in December 2020 for control of the pandemic.[47] Many other vaccines are in the research pipeline and under investigation for use in children.

Table 2 General guidance for care of patients with asthma during the COVID-19 pandemic[36]	
Asthma Medications	• Continue daily controller (inhaled corticosteroids) as prescribed • Step down in treatment only in cases risk/benefit is carefully evaluated • For severe asthma: continue biologic therapy or oral corticosteroids if prescribed. • Close monitoring—use control tests such as the ACT, peak flow meter, and periodic virtual or clinic visits • Provide all patients with a written asthma action plan ○ Recommend that patients do not share inhalers and spacer devices

Acute Exacerbations	• Use a short course of OCS when appropriate for severe asthma exacerbations
	• Avoid nebulizers where possible to reduce the risk of spreading virus.
	  ○ Nebulizers may be required for:
	    ■ Severe or life-threatening exacerbation
	    ■ Young children (<4 y)
	    ■ Patients who are unable to use MDIs even with a valved holding chamber.
	  ○ Strict infection control procedures if aerosol-generating procedures are needed
	• A pressurized metered dose inhaler (MDI) via a spacer is preferred for mild to moderate asthma exacerbation.

Spirometry	• Avoid in patients with confirmed or suspected COVID-19 or if COVID-19 cases are high in community ○ Practice appropriate aerosol, droplet, and contact precautions if spirometry is needed. • Consider home peak flow monitoring • Follow local public health measures to control spread of infection—including personal hygiene and use of PPE.
Vaccination	• Recommend the annual influenza vaccine. • Follow CDC guidelines for COVID-19 vaccination. • After obtaining COVID-19 vaccines, continue to wear a mask and avoid close contact with others.

Abbreviations: ACT, asthma control test; OCS, oral corticosteroid; PPE, personal protection equipment.

SUMMARY

The COVID-19 pandemic has had a severe economic and health impact all over the world, including the United States, in particular. The available data, albeit limited, suggest that the initial concerns of the serious impact of COVID-19 illness in children with asthma are not evident to date. The reduction in asthma morbidities is likely due to a combination of improved adherence and decreased exposure to both allergens and viral infections in children. International guidelines are updated to guide physicians in the midst of the pandemic. In the face of unprecedented time, it is important to be vigilant, adhere to treatment guidelines, and implement preventive measures to eradicate the virus and improve outcomes for children with asthma.

CLINICS CARE POINTS

- The COVID-19 pandemic has caused catastrophic impact on health and well-being of humans globally.
- Unlike children, adults with chronic illnesses and other health risk factors had poorer outcomes.
- Current evidence suggests most children with chronic asthma were able to maintain asthma control during the pandemic.
- It is important to adhere to recommendations of international and national asthma guidelines for treatment of both acute exacerbation and chronic asthma.
- A multipronged measure including stepped pharmacotherapy based on asthma severity is necessary to maintain asthma control in children during the pandemic.
- Current evidence suggests favorable outcomes with inhaled corticosteroids and biologics used in treatment of asthma.
- It is important to implement CDC guidelines on SARS-CoV-2 infection control and vaccinations when available.

DISCLOSURE

The authors have nothing to disclose.

REFERENCES

1. Kahn JS, Mcintosh K. History and recent advances in coronavirus discovery. Pediatr Infect Dis J 2005;24(Suppl):S223–6.
2. Platto S, Xue T, Carafoli E. COVID-19: an announced pandemic. Cell Death Dis 2020;11:799–812.
3. COVID-19 Stats. COVID-19 Incidence, by Age Group -United States, March 1– November 14, 2020. MMWR Morb Mortal Wkly Rep 2021;69:1664.
4. Centers for Disease Control and Prevention. Coronavirus disease 2019 (COVID-19): people who are at high risk 2020. Available at: https://www.cdc.gov/coronavirus/2019-ncov/need-extra-precautions/asthma.html.
5. Novak N, Cabanillas B. Viruses and asthma: the role of common respiratory viruses in asthma and its potential meaning for SARS-CoV-2. Immunology 2020; 161(2):83–93.
6. Singh SP, Pritam M, Pandey B, et al. Microstructure, pathophysiology, and potential therapeutics of COVID-19: A comprehensive review. J Med Virol 2020.

7. Camiolo M, Gauthier M, Kaminski N, et al. Expression of SARS-CoV-2 receptor ACE2 and coincident host response signature varies by asthma inflammatory phenotype. J Allergy Clin Immunol 2020;146(2):315–24.e7.
8. Wakabayashi M, Pawankar R, Narazaki H, et al. Coronavirus disease 2019 and asthma, allergic rhinitis: molecular mechanisms and host-environmental interactions. Curr Opin Allergy Clin Immunol 2021;21(1):1–7.
9. Jackson DJ, Busse WW, Bacharier LB, et al. Association of respiratory allergy, asthma, and expression of the SARS-CoV-2 receptor ACE2. J Allergy Clin Immunol 2020;146(1):203–6.e3.
10. Bunyavanich S, Do A, Vicencio A. Nasal gene expression of angiotensin-converting enzyme 2 in children and adults. JAMA 2020;323(23):2427–9.
11. Yamaya M, Nishimura H, Deng X, et al. Inhibitory effects of glycopyrronium, formoterol, and budesonide on coronavirus HCoV-229E replication and cytokine production by primary cultures of human nasal and tracheal epithelial cells. Respir Investig 2020;58(3):155–68.
12. Peters MC, Sajuthi S, Deford P, et al. Covid-19-related genes in sputum cells in asthma. Relationship to demographic features and corticosteroids. Am J Respir Crit Care Med 2020;202(1):83–90.
13. Skevaki C, Karsonova A, Karaulov A, et al. Asthma-associated risk for COVID-19 development. J Allergy Clin Immunol 2020;146(6):1295–301.
14. Papadopoulus NG, Custovic A, Deschildre A, et al. Pediatric Asthma in Real Life collaborators. Impact of COVID-19 on pediatric burden of asthma: Practice adjustments and disease burden. J Allergy Clin Immunol Pract 2020;8:2594–9.
15. Green I, Merzon E, Vinker S, et al. Covid-19 susceptibility in bronchial asthma. J Allergy Clin Immunol Pract 2021;9(2):684–92.e1.
16. Abe K, Miyawaki A, Nakamura M, et al. Trends in hospitalizations for asthma during the COVID-19 outbreak in Japan. J Allergy Clin Immunol Pract 2021;9(1):494–6.e1.
17. Ruano FJ, Somoza Álvarez ML, Haroun-Díaz E, et al. Impact of the COVID-19 pandemic in children with allergic asthma. J Allergy Clin Immunol Pract 2020;8(9):3172–4.e1.
18. Robinson LB, Fu X, Bassett IV, et al. COVID-19 severity in hospitalized patients with asthma: A matched cohort study. J Allergy Clin Immunol Pract 2021;9(1):497–500.
19. Lieberman-Cribbin W, Rapp J, Alpert N, et al. The impact of asthma on mortality in patients with covid-19. Chest 2020;158(6):2290–1.
20. Zheng F, Liao C, Fan Q-H, et al. Clinical characteristics of children with coronavirus disease 2019 in hubei, china. Curr Med Sci 2020;40(2):275–80.
21. Sun D, Li H, Lu X-X, et al. Clinical features of severe pediatric patients with coronavirus disease 2019 in Wuhan: a single center's observational study. World J Pediatr 2020;16(3):251–9.
22. Castro-Rodriguez JA, Forno E. Asthma and COVID-19 in children: A systematic review and call for data. Pediatr Pulmonol 2020;55(9):2412–8.
23. Wisniewski JA, McLaughlin AP, Stenger PJ, et al. A comparison of seasonal trends in asthma exacerbations among children from geographic regions with different climates. Allergy Asthma Proc 2016;37(6):475–81.
24. Larsen K, Zhu J, Feldman LY, et al. The annual september peak in asthma exacerbation rates. Still a reality? Ann Am Thorac Soc 2016;13(2):231–9.
25. Castro CR, Tarabichi Y, Gunzler DD, et al. Seasonal trends in asthma exacerbations: Are they the same in asthma subgroups? Ann Allergy Asthma Immunol 2019;123(2):220–2.

26. Van Bever HP, Chng SY, Goh DY. Childhood severe acute respiratory syndrome, coronavirus infections and asthma. Pediatr Allergy Immunol 2004;15(3):206–9.

27. Kenyon CC, Hill DA, Henrickson SE, et al. Initial effects of the COVID-19 pandemic on pediatric asthma emergency department utilization. J Allergy Clin Immunol Pract 2020;8(8):2774–6.e1.

28. Taquechel K, Diwadkar AR, Sayed S, et al. Pediatric asthma health care utilization, viral testing, and air pollution changes during the covid-19 pandemic. J Allergy Clin Immunol Pract 2020;8(10):3378–87.e11.

29. Bandi S, Nevid MZ, Mahdavinia M. African American children are at higher risk of COVID-19 infection. Pediatr Allergy Immunol 2020;31(7):861–4.

30. Bailey LC, Razzaghi H, Burrows EK, et al. Assessment of 135 794 pediatric patients tested for severe acute respiratory syndrome coronavirus 2 across the united states. JAMA Pediatr 2021;175(2):176–84.

31. Secord E, Poowuttikul P, Pansare M, et al. Pediatric emergency visits for asthma drop significantly with covid 19 school closure. J Allergy Clin Immunol 2021; 147(2):AB150.

32. Leeb RT, Price S, Sliwa S, et al. Covid-19 trends among school-aged children - united states, march 1-september 19, 2020. MMWR Morb Mortal Wkly Rep 2020;69(39):1410–5.

33. American Telemedicine Association. ATA commends. Congress for giving HHS authority to waive restrictions on telehealth for Medicare beneficiaries in response to the COVID-19 outbreak. Arlington (VA): American Telemedicine Association; 2020. Available at: www.americantelemed.org/press-releases/ata-commends-congress-for-waiving-restrictionson-telehealth-for-medicare-beneficiaries-in-res ponse-to-the-covid-19-outbreak/. Accessed March 16, 2020.

34. Centers for Medicare & Medicaid Services. Coverage and payment related to COVID-19 Medicare. 2020. Available at: https://www.cms.gov/files/document/ 03052020-medicare-covid-19-fact-sheet.pdf. Accessed: March 15, 2020.

35. Hollander JE, Carr BG. Virtually perfect? Telemedicine for Covid-19. N Engl J Med 2020;382:1679–81.

36. Shaker MS, Oppenheimer J, Grayson M, et al. COVID-19: pandemic contingency planning for the allergy and immunology clinic. J Allergy Clin Immunol Pract 2020;8:1477–88.e5.

37. Cardinale F, Ciprandi G, Barberi S, et al. Consensus statement of the Italian society of pediatric allergy and immunology for the pragmatic management of children and adolescents with allergic or immunological diseases during the COVID19 pandemic. Ital J Pediatr 2020;46:84.

38. Kaye L, Theye BA, Smeenk I, et al. Changes in medication adherence among patients with asthma and COPD during the COVID-19 pandemic. J Allergy Clin Immunol Pract 2020;8:2384–5.

39. Oreskovic NM, Kinane TB, Aryee E, et al. The unexpected risks of covid-19 on asthma control in children. J Allergy Clin Immunol Pract 2020;8(8):2489–91.

40. Cazeiro C, Silva C, Mayer S, et al. Inhaled corticosteroids and respiratory infections in children with asthma: a meta-analysis. Pediatrics 2017;139(3).

41. Bradding P, Richardson M, Hinks TSC, et al. ACE2, TMPRSS2, and furin gene expression in the airways of people with asthma-implications for COVID-19. J Allergy Clin Immunol 2020;146(1):208–11.

42. GINA interim guidance on COVID-19 and asthma. Available at: https://ginasthma. org/wp-content/uploads/2020/12. Accessed: January12, 2020.

43. AAAAI. Asthma and COVID-19 2020. Available at: https://www.aaaai.org/ask-the-expert/covid. Accessed: December 20, 2020.

44. Morais-Almeida M, Aguiar R, Martin B, et al. COVID-19, asthma, and biological therapies: What we need to know. World Allergy Organ J 2020;13:100–26.
45. Cazzola M, Ora J, Bianco A, et al. Guidance on nebulization during the current COVID-19 pandemic. Respir Med 2020;176:106236.
46. Mei-Zahav M, Amirav I. Aerosol treatments for childhood asthma in the era of COVID-19. Pediatr Pulmonol 2020;55(8):1871–2.
47. Camargo CA Jr, Rachelefsky G, Schatz M. Managing asthma exacerbations in the emergency department: Summary of the National Asthma Education and Prevention Program Expert Panel Report 3 guidelines for the management of asthma exacerbations. J Allergy Clin Immunol 2009;124(2):S5–14.
48. Crimi C, Impellizzeri P, Campisi R, et al. Practical considerations for spirometry during the COVID-19 outbreak: Literature review and insights. Pulmonology 2020.

Health Disparities and Their Effects on Children and Their Caregivers During the Coronavirus Disease 2019 Pandemic

Lynn C. Smitherman, MD[a],*, William Christopher Golden, MD[b],
Jennifer R. Walton, MD, MPH[c]

KEYWORDS

- COVID-19 pandemic • Health disparities in children • Systemic racism

KEY POINTS

- COVID-19 disproportionately affects children of color, and children considered vulnerable due to their living situations or underlying health conditions.
- Children of color have higher rates of hospitalization and more serious disease from COVID-19 than white children, mirroring the demographics of adult patients with COVID-19.
- Health disparities of children uncovered during the COVID-19 pandemic are due to structural racism, underlying medical problems, limited access to care, the occupations/employment of their caregivers, and the limited ability to minimize exposure/transmission in their home environments.
- To reduce health disparities among vulnerable populations of children during this pandemic and in the future, an intensified effort must be initiated and sustained to dismantle the social determinants of health, particularly measures to provide economic stability for families and access to health care and community infrastructure to support technology needed for education and telemedicine to achieve health equity.

[a] Department of Pediatrics, Wayne State University School of Medicine, 400 Mack Avenue, Suite 1 East, Detroit, MI 48201, USA; [b] Eudowood Neonatal Pulmonary Division, Department of Pediatrics, Johns Hopkins University School of Medicine, 1800 Orleans Street, Bloomberg 8523, Baltimore, MD 21287, USA; [c] Division of Developmental Behavioral Pediatrics, Department of Pediatrics, Nationwide Children's Hospital, The Ohio State University College of Medicine, 700 Children's Drive, Columbus, OH 43205, USA
* Corresponding author.
E-mail address: lsmither@med.wayne.edu

Pediatr Clin N Am 68 (2021) 1133–1145
https://doi.org/10.1016/j.pcl.2021.05.013
pediatric.theclinics.com
0031-3955/21/© 2021 Elsevier Inc. All rights reserved.

INTRODUCTION

As of the end of January 2021, there have been more than 26,000,000 infections and more than 435,000 deaths attributable to COVID-19.[1] Unfortunately, racial and ethnic minorities have been affected most significantly by this pandemic, particularly African Americans, Latinx Americans, and Indigenous Americans.[2] For example, African Americans compose 13.4% of the US population but represent 15.5% of COVID-19-related deaths.[1] In addition, although severe acute respiratory syndrome corona-virus 2 (SARS-CoV-2) affects children to a lesser extent than adults, non-Hispanic black and Hispanic children are hospitalized at a higher rate than white children and have more serious disease.[3,4] Finally, children with underlying health conditions, including obesity, chronic lung disease, and prematurity are hospitalized with COVID-19 at a higher rate than those without chronic medical conditions.[3] This disproportionate impact of COVID-19 in minoritized communities has been linked to pre-existing health disparities.[5–7]

Health disparities are defined as differences among specific populations in the ability to achieve full health potential (as measured by differences in incidence, prevalence, mortality, burden of disease, and other adverse health conditions).[5] Among children, multiple factors contribute to these disparities, including economic stability, and access to health care. According to the Annie E. Casey Foundation, before the current pandemic, 12 million children in the United States were living in poverty in 2019, including one-third of African American and Native American children and 25% of Latinx children.[8] During the same period, of the 4.4 million children without health insurance, 14% were Native American, 9% were of Hispanic descent, and 18% were immigrants.[8] At present, owing to the impact of the pandemic on job security, more than 50% of African American, Latinx, and multiethnic adults are now without medical insurance, directly affecting the health security of their children.[8] With the onset of the pandemic and the social and political upheaval felt by many disenfranchised communities, these well-documented disparities (and the importance of addressing them) have again been brought to the attention of the medical community.[2–8]

This overview will examine the effects of these health disparities in various populations of children in this country. We will first examine the historical context of health disparities, how they developed, and why they still exist. We will then examine how specifically the COVID-19 pandemic impacted these disparities among children and adolescents, both directly and indirectly. Finally, we hope to provide some recommendations to reduce these disparities.

Historical Review of Health Care Disparities

Health care disparities have been described in the medical literature over the decades. Unequal distribution of resources along with the social determinants of health (economic stability, education, social and community context, health and health care and neighborhood) all contribute to the overall health and well-being of individuals in our society.[9]

A well-established reason for inequitable distribution of resources is systemic racism (racial bias across institutions and society), which has operated over centuries and has impacted generations of citizens in this country. This form of racism is more subtle than interpersonal racism and is unattributable to a particular individual or group of individuals. Examples include "red-lining" (restricting financial services, including loans and mortgages, to persons living in certain neighborhoods based on race), denying land ownership to ethnic/racial minorities, and minimizing access to resources such as healthy foods and transportation in communities where racial/ethnic minorities tend to live. Systemic racism has also contributed to decreased property values in communities of color, reducing federal, state, and local services (such as school funding and community resources) to impoverished communities. These policies have become embedded into the fabric of our society, and over time have become the status quo.[9,10]

Systemic racism has resulted in devastating effects on communities of color. Over centuries, policies endorsed and supported by systemic racism have limited opportunities where racial/ethnic minorities live, work, and obtain an education.[9] A long-standing history of the denial of basic rights and resources has burdened African Americans with lower socioeconomic status relative to whites, along with underresourced communities, which over time has contributed to comorbid conditions leading to vulnerability to poor health outcomes.[11] In addition, migrants from certain countries were not automatically granted citizenship, resulting in diminished opportunities to improve their economic status. Citizens of Hispanic descent, particularly those whose families emigrated from Mexico and Central America, have been denied home ownership and have lived under the scrutiny of immigration laws and policies.[12] Indigenous Americans have suffered forced migration and forced assimilation under racist laws and policies. Therefore, based on the policies, laws, and social structure of the United States, structural racism was successful in preventing communities of color to thrive. Structural racism also significantly accounts for the differences in health and well-being among ethnic and racial minorities in this country.[13,14] In effect, centuries of discrimination and racial trauma have negatively impacted the overall health of people of color.[11–14]

While racism has played a major role in health disparities, poorer health outcomes also have been demonstrated in patients with other medical and social constraints. Homelessness,[15] physical disability and/or special care needs,[16–19] and geography[20] all have been implicated in disparate health outcomes among adults and children. Recent work has suggested that vulnerable populations warrant close attention to ensure receipt of appropriate health care during the current COVID-19 pandemic.[21]

Health Disparities and Pandemics, Including Coronavirus Disease 2019

Historically, communities that are most impacted by new epidemics are often facing other threats to health and overall well-being.[7] Looking back at the Spanish flu in 1918 and the AIDS epidemic in the 1980s to the 1990s, marginalized communities were hit the hardest.[7]

Evidence demonstrates that although whites may have higher cases of COVID-19 based on raw numbers, blacks and Hispanics have higher rates and mortality based on percentage of the population.[1] There are many reasons for these discrepancies, most of which surround social determinants of health. Access to health care, immigration status, and language barriers all contribute to health inequity among Hispanics. For example, currently, Hispanics have the lowest rates of medical insurance coverage of all racial/ethnic groups in the United States (19.8% compared with 5.4% non-Hispanic whites). Compounding this statistic is that immigration status might impede eligibility to access health care, and almost 30% of this population is not fluent in English, thus posing additional barriers.[12] In addition, underfunding of the American Indian health system along with the additional burden of chronic disease predisposes this population to poorer outcomes secondary to COVID-19.[14]

Historically, blacks and Hispanics have higher disease burdens in the case of chronic lung disease, heart disease, diabetes, and obesity, conditions that also are risk factors of higher risk of mortality due to COVID-19.[11,12] These disparities extend to children as well. For children hospitalized with COVID-19-related illnesses, 45.7% of Hispanic children and 29.8% of black children had an underlying medical condition (obesity, chronic lung disease, or prematurity) compared with 14.9% of white children.[3] However, when social determinants of health, including neighborhood conditions, employment, and access to healthy foods are superimposed on these biological risks, the reasons for the higher case load and mortality become clear.[7] Many African Americans, Hispanic Americans, and Indigenous Americans live in dense housing (often in multigenerational families) and therefore are unable to socially distance. Strategies to minimize risk, such as facial coverings and frequent handwashing, may not always be attainable if someone in the household tests positive for COVID-19, making appropriately quarantining/isolation impossible.[6,11–14] In addition, essential workers typically tend to be people of color, who, despite the pandemic, must interact daily with the public (as opposed to telecommuting), increasing their risk of exposure.[6]

Impact of Health Disparities and Coronavirus Disease 2019 on Specific Pediatric Populations

Newborns

Amid this pandemic, important attention must be directed to the medical outcomes of neonates. The effects of SARS-CoV-2 extend across the antenatal to neonatal continuum, particularly affecting communities that traditionally have been marginalized. Studies of pregnant and parturient women in major US cities have demonstrated increased SARS-CoV-2 infection and/or seroprevalence among ethnic/racial minorities, and national data indicate an increased risk of death among infected Hispanic and non-Hispanic black women.[22–25] Additionally, pregnant women infected with SARS-CoV-2 have an increased risk of preterm delivery,[26,27] which may exacerbate the known disparity in such deliveries among African American women in the United States.[28,29] Finally, Niles and colleagues[30] argue that care and non–evidence-based policies implemented during the outbreak, including early inductions and elective cesarean deliveries (to manage hospital volumes) and limiting care partners during labor and delivery, disproportionately affect outcomes among women of color. These factors may reduce or eliminate opportunities for establishment of the maternal-neonatal dyad.

Data indicate rates of neonatal acquisition of SARS-CoV-2 at approximately 2% to 7%, with newborns presenting predominately with respiratory symptoms and being more significantly ill than older children.[31,32] Intrauterine and postnatal acquisition of SARS-CoV-2 infection in newborns has been described, although the mechanisms and risk factors for neonatal infection are not completely clear.[31,33–35] Additionally, specific data on racial disparities among SARS-CoV-2-infected newborns still are being investigated.

Further challenges remain in hospital-based newborn care during the pandemic, which may directly impact minoritized communities. In April, 2020, the American Academy of Pediatrics (AAP) recommended temporary separation of SARS-CoV-2-positive mothers from their newborns after birth to minimize the risk of neonatal infection.[36] Subsequent data demonstrated decreased rates of immediate and long-term breastfeeding among separated maternal-neonatal dyads.[37] These results, along with data showing no increased risk of neonatal infection with rooming-in, led the AAP in July 2020 to endorse room sharing (with appropriate infection control practices) for healthy babies with their nonacutely ill mothers.[36] However, the previous restrictions may have impaired nursing practices among African American mothers, who are less likely to initiate and continue breastfeeding through infancy.[38]

Additional stressors may occur at home and in outpatient settings. Newborn care (and provision of discharge instructions) to nonmaternal caregivers may be required, especially if an ill mother remains hospitalized. However, as a disproportionate number of cases of SARS-CoV-2 occur in racial/ethnic minorities,[39] these additional caretakers may place the baby at risk for postnatal viral acquisition and illness. Furthermore, hand hygiene and mask wearing (with breastfeeding and other components of neonatal care) still are recommended for mothers and family members convalescing from SARS-CoV-2 illness,[36] which may represent an additional expense for families. Finally, routine newborn appointments (for state newborn screening, hyperbilirubinemia monitoring, and weight/feeding assessment) may be delayed due to limitations in physical space (for isolating infected or at-risk patients) and personal protective equipment (for providers) in primary care offices. Telemedicine and home health nursing visits, evolving alternatives to traditional office appointments, seem to be attractive models for pediatric primary care in the midst of the pandemic. However, minoritized communities, many with limited financial resources and technology access, residua of racial residential segregation, and existent language barriers, may be unable to use these opportunities, possibly worsening disparities in short-term neonatal outcomes.

School-aged children and adolescents

Almost 60 million students have been significantly affected from school closures due to COVID-19.[40] Evidence has grown about the adverse effects on the physical, developmental, socioemotional, and environmental health of children before the COVID-19 pandemic by various social determinants of health, including poverty and racism. The impact has exponentially increased since the pandemic's arrival.

One example of these effects on children is the growth of the nation's digital divide. Before the pandemic, underserved and marginalized populations already had difficulty accessing stable telephone and Internet connections. Per the Pew Research Center, in 2019, 79% of white households had home broadband connection, compared with 66% of black households and 61% of Hispanic households.[41] Financial disparities also impact this divide; 92% of those who make $75,000 or more had home broadband compared with 87% who make $50,000 to $74,999, 72% who make $30,000 to $49,999, and 56% who make $30,000 or less.[41] The pandemic has intensified this inequity, and as health care systems nationwide converted to telehealth options to continue to provide care, so did the amplification of the digital divide. Social determinants of health fostered this negative impact, in mechanisms ranging from limited or lack of Internet access, patients' level of literacy on use of technology, building rapport and trust with patients, and cost.[42] This divide leads to families trying to access the Internet in not ideal ways via public spaces, such as parking lots.[43] Those individuals who come from a lower socioeconomic status, elderly, racial/ethnic minority, and/or with disabilities, need to be considered as the digital divide is addressed.[44] Cities (such as Baltimore, Philadelphia, and San Antonio) and organizations have become creative in delivering secure Internet connections to underserved communities. The need for continued advocacy nationwide on this effort is imperative.[43]

The COVID-19 pandemic may also have impacted childhood obesity. One study using a microsimulation model of students followed from kindergarten through fifth grade showed that mean body mass indices and childhood obesity prevalence increased as the time of the school closure increased (based on different scenarios of school closures due to COVID-19).[45] A 0.640% change in childhood obesity was noted from a 2-month closure alone for kindergarten students (closed April and May 2020), and a 2.373% change was noted from closures and decreased activity from April 2020 through December 2020.[45] More of an impact on childhood obesity was noted in male, non-

Hispanic black and Hispanic children.[45] Another study demonstrated that decreased physical activity and increased sedentary behavior were noted in children in the United States, early in the COVID-19 pandemic, and specifically more among children aged 9 to 13 years compared with children aged 5 to 8 years.[46] There is guidance from the AAP on identifying children at risk for obesity, acknowledging and addressing the inequities in accessing opportunities and obesity rates, and supporting families on the importance of healthy eating and physical activity during the COVID-19 pandemic.[47]

Unique childhood populations

During the 2018 to 2019 academic year, more than 7 million children in the nation received special education services in school, with the highest percentage for American Indian/Alaska Native students at 18%.[48] It was reported that 16% of Black students, 14% of white students, 14% of students of 2 or more races, and 13% of Hispanic students were reported to have disabilities requiring special education services.[48] Jeste and colleagues,[49] in evaluating how access to educational and health care services have changed since the pandemic, noted that 74% of parents of children with disabilities reported their children lost at least one therapy or educational service, 56% reported their children received "at least some" services, and 36% reported losing access to a health care provider. These data indicate that the pandemic has adversely affected daily functioning and routine of children with special needs. Depending on the type of disability (for example, autism spectrum disorder), this decrease in support may lead to an increase in challenging behaviors by frequency and/or intensity.[50] Guidance to support children with disabilities and their families receiving their educational services exist at federal and state levels, including virtual options. Although some virtual options have shown success for some students with disabilities, addressing the barriers to access and education (as previously discussed) to those options are vital for true equitable academic success for students from all backgrounds.

Before the pandemic, cases of pediatric mental illness and suicide trends have been on the rise and are concerning, as children as young as 5 years have been identified with mental health problems.[51] COVID-19 has gravely affected pediatric mental health, both directly and indirectly. This pandemic is traumatizing, leading to children becoming fearful of having COVID-19 or a family member becoming ill or dying. In addition, children realize this pandemic has affected their ability to interact with peers, celebrate birthdays (or other holidays), and attend school. Parents and caregivers are also enduring this trauma and the difficulties navigating employment, providing for their families, and keeping everyone healthy. These stressors have led to missed appointments with health care providers, and for some families, worsening housing and food insecurity, significantly increasing adverse childhood experiences.

Researchers reviewed the mental health effects in children impacted by the pandemic and noted abuse, neglect, and a variety of psychiatric disorders, including suicidal ideations.[52] Leeb and colleagues[53] found that starting in April 2020, pediatric mental health-related emergency department visits increased 24% in children aged 5 to 11 years, and increased 31% in children aged 12 to 17 years, when compared with 2019 data. Additionally, given the importance of schools as an option for health care delivery (specifically for mental health treatment), closures significantly disrupted these services, particularly for racial and ethnic minority students.[54] Leff and colleagues[55] further noted that black children were more than 50% less likely to come to the emergency department (ED) with a mental health condition compared with before the pandemic, possibly for a few reasons, such as unequal access to care (especially with school closures) and COVID-19 disproportionately affecting black communities and delaying seeking care.[55]

Children with medical complexity are at risk of reduced health care access during the pandemic due to decreased care from home health aides and school closures, where medical care was provided during the day.[56] Because of the increased vulnerability of these children, parents were at risk for unemployment if they were not able to work from home and at risk for mental/emotional stress without respite and in-home support[56]; this further increases the isolation of these families and increases the vulnerability of children with medical complexity. Medical visits may be reduced as parents/caregivers fear exposure to COVID-19.[8,56]

During this time of the pandemic, children are at a higher risk for maltreatment.[56,57] With school closures the number of mandatory reporters that see children on a regular basis is significantly reduced. The more than 400,000 children in the foster care system during the pandemic are particularly vulnerable because of the shelter-in-place and social distancing executive orders that were placed to decrease the transmission of COVID-19.[56,57] Many children in foster care have experienced adversity and trauma, which led to their initial placement.[56–58] Compounding this is that social distancing in many areas meant that these children were not able to have face-to-face visits with their birth families, which may contribute to their emotional stress.[56] In some states, case workers have been either furloughed or unable to make home visits with children in care for routine safety checks, delaying the potential for reunification with birth families. In addition, delays in court proceedings delay adoptions for children in care.[56] Furthermore, children who age out of the system during the pandemic are left in a more vulnerable state as they try to navigate life as adults during a public health and economic crisis.[56]

Homeless families with children do not have the privilege of adhering to the public health recommendations to decrease the spread of COVID-19.[56] Sheltering in place, access to hygiene supplies, and practicing social distancing are not always possible or practical for families with housing insecurity.[55] Of those families, approximately 75% are "doubling up," that is, living with another family; approximately 14% live in shelters, 7% live in hotels or motels, and approximately 3% are unsheltered.[56,57] During the pandemic, 78% of families experiencing homelessness are Hispanic, again in line with the health disparities seen during the pandemic.[56] Unaccompanied youth who are homeless are more likely to be African American; identify as lesbian, gay, bisexual, transgender, and gender or sexual orientation questioning (LGBTQ), or have less than a high school education.[57] According to the Annie E. Casey Foundation, 18% of families are concerned that they will not be able to pay for their rent on time during the pandemic, with higher proportions of African American families (31%) and Hispanic families (26%) compared with white families (12%).[8] Families who are doubling up are frequently under the threat of being asked to leave due to financial or safety reasons.[56] Those living in shelters use communal bathrooms and kitchens, again making social distancing and hygiene difficult.[56] In general, contact tracing, prevention, and treatment are more difficult for families that are homeless.[56]

Impact of Coronavirus Disease 2019 on Caregivers

Children depend on their parents, guardians, and/or caregivers for basic needs (food, shelter, clothing) as well as transportation, education, and health care access (ie, insurance). Any condition that impacts the caregivers' ability to provide these needs negatively impacts the overall well-being of the child. For example, a caregiver employed as an essential worker during this pandemic might be unable to provide supervision of children at home as they attend school virtually. Caregivers may be at a greater risk of exposure to COVID-19 depending on his or her employment status and might not adequately be able to quarantine upon exposure, thus increasing the risk of infection to the entire family.[6] In addition, many frontline jobs do not compensate workers who have to stay home due to illness, placing workers at risk of losing their source of income.[6,8] Furthermore, many of these workers have inadequate health insurance coverage and may delay care once symptomatic, risking their own health and the health of their family and community.[6,8]

Although the percentage of whites working essential jobs was only slightly lower than nonwhites (Hispanics, blacks, and Asians), job characteristics of essential workers varies with race/ethnicity.[6] Approximately 12% of Whites and 17% of Asians are essential workers able to work from home, compared with 10% blacks and 9% Hispanics.[6,8] A higher proportion of blacks tend to work in health care (eg, nursing assistants, home health care aides, ambulance drivers, housekeeping) and public safety (eg, police officers, firefighters, security guards, corrections officers, postal employees, public transportation workers, and those who work in funeral homes and crematoriums).[6,59] Hispanics are overrepresented in the foodservice industry.[6,60] These occupations increase the exposure risk to COVID-19 among minorities.

Impact of Coronavirus Disease 2019 on Physicians and Other Health Care Workers of Color

The COVID-19 pandemic has also had a significant effect on physician and skilled health workers of color. Of the 18.6 million health care workers in the United States, 40% are people of color (16% blacks, 13% Hispanic, and 7% Asian).[60,61] At present, African Americans, Hispanics, and Native American constitute 5%, 5.8%, and 0.4% of practicing physicians, respectively.[60,61] These discrepancies in themselves have led to some of the health disparities seen in minority communities, and one of the interventions to counteract this is to increase the pipeline to include more physicians of color into the profession.[61] However, this pandemic has caused a disparate toll on these physicians of color. Many disproportionately practice in communities with higher rates of COVID-19 and thus are at a higher risk of exposure.[60,61] In addition, these physicians are more likely to have chronic health conditions, placing them at higher risk for severe morbidity and mortality from COVID-19.[60,61] Also, those physicians in private practice have witnessed the economic impact of the pandemic on their livelihood, and those who serve their communities in safety net health care institutions have had to deal with understaffed and underresourced personnel.[61] Furthermore, when African Americans enter the health care system as patients, they are at a higher risk of receiving lower-quality care, particularly if they are treated using diagnostic criteria and clinical pathways embedded with racial bias.[61] Finally, physicians of color in general are at a greater risk of developing mental health problems including anxiety, depression, posttraumatic stress disorder, imposter syndrome, and survivor guilt.[12,61]

SUMMARY
Steps to Minimize Health Disparities and Their Impact on Children, Caregivers, and Health Care Workers During the Coronavirus Disease 2019 Pandemic and Beyond

COVID-19 has illuminated the areas of needed improvement in the delivery of equitable child health and education. Several agencies and organizations are providing guidelines on how to support families, schools, and health care systems in this effort. The Economic Policy Institute has highlighted the lessons learned and suggested a plan through "relief, recovery, and rebuilding,"[62] where this nation critically reviews its resources and interest in child development. The Centers for Disease Control and Prevention created a resource kit to support child behavioral and mental health, categorized by age groups.[63] Pediatric providers must continue to check in with their families and keep open communication. A resource to assist providers is the Roadmap to Resilience, Emotional, and Mental Health from the American Board of Pediatrics.[64]

For parents and caregivers who are unable to secure economic stability and health care through employment, there must be mechanisms available to assist with access to safety net resources easily and without the threat of legal action or deportation.[12–14,56–60]

For children of unique populations, steps to minimize the impact of COVID-19 include:

- Providing access to telehealth visits
- Endorsing caregiver support groups
- Ensuring respite care for children with complex medical conditions and their families
- Heightening awareness among other mandatory reporters
- Providing paid leave and economic assistance to foster families
- Enhancing technical support and connectivity for parents for telemedicine visits and resource acquisition
- Increasing state funding for family preservation services for children in foster care
- Offering emergency rental assistance and upholding a moratorium on evictions and foreclosures for homeless children[55–58]

Whatever obstacle may come, be it COVID-19 or another global disaster, steps must be taken to ensure the resilience of children and adolescents and their families. In addition to those efforts, we must also ensure that our health care system has the resources and personnel needed to ensure the equitable delivery of health care services to everyone. Policies to promote the overall health and well-being of children, adolescents, and their families, including the promotion and sustaining of safety net resources, access to health care, safe living environments, and economic security, should continue to be this nation's top priority.

CLINICS CARE POINTS

- Compared with the general population, non-Hispanic blacks, indigenous Americans/Alaskan Natives, and Hispanics have higher rates of COVID-19 infection and deaths, because of several factors including:
  - Timely access to medical care
  - Poverty
  - Occupation
  - Systemic racism

- Although children in general have lower rates of COVID-19 infection and hospitalization, non-Hispanic black and Hispanic children have higher rates of hospitalization due to COVID-19 infection.

- In addition to people of color, unique populations of children at higher risk of medical complications of COVID-19 due to health disparities include:
  - Children who are immigrants
  - Children who are obese
  - Children with chronic illnesses and/or disabilities
  - Children who are homeless
  - Children who are impoverished
  - Children who are in foster care

- Health disparities during the COVID-19 pandemic have also been demonstrated in education, safety net programs, and mental health support services.

- Recommendations to decrease these disparities include addressing social determinants of health:
  - Education: providing schools and families with appropriate resources to stabilize and enhance virtual learning, offering individualized instruction for students falling behind, and redesigning the educational system to focus on the whole child
  - Health and health care: monitoring and addressing the physical and mental health of patients and families during the pandemic, advocating for the elimination of barriers to COVID-19 testing and vaccines, and recommending appropriate compensation for telemedicine care
  - Economic stability: providing personal protective equipment (PPE) for all essential workers, supporting fair housing practices (rental assistance, eviction moratoria) during the pandemic, and promoting affordable/free PPE supplies to families with high-risk household members.

DISCLOSURE

Dr L.C. Smitherman and Dr W.C. Golden have no disclosures relevant to the material presented.

REFERENCES

1. Center for Disease Control. Available at: https://covid.cdc.gov/covid-data-tracker/#cases_casesper100klast7days. Accessed January 17, 2021.
2. Abedi v. Olulana O, Avula V, Chaudhary D, Khan A, Shahjouei S, Li J, and Zand R. Racial, Economic and Health Inequality and COVID-19 Infection in the United States. J Racial Ethn Health Disparities 2020;1–11.
3. Kim L, Whitaker M, O'Halloran A, et al. Hospitalization Rates and Characteristics of Children Aged <18 Years Hospitalized with Laboratory-Confirmed COVID-19-COVID-NET, 14 States, March 1-25, 2020. MMWR Morb Mortal Wkly Rep 2020; 69:1081–8.
4. Lee EH, Kepler KL, Geevarughese A, Paneth-Pollak R, Dorsinville MS, Ngai S, Reilly KH. Race/Ethnicity Amoung Children with COVID-19-Associated Multisystem Inflammatory Syndrome. JAMA Netw Open 2020;3(11):e20302800.
5. Baciu A, Negussie Y, Geller A, et al, editors. The state of health disparities in the United States in communities in action: pathways to health equity. National Academies of Sciences, Engineering, and medicine; health and medicine Division; board on population health and public health practice; Committee on community-based Solutions to promote health equity in the United States. Washington (DC): National Academies Press; 2017.
6. Selden TM, Berdahl TA. COVID-19 and Racial/Ethnic Disparities in Health Risk, Employment, and Household Composition. Health Aff 2020;39(9):1624–32.
7. Gravlee C. Systemic racism, chronic health inequities, and COVID-19: A syndemic in the making? Am J Hum Biol 2020;e23482.
8. Kids, Families and COVID-19: Pandemic Pain Points and the Urgent Need to Respond. Annie E. Casey Foundation. December 2020;14.
9. Jones CP. Confronting Institutional Racism. Phylon 2002;50(1–2):7–22, 1960.
10. Johnson T. Intersection of Bias, Structural Racism and Social Determinants with Health Care Inequities. Pediatrics 2020;146(2). e2020003657.
11. Yancy CW. COVID-19 and African Americans. JAMA 2020;323(19):1891–2.
12. Gil R, Marcelin JR. Zuniga-Blanco, Marquez C, Mathew T, Piggott D. COVID-19 Pandemic: Disparate Health Impact on the Hispanic/Latinx Population in the United States. J Infect Dis 2020;222(10):1592–5.

13. Fingling MG, Casey LS, Fryberg SA, Hafner S, Blendon RJ, Benson JM, Sayde JM, Miller C. Discrimination in the US: Experiences of Native Americans. Health Serv Res 2019;54:1431–41.
14. Hatcher SM, Agnew-Brune C, Anderson M, et al. COVID-19 Among American Indian and Alaska Native Persons-23 States, January 31-July 3, 2020. MMWR Morb Mortal Wkly Rep 2020;69:1166–9.
15. Oppenheimer SC, Nurius PS, Green S. Homelessness history impacts on health outcomes and economic and risk behavior intermediaries: new insights from population data. Fam Soc 2016;97(3):230–42.
16. Na L, Singh S. Disparities in mental health, social support and coping among individuals with mobility impairment. Disabil Health J 2021;14(2):101047.
17. Minnaert J, Kenney MK, Ghandour R, et al. CSHCN with hearing difficulties: Disparities in access and quality of care. Disabil Health J 2020;13(1):100798.
18. Jolles MP, Thomas KC. Disparities in self-reported access to patient-centered medical home care for children with special health care needs. Med Care 2018;56(10):840–6.
19. Acharya K, Meza R, Msall ME. Disparities in life course outcomes for transition-aged youth with disabilities. Pediatr Ann 2017;46(10):e371–6.
20. Morales DA, Barksdale CL, Beckel-Mitchener A. A call to action to address rural mental health disparities. J Clin Transl Sci 2020;4(5):463–7.
21. Verduzco-Gutierrez M, Lara AM, Annaswamy TM. When Disparities and Disabilities Collide: Inequities during the COVID-19 Pandemic. PM&R 2021;13(4):412–4.
22. Emeruwa UN, Spiegelman J, Ona S, et al. Influence of race and ethnicity on severe acute respiratory syndrome coronavirus 2 (SARS-CoV-2) infection rates and clinical outcomes in pregnancy. Obstet Gynecol 2020;136(5):1040–3.
23. Sakowicz A, Ayala AE, Ukeje CC, et al. Risk factors for severe acute respiratory syndrome coronavirus 2 infection in pregnant women. Am J Obstet Gynecol MFM 2020;2(4):100198.
24. Flannery DD, Gouma S, Dhudasia MB, et al. SARS-CoV-2 seroprevalence among parturient women in Philadelphia. Sci Immunol 2020;5(49):eabd5709.
25. Zambrano LD, Ellington S, Strid P, et al. Update: characteristics of symptomatic women of reproductive age with laboratory-confirmed SARS-CoV-2 infection by pregnancy status - United States, January 22-October 3, 2020. MMWR Morb Mortal Wkly Rep 2020;69(44):1641–7.
26. Marín Gabriel MA, Vergeli MR, Carbonero SC, et al. Maternal, perinatal and neonatal outcomes with COVID-19: a multicenter study of 242 pregnancies and their 248 infant newborns during their first month of life. Pediatr Infect Dis J 2020;39(12):e393–7.
27. Allotey J, Stallings E, Bonet M, et al. Clinical manifestations, risk factors, and maternal and perinatal outcomes of coronavirus disease 2019 in pregnancy: living systematic review and meta-analysis. BMJ 2020;370:m3320.
28. Johnson JD, Green CA, Vladutiu CJ, et al. Racial disparities in prematurity persist among women of high socioeconomic status. Am J Obstet Gynecol MFM 2020;2(3):100104.
29. Kistka ZA, Palomar L, Lee KA, et al. Racial disparity in the frequency of recurrence of preterm birth. Am J Obstet Gynecol 2007;196(2):131.e131–6.
30. Niles PM, Asiodu IV, Crear-Perry J, et al. Reflecting on equity in perinatal care during a pandemic. Health Equity 2020;4(1):330–3.
31. Barrero-Castillero A, Beam KS, Bernardini LB, et al. COVID-19: neonatal-perinatal perspectives. J Perinatol 2021;41(5):940–51.

32. Liguoro I, Pilotto C, Bonanni M, et al. SARS-COV-2 infection in children and newborns: a systematic review. Eur J Pediatr 2020;179(7):1029–46.

33. Naz S, Rahat T, Memon FN. Vertical transmission of SARS-CoV-2 from COVID-19 infected pregnant women: a review on intrauterine transmission. Fetal Pediatr Pathol 2021;40(1):80–92.

34. Wang W, Xu Y, Gao R, et al. Detection of SARS-CoV-2 in different types of clinical specimens. JAMA 2020;323(18):1843–4.

35. Kimberlin DW, Stagno S. Can SARS-CoV-2 Infection be acquired in utero?: More definitive evidence is needed. JAMA 2020;323(18):1788–9.

36. American Academy of Pediatrics. FAQ: Management of Infants Born to Mothers with Suspected or Confirmed COVID-19. Available at: https://services.aap.org/en/pages/2019-novel-coronavirus-covid-19-infections/clinical-guidance/faqs-management-of-infants-born-to-covid-19-mothers/. Accessed January 18, 2020.

37. Popofsky S, Noor A, Jill Leavens-Maurer J, et al. Impact of maternal severe acute respiratory syndrome coronavirus 2 detection on breastfeeding due to infant separation at birth. J Pediatr 2020;226:64–70.

38. Beauregard JL, Hamner HC, Chen J, et al. Racial disparities in breastfeeding initiation and duration among U.S. infants born in 2015. MMWR Morb Mortal Wkly Rep 2019;68(34):745–8.

39. COVID-19 Racial and Ethnic Health Disparities. Available at: www.cdc.gov/coronavirus/2019-ncov/community/health-equity/racial-ethnic-disparities/increased-risk-illness.html. Accessed January 18, 2021.

40. Masonbrink AR, Hurley E. Advocating for Children During the COVID-19 School Closures. Pediatrics 2020;146(3):e20201440.

41. Internet Broadband Fact Sheet. Pew Research Center Internet & Technology. 2019. Available at: https://www.pewresearch.org/internet/fact-sheet/internet-broadband/#who-has-home-broadband. Accessed January 17, 2021.

42. Ramsetty A, Adams C. Impact of the digital divide in the age of COVID-19. J Am Med Inform Assoc 2020;27(7):1147–8.

43. Flaherty C, Wood SM, Chen K. Broadband Internet Access, Education & Child Health: From Differences to Disparities, Part 1. PolicyLab Blog post September 2020 Notes. Available at: https://policylab.chop.edu/blog/broadband-internet-access-education-child-health-differences-disparities-part-1. Accessed January 17, 2021.

44. Gray DM, Joseph JJ, Olayiwola JN. Strategies for Digital Care of Vulnerable Patients in a COVID-19 World—Keeping in Touch. JAMA Health Forum Published Online 2020. https://doi.org/10.1001/jamahealthforum.2020.0734.

45. An R. Projecting the impact of the coronavirus disease-2019 pandemic on childhood obesity in the United States: A microsimulation model. J Sport Health Sci 2020;9:302–12.

46. Dunton GF, Do B, Wang SD. Early effects of the COVID-19 pandemic on physical activity and sedentary behavior in children living in the U.S. BMC Public Health 2020;20:1351.

47. Supporting Healthy Nutrition and Physical Activity During the COVID-19 Pandemic. American Academy of Pediatrics; 2020. Available at: https://services.aap.org/en/pages/2019-novel-coronavirus-covid-19-infections/clinical-guidance/supporting-healthy-nutrition-and-physical-activity-during-the-covid-19-pandemic/. Accessed January 27, 2021.

48. The Condition of Education: Students with Disabilities. National Center for Education Statistics, May 2020. Available at: https://nces.ed.gov/programs/coe/indicator_cgg.asp. Accessed January 17, 2021.

49. Jeste S, Hyde C, Distefano C, Halladay A, Ray S, Porath M, Wilson RB, Thurm A. Changes in access to educational and healthcare services for individuals with intellectual and developmental disabilities during COVID-19 restrictions. J Intellect Disabil Res 2020;64:825–33.
50. Eshraghi AA, Li C, Alessandri M, Messinger DS, Eshraghi RS, Mittal R, Armstrong FD. COVID-19: overcoming the challenges faced by individuals with autism and their families. The Lancet Psychiatry 2020;7(6):481–3.
51. Bridge JA, Asti L, Horowitz LM, et al. Suicide Trends Among Elementary School–Aged Children in the United States From 1993 to 2012. JAMA Pediatr 2015; 169(7):673–7.
52. de Figueiredo CS, Sandre PC, Portugal LCL, et al. COVID-19 pandemic impact on children and adolescents' mental health: Biological, environmental, and social factors. Prog Neuro-psychopharmacology Biol Psychiatry 2021;106:110171.
53. Leeb RT, Bitsko RH, Radhakrishnan L, Martinez P, Njai R, Holland KM. Mental Health–Related Emergency Department Visits Among Children Aged <18 Years During the COVID-19 Pandemic — United States, January 1–October 17, 2020. MMWR Morb Mortal Wkly Rep 2020;69:1675–80.
54. Golberstein E, Wen H, Miller BF. Coronavirus Disease 2019 (COVID-19) and Mental Health for Children and Adolescents. JAMA Pediatr 2020;174(9):819–20.
55. Leff RA, Setzer E, Cicero MX, Auerbach M. Changes in pediatric emergency department visits for mental health during the COVID-19 pandemic: A cross-sectional study. Clin Child Psychol Psychiatry 2021;26(1):33–8.
56. Wong CA, Ming D, Maslow G, Gifford EJ. Mitigating the Impacts of the COVID-19 Pandemic Response on At-Risk Children. Pediatrics 2020;146(1):e20200973.
57. Annie E. Casey Foundation. Foster Care. Available at: https://www.aecf.org/topics/foster-care/?gclid=Cj0KCQiAmL-ABhDFARIsAKywVafrrw_UzGo3vVK7-wiDLkeYCl7xnGDkenDz4LX4Ge3Lli8kfNx5SCUaAgc_EALw_wcB. Accessed January 26, 2021.
58. Hilavinka E, Firth S. CCOVID-19 Strips Safety Net for Foster Youth "Aging Out' During Pandemic. Medpage Today 12/8/20. Available at: https://www.medpagetoday.com/special-reports/exclusives/90072?vpass=1. Accessed January 24, 2021.
59. Beharry MS, Christensen R. Homelessnes in pediatric populations: strategies for prevention, assistance and advocacy. Pediatr Clin North Am 2020;67(2):357–72.
60. Artiga S, Rae M, Pham O, Hamel L, Munan C. COVID-19 Risks and Impacts Among Health Care Workers by Race and Ethnicity. 2020. Available at: https://www.kff.org/racial-equity-and-health-policy/issue-brief/covid-19-risks-impacts-health-care-workers-race-ethnicity/. Accessed January 17, 2021.
61. Filut A, Carnes M. Will Losing Black Physicians be a Consequence of the COVID-19 Pandemic? Acad Med 2020;95(12):1796–8.
62. Garcia E, Weiss E. COVID-19 and student performance, equity, and U.S. education policy. Economic Policy Institute. 2020. Available at: https://www.epi.org/publication/the-consequences-of-the-covid-19-pandemic-for-education-performance-and-equity-in-the-united-states-what-can-we-learn-from-pre-pandemic-research-to-inform-relief-recovery-and-rebuilding/. Accessed January 17, 2021.
63. COVID-19 Parental Resources Kit. Center for Disease Control and Prevention. 2020. Available at: https://www.cdc.gov/coronavirus/2019-ncov/daily-life-coping/parental-resource-kit/index.html. Accessed January 17, 2021.
64. Roadmap to Resilience. Emotional, and Mental Health. The American Board of Pediatrics. 2020. Available at: https://www.abp.org/foundation/roadmap. Accessed January 17, 2021.

UNITED STATES POSTAL SERVICE ® Statement of Ownership, Management, and Circulation (All Periodicals Publications Except Requester Publications)

1. Publication Title	2. Publication Number	3. Filing Date
PEDIATRIC CLINICS OF NORTH AMERICA	424 – 66	9/18/2021

4. Issue Frequency	5. Number of Issues Published Annually	6. Annual Subscription Price
FEB, APR, JUN, AUG, OCT, DEC	6	$240.00

7. Complete Mailing Address of Known Office of Publication (Not printer) (Street, city, county, state, and ZIP+4®)
ELSEVIER INC.
230 Park Avenue, Suite 800
New York, NY 10169

Contact Person
Malathi Samayan
Telephone (Include area code)
91-44-4299-4507

8. Complete Mailing Address of Headquarters or General Business Office of Publisher (Not printer)
ELSEVIER INC.
230 Park Avenue, Suite 800
New York, NY 10169

9. Full Names and Complete Mailing Addresses of Publisher, Editor, and Managing Editor (Do not leave blank)

Publisher (Name and complete mailing address)
TAYLOR BALL, ELSEVIER INC.
1600 JOHN F KENNEDY BLVD. SUITE 1800
PHILADELPHIA, PA 19103-2899

Editor (Name and complete mailing address)
KERRY HOLLAND, ELSEVIER INC.
1600 JOHN F KENNEDY BLVD. SUITE 1800
PHILADELPHIA, PA 19103-2899

Managing Editor (Name and complete mailing address)
PATRICK MANLEY, ELSEVIER INC.
1600 JOHN F KENNEDY BLVD. SUITE 1800
PHILADELPHIA, PA 19103-2899

10. Owner (Do not leave blank. If the publication is owned by a corporation, give the name and address of the corporation immediately followed by the names and addresses of all stockholders owning or holding 1 percent or more of the total amount of stock. If not owned by a corporation, give the names and addresses of the individual owners. If owned by a partnership or other unincorporated firm, give its name and address as well as those of each individual owner. If the publication is published by a nonprofit organization, give its name and address.)

Full Name	Complete Mailing Address
WHOLLY OWNED SUBSIDIARY OF REED/ELSEVIER, US HOLDINGS	1600 JOHN F KENNEDY BLVD. SUITE 1800 PHILADELPHIA, PA 19103-2899

11. Known Bondholders, Mortgagees, and Other Security Holders Owning or Holding 1 Percent or More of Total Amount of Bonds, Mortgages, or Other Securities. If none, check box ► ☐ None

Full Name	Complete Mailing Address
N/A	

12. Tax Status (For completion by nonprofit organizations authorized to mail at nonprofit rates) (Check one)
The purpose, function, and nonprofit status of this organization and the exempt status for federal income tax purposes:
☒ Has Not Changed During Preceding 12 Months
☐ Has Changed During Preceding 12 Months (Publisher must submit explanation of change with this statement)

PS Form 3526, July 2014 [Page 1 of 4 (see instructions page 4)] PSN: 7530-01-000-9931 PRIVACY NOTICE: See our privacy policy on www.usps.com

13. Publication Title	14. Issue Date for Circulation Data Below
PEDIATRIC CLINICS OF NORTH AMERICA	JUNE 2021

15. Extent and Nature of Circulation		Average No. Copies Each Issue During Preceding 12 Months	No. Copies of Single Issue Published Nearest to Filing Date
a. Total Number of Copies (Net press run)		568	483
b. Paid Circulation (By Mail and Outside the Mail)	(1) Mailed Outside-County Paid Subscriptions Stated on PS Form 3541 (Include paid distribution above nominal rate, advertiser's proof copies, and exchange copies)	276	264
	(2) Mailed In-County Paid Subscriptions Stated on PS Form 3541 (Include paid distribution above nominal rate, advertiser's proof copies, and exchange copies)	0	0
	(3) Paid Distribution Outside the Mails Including Sales Through Dealers and Carriers, Street Vendors, Counter Sales, and Other Paid Distribution Outside USPS®	220	180
	(4) Paid Distribution by Other Classes of Mail Through the USPS (e.g., First-Class Mail®)	0	0
c. Total Paid Distribution (Sum of 15b (1), (2), (3), and (4))	►	496	444
d. Free or Nominal Rate Distribution (By Mail and Outside the Mail)	(1) Free or Nominal Rate Outside-County Copies included on PS Form 3541	51	22
	(2) Free or Nominal Rate In-County Copies Included on PS Form 3541	0	0
	(3) Free or Nominal Rate Copies Mailed at Other Classes Through the USPS (e.g., First-Class Mail)	0	0
	(4) Free or Nominal Rate Distribution Outside the Mail (Carriers or other means)	51	22
e. Total Free or Nominal Rate Distribution (Sum of 15d (1), (2), (3) and (4))	►	547	466
f. Total Distribution (Sum of 15c and 15e)	►	21	17
g. Copies not Distributed (See Instructions to Publishers #4 (page #3))	►	568	483
h. Total (Sum of 15f and g)	►		
i. Percent Paid (15c divided by 15f times 100)		90.67%	95.27%

* If you are claiming electronic copies, go to line 16 on page 3. If you are not claiming electronic copies, skip to line 17 on page 3.

PS Form 3526, July 2014 (Page 2 of 4)

16. Electronic Copy Circulation		Average No. Copies Each Issue During Preceding 12 Months	No. Copies of Single Issue Published Nearest to Filing Date
a. Paid Electronic Copies	►		
b. Total Paid Print Copies (Line 15c) + Paid Electronic Copies (Line 16a)	►		
c. Total Print Distribution (Line 15f) + Paid Electronic Copies (Line 16a)	►		
d. Percent Paid (Both Print & Electronic Copies) (16b divided by 16c × 100)	►		

☒ I certify that 50% of all my distributed copies (electronic and print) are paid above a nominal price.

17. Publication of Statement of Ownership
☒ If the publication is a general publication, publication of this statement is required. Will be printed in the OCTOBER 2021 issue of this publication. ☐ Publication not required.

18. Signature and Title of Editor, Publisher, Business Manager, or Owner

Malathi Samayan - Distribution Controller   *Malathi Samayan*   Date 9/18/2021

I certify that all information furnished on this form is true and complete. I understand that anyone who furnishes false or misleading information on this form or who omits material or information requested on the form may be subject to criminal sanctions (including fines and imprisonment) and/or civil sanctions (including civil penalties).

PS Form 3526, July 2014 (Page 3 of 4) PRIVACY NOTICE: See our privacy policy on www.usps.com